A Catalogue of the Manuscripts and Archives of the
Library of the College of Physicians of Philadelphia

Frontispiece. 399. Gilbert Collection. Letter on vaccination by Thomas Jefferson to Redman Coxe.

A Catalogue of the Manuscripts and Archives of the Library of The „College of Physicians of Philadelphia

Prepared by the
Francis Clark Wood Institute
for the History of Medicine

Rudolf Hirsch, Editor

Assisted by Timothy L. Bratton and
Ericka Thickman Miller, Archivist

With an Introduction by
Whitfield J. Bell, Jr.

University of Pennsylvania Press
Francis Clark Wood Institute
College of Physicians of Philadelphia

Philadelphia / 1983

Contents

List of Illustrations   vii

Acknowledgment   ix

List of Donors   xi

Introduction   xv

Note to Reader   xix

Manuscripts and Archives   1

Indices   233

List of Illustrations

Frontispiece. 399. Gilbert Collection. Letter on vaccination by Thomas Jefferson to Redman Coxe.

Plate 1. 28. Arnoldus de Villanova. *De Infirmitatibus occulorum,* 14th century *(page 7).*

Plate 2. 165. Autopsy report of Charles II, 1684 *(page 33).*

Plate 3. 185.11 College of Physicians of Philadelphia *Charter.* Draft by Benjamin Rush, 1788 *(page 37).*

Plate 4. 190. Astrological Calendar appended to *Viaticum, Libri I-VII* by Constantinus Africanus, first half 13th century *(page 54).*

Plate 5. 624. Donald McNeil. *Of Natural Philosophy, 178 (page 133).*

Plate 6. 810. V. Philippe. *Observations de practique chirurgicale.* 1760-90 *(page 172).*

Plate 7. 1038. Sketch of James Tyson from the student notes of Joseph McFarland,1888 *(page 210).*

Acknowledgment

The Francis Clark Wood Institute for the History of Medicine is deeply indebted to the American Philosophical Society and the Commonwealth Fund for their generous contributions that have made possible the appearance of this catalogue of manuscripts. We all wish especially to extend our thanks to Carleton B. Chapman of the Commonwealth Fund for the interest he has taken in the creation of this book and of the Institute itself.

Others who have made important contributions to the planning and completion of this catalogue are Whitfield J. Bell, Jr.; Rudolf Hirsch; W. D. McDaniel, 2nd; Edith Wright; Lisabeth Holloway; Stephanie Morris; Ellen B. Gartrell; Christine Ruggere; Timothy L. Bratton; Martha Jamison; Marita Krivda; and Ericka Thickman Miller.

Ronald F. Kotrc
Director
Francis Clark Wood Institute

List of Donors

Many persons have generously contributed to the growth of the College's collection of manuscripts and archival materials. In recognition their names are here recorded. Not all donors may be known to the compilers; for omissions we apologize.

Actee, W.F., 582
Allen, Lewis H., 77
Allison, Samuel D., 310
Allyn, Herman B. (heirs), 329
American Philosophical Society, 863
Arrow, G.H.,902
Ashhurst, Astley Paston Cooper, 32, 192, 804, 924
Ashhurst, John Jr., 604
Atkinson, William Biddle, 18
Atlee, Walter Franklin, 280, 928
Bache, Franklin, 42
Bahl, J.R., 955
Barnshaw, Harold D., 1024
Batson, Oscar V., 588, 1052
Baum, Charles, 779
Bechet, Paul Esnard (Mrs.), 58
Binkley, George Webster, 748
Blackmore, C.T.(Mrs.), 364
Blayley, William H., 76
Bluefarb, Smauel M., 840, 841
Bookhammer, Robert, 109
Brown, T. Wistar (Mrs.), 198, 199
Cadwalader, Charles, 84
Cadwalader, John, 671
Carnett, John B., 272
Carson, John, 9, 111
Carson, Joseph, 53
Carson, Joseph (heirs), 123-27, 447
Chance, Burton, 1015, 1023
Chapman, Henry Cadwalader, 84, 140, 144
Charles, Stephen Tudor, 166
Chester County Medical Society, 815, 907
Clark, Leonardo S., 824, 913
Clarke, Mary A., 176
Cole, Charles S., Jr., 690
Coles, Harold Newton, 180

Coles, Stricker, 929
Cooper, David A. (Mrs.), 287
Craven, Anna R., 908
Craven, John V., 924
Creese, James (Mrs.), 709
Da Costa, Jacob Mendez, 444, 477
Daland, Judson, 231
Daniel, Emily, 850
Darrach, James, 298, 822
Davis, Edward, 830
Deaver, J. Montgomery, 506
Dercum, Francis X., 305
Dewey, S.C. (Miss), 82
Dixon, Samuel Gibson, 680
Dulles, Charles Winslow, 266
Dunglison, Richard James, 275
Dunglison, Violette Fisher, 270
Du Pont, B.G. (Mrs.), 255, 256, 258, 259
Durant, Thomas Morton, 351
Ellicott, Valcoulon Le Moyne, 597, 823
Elmer, Walter G., 819
Emlen, John Thompson, 289
Episcopal Hospital, Philadelphia, 605
Evans, Edwin L., 38
Fisher, Charles Percy, 270, 302
Flick, John Bernard, 915
Foster, Richard W., 131, 816, 935
Fox, Herbert, 641
Frazier, Charles Harrison, 315
Free Library of Philadelphia, 97, 106
Gellhorn, Ernst, 328
Gelwix, John M., 791
Gerhard, William Wood, 21
Girvin, Helen, 340
Goodman, Edward B., 998
Greene, Herbert A., 76
Guthrie, Douglas James, 336

Gwyn, Norman Beechley, 753
Hall, William Kearney, 370
Harris, Montgomery, 262, 1027
Hartshorne, Edward, 1061
Harvey, Edward F. (Mrs.), 756
Haverford College, 471
Hays, Issac Minis, 18, 257, 362, 775, 992
Helfand, Willliam, 969
Henry, Frederick Porteous, 964
Hirsh, Joseph, 466
Historical Society of Pennsylvania, 181, 435
Hodge, Edward Blanchard, 416, 1057
Hodge, Hugh Lenox, 46, 148, 279, 319, 403, 472, 717, 790, 847, 901, 967
Hoffman, B. (Mr. & Mrs.), 104
Hoffman, Syd (Mrs.), 104
Holt, William L., 250
Howell, Josephine, 864
Huber, John F., 104
Huston, H.L. (Mrs.), 260
Hyde, A.P. (Mr. & Mrs.), 450
Issacs, Raphael, 457
Ivy, Robert Henry, 990
Johnston, George B., 654, 663 '
Kane, Francis Fisher, 155, 937
Kates, Jerome S., 483
Keen, Florence, 487
Keen, William Williams, 489-91
King, Charles Ray, 494
Krumbhaar, Edward Bell, 7, 183, 308, 402, 458, 507, 697, 715, 793, 930, 956, 989, 1037
Leidy, Joseph, Jr., 338, 587
Lewis, Fraser, 601
Lewis, Howard L. (Mrs.), 431
Lewis, Samuel, 743, 921
Light, Arthur Bomberger, 798
McClendon, Jesse F., 249
MacDonnough (Mrs.), 681
McGuire, Hunter Holmes, 918
Make, Sydney (Mrs.), 104
Manson, Clara, 104
Marshall, John, 629-31
Martin, Thomas S., 167
Meigs, Arthur V., 96
Melnick, Theodore (Mrs.), 652
Miller, Thomas Grier, 455
Mills, Charles Karsner, 669, 670

Mitchell, Silas Weir, 17, 28, 105, 143, 147, 200, 300, 339, 342, 477, 674, 686, 687, 703, 825, 861, 1045
Montgomery, E.E., 916
Morgan, John, 694
Morris, Edward Shippen, 909
Moyerman, Samuel, 934
Musser, John H., 698
Myers, Leonard S., 242
Nebinger, Robert, 291
Nicholson, John Page, 686
Nicholson, William R., 225
Norris, George William, 468, 479, 721, 722, 724, 730, 732
Norris, Robert F. (Mrs.), 1092
Norris, William Fisher (family), 728
Osler, William, 66, 306, 752, 951
Packard, Francis Randolph, 686
Packard, John H., 567, 569, 571
Pancoast, Henry K., 440
Pancoast, William Henry, 12, 820
Peitzman, Steven J., 104
Pelouze, Percy Starr, 770
Pepper, William, 179, 839, 954, 1037
Percival, Milton Fraser (Mrs.), 622
Perkins, William (Mrs.), 785
Pitfield, Robert Lucas, 69
Potts, Clara Ethel, 1071
Radbill, Samuel X, 81, 135, 715, 798, 816, 842-44
Randall, Burton Alexander, 846
Ridley, William P. (Mrs.), 459
Risley, Samuel D., 747
Roberts, John Bingham, 868-74
Rogers, Fred Baker, 49, 104, 151, 879
Rosenberg, Charles E., 350, 1062, 1070
Sayre, Francis B., 939
Schaeffer, William Ashmead, 171, 222, 791, 817
Schofield, Frederick S., 770
Schweinitz, George Edmund de, 632
Shelley, Walter B., 1054
Shippen, Edward, 909
Smith, Henry Lee, 1022
Smith, Kline & French, 316, 473, 960
Snodgrass, Leeman Espy, 32, 972
Solis-Cohen, Jacob da Silva, 426, 639, 976, 977, 979, 980
Solis-Cohen, Myer, 1120
Solis-Cohen, Solomon (Mrs.), 831
Spiller, William Gibson, 676, 677, 808, 985

Stengel, Alfred, 261
Stewart, Harold L., 281
Stille, Alfred, 995
Stoddart, F.S.Janney, 294
Strawbridge, Francis (Mrs.), 852
Sturgis, Katharine Rosenbaum Guest Boucot, 1005
Sturgis, Samuel Booth, 100, 1006, 1008
Swan, John Mumford, 668
Taylor, William Johnson, 456
Thorington, J. Monroe, 1025
Tilden, Marmaduke (Mrs.), 708
University of Pennsylvania, School of Medicine, 827
Wadsworth, William Scott, 1059
Walsh, Joseph Patrick, 324, 325
Webb, Louise (heirs), 495
Weiss, Warren, 128

Wells, M. Henry (Mrs.), 98, 99
Westcott, Thompson Seiser (Mrs.), 11, 1077-81
Wharton, Henry Redwood, 161, 851
Wickersham, M.S., 647, 947
Wilcox, Mark, Jr., 994
Wistar, Esther F. (Mrs. Mifflin W.), 1091
Wistar, Mifflin, 73, 445, 448, 693
Wood, Emlen, 876
Wood, Francis Clark, 634, 816, 862
Wood, George Bacon, 1114
Wood, George Bacon (Mrs.), 1107
Wood, Harold Bacon, 1107
Wood, Horatio C., 336, 789, 1114
Wood, Howland (Mrs.), 884
Woodhouse, Samuel Washington (Mrs.), 1125
Ziegler, Samuel Lewis, 245

Introduction

Like other old cities, Philadelphia contains a number of institutions whose history and records go back several centuries; and many have accumulated archives, libraries, and artifacts that are hardly known to their own members and staffs, much less the public. Thus it happens in such places that scholars are constantly making "discoveries." Nowhere in the past twelve to twenty years has the excitement of fresh revelations been sustained at so high a pitch as in Philadelphia. No year passes that the Library Company of Philadelphia does not turn up some single volume or whole collection of singular interest and importance. The Pennsylvania Hospital, when it began to organize its archives, found them in closets, attics, and cellars — even in a laundry hamper — that had not been visited for years. And only two or three years ago a bundle of bills and receipts for the construction of its hall in 1785-89 was found on a shelf in a storage room in the American Philosophical Society; they had been tied up in 1801 and not looked at since. With the preparation of this guide to its archives and manuscript collections the College of Physicians entered the discovery lists.

To be sure, the College archives and manuscripts were not totally unknown. Historians from S. Weir Mitchell onwards, including a good many who prepared papers for the Section on Medical History, had found their way or been led to the treasures; and in recent years the College's scholarly librarian Walton B. McDaniel, II, revealed bits of the astonishingly rich and varied collection in the modest mimeographed occasional sheets he called "Fugitive Leaves." Although many individual manuscripts and manuscript collections were catalogued, if only after a fashion, others were not. Only chance could have uncovered the papers of the eighteenth century physician Thomas Ruston or the fifty letters from Colonel Fielding Garrison to Dr. Burton Chance. This guide displays the holdings of the College and puts them within reach of every serious scholar.

Some important single pieces are described here — the manuscript of Dr. Thomas Cadwalader's "Essay on the West-India Dry-Gripes," which Franklin printed in 1745; John Redman's letter on the yellow fever in 1762, which was useful to physicians coping with the more devastating epidemic of thirty years later; George de Benneville's "Medicina Pensylvania," compiled in 1762-79. There are twenty-eight letters of Osler to Maude Abbott on the medical museum at McGill University, and seventeen from Edward Jenner to Charles Murray about the National Vaccine Establishment. As one would expect, there are letters and papers of such able and famous Philadelphia practitioners as Jacob da Silva Solis-Cohen, Alfred Stillé, James Tyson, John Ashhurst, Robley Dunglison, and George Bacon Wood. And, as one might not expect, the College owns a miscellany of medieval medical and pharmaceutical documents in Latin, Italian, and German.

The College collection contains scores of volumes of lectures and notes of lectures of the eighteenth and nineteenth centuries — by Charles Alston, William Cullen, Joseph Black, James Gregory, Monro *secundus* in Edinburgh; Henry Cline, William and John Hunter in London; by Benjamin Rush, Adam Kuhn, Caspar Wistar, Philip Syng Physick, Benjamin Smith Barton, Nathaniel Chapman, and a dozen more in Philadelphia. Of special value to a great number of biographers are the autograph collections assembled by Joseph Carson and W. Kent Gilbert: they contain hundreds of letters of physicians and medical people such as Elisha Bartlett, Daniel Drake, Oliver W. Holmes, Florence Nightingale, and Josiah C. Nott, and of such scientists as Joseph Henry, Asa Gray, Gotthilf Muhlenberg, Thomas Nuttall, Prince Charles Lucien Bonaparte, and Baron Cuvier.

The papers of a number of professional societies which have come to rest in the College are described in these pages — the American Aesculapian Society, 1805-07, the West Philadelphia Medical Society, 1881-88, the Société médicale américaine de Paris, 1894. There are constitutions, by-laws, membership lists, minutes, accounts, and other records of local societies for laryngology, neurology, pathology, pediatrics, obstetrics, ophthalmology, and a dozen more specialties. There are the archives (in 106 volumes) of the Philadelphia Orthopaedic Hospital and Infirmary for Nervous Diseases, 1867-1942, and personal accounts of service in military hospitals in the first World War. The archives of the College itself are especially valuable, for the Fellows were the leaders of the profession, and the College committees addressed a variety of professional and community concerns. One expects to see a committee on the state of the medical profession, 1839, on a national medical association, 1845, on an anatomy act, 1867; even on the use of tobacco, 1833; but what was the reason for a "Committee on Trolley-Car Gong and Bell," 1894?

That these manuscripts and collections of manuscripts are indispensable for the history of medicine in Philadelphia is clear. They are, however, no less important to students of medicine in the United States generally. The reason is simply that Philadelphia early was and long remained the center of medical education and practice in this country. Even before the medical school was established here in 1765 — the first in the British North American colonies — ambitious young students came to Philadelphia to study with one of the hospital physicians. The number became a flood after independence: scores of young men from New England, after completing apprenticeships at home or attending Harvard Medical School, sought further education and experience from Benjamin Rush or Benjamin Smith Barton and in the wards of the Pennsylvania Hospital. This procession continued until the Massachusetts General Hospital was opened for patients. Similarly, Benjamin Silliman and Jonathan Knight, both members of the first faculty of the Medical Institution of Yale College, were sent to Philadelphia to receive the medical and scientific education not available to them at home. No small part of the history of medicine in America was made in Philadelphia, and a good deal of it must be written from records preserved in this city and in the College of Physicians, which, thanks to this guide, are now laid open. The correspondence of Edward B. Krumbhaar, for example, encompassed, among others, Sir Frederick Banting, Alexis Carrel, Fielding Garrison, William W. Keen, Sir William Osler, Peyton Rous, William W. Welch, William Howard Taft, and Franklin Delano Roosevelt.

It is worth remarking that a great many of the medical manuscripts described here are of distinguished clinical teachers and medical practitioners. From the lecture notes, commonplace books, account books like the "Co-partnership Ledgers" of Thomas and Phineas Bond; from letters and papers on the great epidemics of yellow fever in the 1790s, cholera in 1832, and influenza in 1918 the historian can learn — not without effort — what the actual state of practice was. And, notably in the papers of William W. Keen, there are echoes of old wars and battles — of anti-vivisection and anti-vaccination (the anti-vaccinationists fought to prevent typhoid inoculation of American soldiers in the first World War), and of the rivalry and ill-feeling that vexed relations between the University of Pennsylvania and Jefferson Medical College.

Philadelphia medicine has been well served through the years by a succession of able historians — by Carson and Corner on the University of Pennsylvania School of Medicine, by Ruschenberger on the College of Physicians, by Packard, Morton, and Woodbury on the Pennsylvania Hospital, by biographers and editors of Rush, Shippen, Morgan, and Mitchell. Thanks to this guide one may confidently predict that the next generation of historians will prepare fuller and more refined stories of men, institutions, and events; they will even be led to unsuspected topics — surely there must be matter for at least *one* instructive paper in the thirty-two volumes of the Philadelphia Committee for Clinical Study of Opium Addiction, 1925-29.

As one turns the pages of Dr. Hirsch's guide one concludes that the College's collection has grown through nearly two centuries without systematic or sustained effort. It contains important, even magnificent, pieces; but there are also astonishing omissions. Where are the papers, in the quantities that must once have existed, of William Wood Gerhard, Samuel D. Gross, Isaac Hays, the Meigses, the Peppers, and of Weir Mitchell, who was so eager to preserve the papers of others? This guide will perform another service to history if it notifies the Fellows of the College and other physicians, their widows and descendants, that the archives and collections of the College are ready to receive manuscript letters and documents of every kind, and that the library and historical collections of the College have a staff that intends to solicit, collect, and catalogue them. If this comes to pass, the holdings of the College will increase; we may expect to see, some fifteen to twenty years hence, the publication of a supplement; and the history of Philadelphia and American medicine will be enriched.

Whitfield J. Bell, Jr.
Executive Officer
American Philosophical Society

Note To Reader

The College of Physicians of Philadelphia is a private medical society founded in 1787 by a group of physicians which included Benjamin Rush, John Morgan, John Redman, and William Shippen. It is the oldest extant medical society not established as a licensing agency. Among its founding goals were the provision of a forum for the exchange of information and the promotion of research at the time when medical journalism was in its infancy. To these ends, monthly meetings were organized from the very beginning, a library was founded in 1788 with the gift of books and manuscripts from John Morgan, and publication of the *Transactions* began in 1793. A glance at the "List of Donors" will show the many other Fellows and friends of the College who have generously contributed to the collection's growth since that time.

Anyone unfamiliar with the collections will be made aware quickly of its treasures by the "Introduction" kindly provided by Whitfield J. Bell, Jr. As would be expected, the College possesses a great deal of material which highlights the progress of medicine in America in the eighteenth and nineteenth centuries. However, it is hoped that this catalogue will be of added use to researchers in other fields, since there are also many manuscripts from other centuries, countries and disciplines. From its medieval manuscripts on, the collection reflects the other areas of intellectual investigation which have influenced or progressed along with medicine through the ages.

Over seventeen years ago, the first Curator of Historical Collections, Walton B. McDaniel II, and the Associate Curator, Lizabeth Holloway, began work on this catalogue. It was an enormous task which many hands through the years helped to bring to completion, but uniformity in cataloguing was a goal which was not possible to achieve given the diverse nature of the collection. However, many cross-references, and the extensive name and subject indices are provided to facilitate the catalogue's use.

It should be noted that the collection contains some nontraditional material such as scrapbooks and duplicated items, e.g. mimeographed syllabi, included because of their limited circulation or unique character. Student lecture notes have been

catalogued under the name of the lecturer unless more than one
is represented in a volume. In the latter case, the notes have
been entered under the name of the transcriber or former owner
of the volume, if known. Anonymous lecture notes have been
entered under their title or subject. Papers presented at the
College and other Societies are found under the names of their
authors or grouped together under the name of the Society or
Section of the College. The enormous amount of correspondence
contained in the collection prohibits the indexing of individual
letters; only correspondents of great frequence or interest are
noted. However, indices to the various collections of correspondence are available in the College's Historical Collections.

The number in brackets at the end of each entry is the
College's classification for that item; "N.D." indicates that the
material is still being processed.

In the desire to produce this long-awaited catalogue, some
material in the collection had to be omitted. These manuscripts,
along with those recently acquired, will be included in a future
supplement. Gifts of manuscripts or funds for their acquisition
are sought from the present Fellows and friends of the College in
keeping with the tradition begun by John Morgan almost two
hundred years ago.

Christine A. Ruggere
Curator, Historical Collections

Editor's Note: Invoking an editor's privilege I add the following two special
acknowledgments.   One to Mr. Timothy Bratton whose accuracy and
patience was of considerable help. Secondly I express sincere thanks to the
curator, Miss Christine Ruggere.   Her knowledge of the College's collections,
her familiarity with medical literature, terminology and history, and her
sound judgement were invaluable in the compilation of this catalogue.
Errors, however, are the sole responsibility of the editor.

Users of the catalogue are urged to report mistakes and emendations.
Communications concerning the catalogue should be addressed to the
curator, Historical Collections, The College of Physicians of Philadelphia,
19 South 22nd Street, Philadelphia, PA., 19103.

Rudolf Hirsch

Manuscripts and Archives

1. **Abbott, Maude Elizabeth Seymour,** 1869-1940. Osler's literary output, with especial reference to his contributions to our knowledge of heart disease and the content of the Osler pathological collections at the Medical Museum of McGill University, with a personal reminiscence. *Montreal, 1934.*

   24, 2, [4] ff., 4 charts. 23.5-30 cm. Typewritten, with manuscript additions, and author's signature. Delivered before the Section on Medical History of the College of Physicians of Philadelphia, February 12, 1934. Summary published in *Trans. & Stud.* ser. 4, v. 2: 195-96 (1934) and *Canadian Medical Assoc. Journal,* v. 30: 556-57 (1934).   *[10d/40]*

   —————. See also no. 752.

2. **Abernethy, John,** 1764-1831. Lectures on surgery. *London, 1823.*

   [100] ff. 21 cm. 29 lectures. Notes taken by Samuel Betton; with his signature and bookplate.   *[10b/1]*

   —————. See also no. 743.

3. **Abrahams, Harold Justin,** b. 1901. Applications, correspondence, forms, etc., relating to his study *Extinct Medical Schools of Nineteenth-Century Philadelphia. Philadelphia, etc., 1963-66.*

   1 box (3 folders). 31 cm.   *[n.c.]*

4. **Academy of Medicine of Philadelphia.** Committee on the Means by Which Absorption is Affected. Unsigned summary of the investigation whether the theory is tenable "that the cavity of the veins and heart was utterly intolerant of the minutest portion of foreign matter." *Philadelphia?, after 1843.*

   8 pp. 25 cm. Experiment on animals under the auspices of the Academy, 1821-23, at the expense of Nathaniel Chapman, by Jason Valentine O'Brien Lawrance, Richard Harlan and Benjamin Horner Lawrance with several references to François Magendie (see also *Phila. J. of the Med. and Phys. Sci.,* v. 3: 273-302 and 5: 327-72, the latter signed only by Lawrance and Benjamin H. Coates and also issued separately under the title *An Account of Some Further Experiments*). The present document contains on pp. 7-8 a bibliographical note, crossed out in pencil, incl. a corrected reference "1830", and a pencilled note. The date "after 1843" is based on the reference to Lawrance and Harlan as "the late." Harlan died in 1843. — Fragile.   *[n.c.]*

5. **Aegidius Columna,** 1243?-1316.   De regimine regum et principum. *Italy, first half 14th cent.*

   1, 257 ff., vellum; written in 2 cols.   23.5 cm.   Illuminated figurated initial at beginning (author presenting text to Prince Philip, later Philip IV, king of France); few illuminated initials in text. Contemp. marginal corrections throughout. Sequence of chapters changed by the scribe in the last quire.
   [10a/212]

6. **Agnew, David Hayes,** 1818-92. Principles and practice of surgery. *Philadelphia, 1870?-82?*

   11 boxes; illus.   39-53 cm.   Handwriting not uniform; some smaller sections are in a different, clearer assistant's or secretarial hand. The extensive material is in approximate, numerical arrangement. The text is not consecutive and may include drafts for sections not belonging to Agnew's *Principles and Practice of Surgery.*   *[10b/24]*

   —————. See also nos. 43, 112, *185.13*, 253, 589, 710, 1037, 1080.

7. **Aix (Pharmacies).** Quatre comptes de remèdes. *Aix (en Provence?), 1710-72.*

   7 ff.   30.5 cm.   1 bill, 1710 (signed Bertier), 2 bills, 1748 (Bertrand, and widow Thérèse Paul Molinar), 1 bill, 1772 (signature undeciphered). — Gift of Dr. E.B. Krumbhaar.   *[Z10/126]*

8. **Albert, Daniel Myron,** b. 1936, comp.   Bibliography (on 3 × 5 cards) of the publications of G.E. de Schweinitz. *N.p.d.*

   1 box (418 cards).   With list of obituaries.   *[10a/436]*

9. **Albinus, Bernhard,** 1653-1721. Materia medica, *inc.*: Materia medica est congeries omnium corporum. — Materia formularum. *Leyden?* (cf. Dutch marginal note on f. 15r), *after 1702* (cf. date on f. 158r), *ca. 1710?*

   292 ff.   27 cm.   Title on spine: Albini Materia Medica. The attribution to Albinus was confirmed by Prof. G.A. Lindeboom, Amsterdam (letter of June 12, 1981): "Albinus the Elder was physician in ordinary of the King [Friedrich I] of Prussia, before he was appointed professor of medicine at Leiden University . . . in 1702." A reference to his connection with the king is found on f. 134r: ". . . ego cum Borussiae Regis essem medicus." The writing is careful and regular, and probably the work of a professional copyist; no other lecture notes of Albinus the Elder are known according to Prof. Lindeboom.
   The Materia medica is arranged in alphabetical order and deals with the terminology, worldwide occurrences and use of simplicia, with numerous references to authorities, incl. Bartholinus, Boyle, Croll, Paracelsus, Sydenham, and frequently to "C.B." (most probably referring to Caspar Bauhin, again courtesy of Prof. Lindeboom). The Materia formularum, beginning with title "Proaemium" (*inc.*: Cum absolvimus historiam simplicium on f. 253) deals

with specific compounds (de electuariis, tabellae, de trochiscis, de pilulis [!], de mixturis, etc.). With some pencilled Latin notes, possibly by John Carson (1752-94), who presented the ms. to the College of Physicians.   [10a/1]

————. See also no. 1061.

10.   **Alison, Benjamin.** Commonplace book. *Philadelphia, 1758-71?*

1 v. 20 cm. Contents: Introductory lecture, n.d. — Two clinical lectures, pleripneumonia notha, the case of John Read, teacher; gravel & rheumatism, case of Mary Veitch, Jan. 14, 1758 (probably not in Alison's hand). Notes on various diseases and surgical lectures. — Stanzas of verse (2, with date Dec. 31, 1771, on final flyleaf). Stamped Benjamin Alison.   [10a/182]

11.   **Allen, Harrison,** 1841-1897. Notes on lectures on physiology.... *Philadelphia, 1884-85.*

Ff. 3-96. 22 cm. Recorded by Thompson S. Westcott. — Presented by Mrs. T.S. Westcott.   [10a/221]

————. See also nos. 936, 1080.

12.   **Allen, Henry B.** The reparative power and processes in the human system; illustrated by a case of necrosis of the humerus. *Philadelphia, 1883.*

[1], 80 ff.; pasted-in photograph (f. 30). 26.5 cm. Thesis of Henry B. Allen (Jefferson Medical College), offered in competition for faculty prize no. 1. — Presented by William H. Pancoast.   [10b/13]

13.   **Alston, Charles,** 1683-1760. A course of publick lectures on the materia medica by Charles Alston Proffessor of the Mat: Med: & Bottany in the Colledge of Edinburgh; taken ... by John Redman . . . . In proprium usum. *Edinburgh, 1746.*

210 pp. 21 cm. Fragile, in defective contemp. binding. Spelling reproduced as found in ms. — Alston's lectures were published in 2 vols. in 1770.   [10a/2]

14.   **Alta Friendly Society.** Application forms. *Philadelphia and Pittsburgh, 1887-1905.*

3 boxes. 26 cm. Completed forms contain applications for sick benefits, certificates of attending physicians and official decisions made by this health insurance society.   [10c/143]

15.   **American Aesculapian Society.** Constitution, by-laws, library regulations. *New York, 1805-07.*

18 ff. 20 cm. Copy corrected by John Watts, Jr. — Among subscribers were several graduates of the Medical School of Columbia College, 1806-16. Mem-

bership included beyond second-year students holders of the A.B.   The Society
lapsed for a time, revived in 1812, and published a series of *Transactions.* — Gift
of the heirs of Joseph Carson.   *[10c/1]*

16.   **American Association for the History of Medicine.** Constitution and by-laws, minutes, reports, correspondence, membership
lists, financial records, misc. printed materials. *V.p., 1922-80.*

10'10" of files and 8 boxes. 29-39 cm. Constitution and by-laws, incl.
revisions (1928-75). Minutes and reports, (1922-80), of annual business
meetings, with some attendance lists. Correspondence (1922-80) of AAHM
officers, especially of presidents F.B. Rogers, S. Jarcho, and G. Miller, and of
secretary-treasurers J. Blake, W.J. Bell, and G. Miller. Correspondence and
membership lists of Council (1958-80). Various committee minutes, correspondence, and misc. records (1971-77); records, incl. correspondence, reports,
and some financial material of annual meetings (1922-80). Membership lists
of Association (1924-76), lists of officers (1954-80), and correspondence (1939-
54), concerning deceased members; and correspondence with constituent
societies (1968-78). Accounts (1922-73) of Association, incl. general and
special funds, and membership dues records. Misc. pamphlets, brochures,
and clippings. — Deposited by Secretary of the Association.   *[Z10d/6]*

— — — — —. See also nos. 29, *185.62*, 560.

American Hospital, Paris, *see* **Paris. American Hospital.**

17.   **American Journal of the Medical Sciences.** Index to the
American Journal of the Medical Sciences and the *Philadelphia Journal
of the Medical and Physical Sciences,* from 1820-48. *Philadelphia,
1820-48.*

3 v. 39 cm. Inscribed on flyleaf of v. 1: "... The Index was made for my father
John K. Mitchell & presented to the College of Physicians October 12, 1877 by
S. Weir Mitchell."   *[Z10/25]*

— — — — —. See also nos. 516, 520.

18.   **American Medical Association.** Constitution, delegate registers. *New York, Philadelphia, etc., 1847-60.*

400+ pp. 28-36 cm. Constitution (1847), and register of delegates, with
signatures (1847-60). The constitution (pp. 1-14) is preceded by a report (pp. i-
ii) of the Committee on the Organization of the National Medical Association,
as ordered by the National Medical Convention held in the City of New York in
the month of May, 1846. Contains lists of delegates to AMA annual
conventions (1847-60); the remainder of the 1860 delegates are listed on pp.
14-23. Registration book (1847), containing 233 (i.e. 235) signatures of
delegates (numbers 14 and 15 are used twice) to the first AMA meeting, held
in Philadelphia. — Constitution and register of delegates, gift of W.B.
Atkinson; registration book, gift of I. Minis Hays.   *[10a/153, 10a/168]*

— — — — —. See also nos. *185.14*, 253, 487, 875, 943, 1103, 1115,
1122.

19. **American Pediatric Society.** Minutes, etc. *V.p., 1888-1916.*

    2 v. 27 cm. Includes constitution and by-laws (handwritten in v. 1, printed in v. 2), lists of lectures and members, printed programs, etc. Deposited by the American Pediatric Society (cf. letter of the secretary treasurer, Dr. A.C. McGuinness, May 27, 1954). *[ZZ10a/3]*

    American Physicians' Fellowship Committee, *see* **Histadruth ha-Refu'ith be-'Yisrael.**

20. **Anders, James Meschter,** 1854-1936. The consolidation of the medical schools of Philadelphia — its advantages. *Philadelphia, ca. 1916.*

    2 ff. 28 cm. Typescript. Concerns the then proposed merger of Jefferson Medical College, Medico-Chirurgical College and the University of Pennsylvania Medical School. Fragile; xerox copy enclosed. *[10d/87]*

21. **Andral, Gabriel,** 1797-1876. Cours de pathologie interne. *Paris, 1831-33?*

    2 v. ([62] ff., pp. 45-371; [1], 377 ff.). 21.5 cm. Presented by William Wood Gerhard (1809-72), who studied in Paris in 1830-33 under Andral. *[10a/3]*

    —————. See also no. 172.

22. **Angeluscheff, Zhivko D.,** b. 1897. Papers and correspondence on hearing, deafness, and ultrasonics. *New York, etc., 1957-65.*

    1 envelope. 28 cm. Contents: 1. Hearing cell and sonic boom, to the 8th International Congress of Oto-rhino-laryngology, Oct. 1965, Tokyo (10 ff.). How we are going deaf, to 2d Extraordinary Congress of the International Society of Audiology, Oct. 1965, Kyoto (10, [2]ff.), with bibliography. 2. Letters to the author from M. Morimoto, Japan, Dec. 1965 (xeroxed copy); Bo Lundberg, Stockholm, 1965 (xeroxed copy). 3. Author's letter, 1965, Feb. 23, New York (typewritten, signed) to Douglas Mcfarlan, and discussion by Douglas Mcfarlan of author's paper on ultrasonics, resonance, and deafness, International Congress of Otolaryngology, Washington, May 1957 (xeroxed copy). *[10a/438]*

23. **Anti-Vaccination League of Pennsylvania.** Membership lists, case reports, receipt book. *Philadelphia, ca. 1900-16.*

    500+ pp. 26.5-35.5 cm. List (ca. 1900-16) of names and addresses of League members, both American and foreign. Cases (ca. 1912) of compulsory smallpox vaccination, some reports submitted by Charles J. Field. Receipt book (1906-13) listing payments of memberships, donation, and sales.
    [10c/97, Z10c/17, ZZ10c/12]

24. **Anti-Vaccination Society of America.** Constitution and by-laws, minutes, reports, correspondence, financial records, printed materials. *New York, etc., 1885-98.*

1 v. (217 pp., pp. 81-217 blank); 1 envelope. 26-37.5 cm. Originals and copies of constitution, by-laws, minutes, reports, correspondence, financial statements, printed items, and clippings of this Society, organized in 1879, and incorporated in 1885 "to investigate the benefits, or evil results" of smallpox vaccination.

[10c/98]

25. **Apostoli, Georges,** 1847-1900. De la galvano-puncture chimique en gynécologie. *Paris, 1886.*

4 ff. 31 cm. Reproduced from handwritten copy. Request to publish the attached resumé, distributed to various journals. — Fragile.   *[n.c.]*

26. **Arnold, Will Ford,** 1862-1921. Hookworm disease in the South; its neglect. *N.p., ca. 1906.*

6 ff. 28 cm. Typescript. Paper "read at the 1906 meeting of the Tri-State Medical Association of Mississippi, Arkansas & Tennessee," and published in *Memphis Medical Monthly*, v. 27 (1907). Stillé Society Library rules pasted inside front cover.   *[Z10a/1]*

27. **Arnoldus de Villanova,** 1240?-1311. De conservatione sanitatis, ff. 1r-26r. — Regimen speciale, ff. 26r-28v. *Catalonia?, ca. 1400.*

28 ff. 19 cm. Description by dealer inside front cover; revised description by Dr. M. Battlori (dated 1950) at end. Alternate title of the De conservatione sanitatis: Regimen sanitatis.   *[10a/210]*

28. ————. De cura sterilitatis mulierum compositus a M[agistro] R[aymundo] de M[oleriis], *inc.:* Sapientis verbum est, data est . . . (*vide* Thorndike & Kibre, col. 638), ff. 1r-7v. — *With* De infirmitatibus occulorum (fragment, Liber quintus *inc.:* Cum de novo accidit malum . . .), ff. 8r-12r, and Alie cure infirmitatum occulorum, *inc.:* Sciendum est quod ungule sunt . . ., ff. 12r-17v. *Italy?, 14th cent.*

17 ff.; illus. 19 cm. The *De cura sterilitatis* has also been attributed to Raymundus de Moleriis and occasionally to Jordanus de Turre. It is incomplete at end and lacks the companion tract *Impedimenta conceptionis ex parte viri.* — The *De infirmitatibus occulorum* is a fragment containing the end of liber quartus (22 lines only) and liber quintus. Folio 11v illustrates instruments (ferramenta) used to deal with disorders of the eye (catharactas, ungulas, palpebras, etc.). Closely cropped with minor loss of text. — Gift of S. Weir Mitchell.   *[10a/135]*

29. **Arons, Walter Leonard,** b. 1920. The note-book of Doctor John Archer (1766-1767) . . . . *Philadelphia, 1944.*

30 ff. 29 cm. Typescript (carbon copy). Submitted by W.L. Arons of the University of Pennsylvania Medical School in competition for the William Osler Medal of the American Association for the History of Medicine.

[Z10/160]

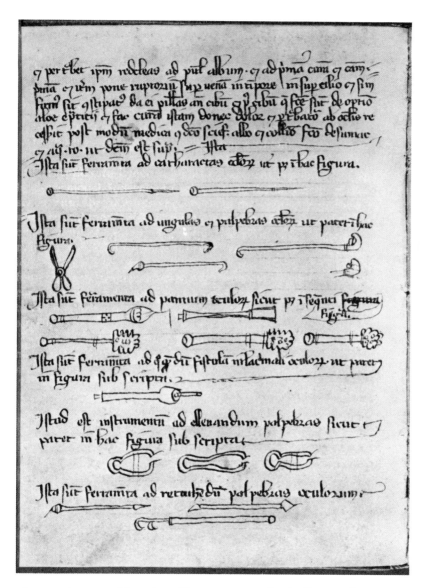

Plate 1. 28. Arnoldus de Villanova. *De Infirmitatibus occulorum*, 14th century.

30.   **Artephius.** Chapitre intitulé De la generation de l'homme. Le vray titre doit être De la regeneration de l'homme . . . . *France, late 18th cent.*

> 391 [i.e. 402] pp. 17 cm. With corrections and marginalia. For information on Artephius and printed editions in various languages (incl. French) see J. Ferguson, *Bibl. Chem.*, v. 1, pp. 50-1. Pages numbered 1-110, 101-110, 112-349, 349-391 and 1 p. on recto of endpaper.   *[10a/162]*

31.   **Artzney Buch.** Collection of prescriptions and remedies. *Germany, 1568-1600.*

> [168] ff. 15 cm. Leaves 50-51, 95 and 104 blank; 1 f. at the beginning (blank?) missing, another, between 145 and 146, torn out. In 3 or more hands. Separate caption titles: Von etlichen Künsten (f. 48r), dated 1568. – Etlich Artzney (f. 51v), dated 1600. – . . . Von gebranthen Wassern (by Michael Schrick?; f. 105r), dated 1568. – Ausz . . . gedruckten Kreuter Büchern (f. 139). With 2 indices: Register über disz Artzenei Buch (ff. 96r-101v). – Register über das letzte Artzney Buech . . . 1600 (f. 168r, ending with letter C, the rest missing). Deals with a great variety of medicines against epilepsy, jaundice, the plague, podagra, stillbirth, strokes, venereal diseases, etc. "Ex libris Johann Christoph Götz Badensis" inside front cover (probably Johann Christoph Goetze, 1688-1733).   *[10a/231]*

– – – – –. See also no. 712.

32.   **Ashhurst, Astley Paston Cooper,** 1876-1932. Papers. *Philadelphia, etc., 1900-30.*

> 3 boxes. 32-39 cm. Contents: *Box 1.* World War I: Organization, correspondence concerning records, etc., of Base Hospital no. 34, Nantes, France. – *Box 2,* envelope 1. Biographies of his father John Ashhurst, jr.; env. 2, Bibliography of J.A., jr.; 3. Accounts of American travel; 4. Correspondence with C.B.G. de Nancrede, 1911-16, concerning the chair of surgery at the Univ. of Michigan; 5. Correspondence, chiefly letters to A.P.C. Ashhurst, incl. typed transcripts, calendars. – *Box 3,* env. 6. European trips, 1905 and 1914; 7. Exhibits: on fracture (College pf Physicians of Philadelphia, March 6, 1928); Lister centenary (*ibid.,* April 5, 1927); 8. The classification and mechanism of fractures of the leg bones involving the ankle, by A.P.C. Ashhurst and Ralph S. Bromer (50, [3] ff.); Roentgen ray studies of the ankle joint by R.S. Bromer (14, [5] ff.), both read before the Amer. Surg. Assoc., 1921, published in extended form in *Arch. Surg.,* v. 4: 51-129 (1922); 9. Operative surgery of the hip joint (95, 5 ff.), presented at the International Soc. of Surg., Warsaw, 1929, published in *Arch. Surg.,* v. 20: 87-144 (1930); 10. Misc. biographical information; 11. Memorandum on Gwilym George Davis. – Presented by various donors, esp. Mrs. A.P.C. Ashhurst and L.E. Snodgrass.   *[10a/322]*

33.   – – – – –. Textbook of surgery. *Philadelphia, ca. 1908-13.*

> 6 boxes. 39 cm. Title from chapter I (box 1, set A; "Institutions" crossed out, "Text Book" substituted in ink). Published under title *Surgery, its Principles and Practice* (Philadelphia, Lea & Febiger, 1914). Letter from publisher on illustrations (box 1) dated January 1909 indicates that work on the text must have

begun in 1908 or earlier. Three sets: A. typed chapters I-XIV. — B. handwritten with corrections, chapters I-VIII. — C. handwritten, chapters I-XXVIII. — No attempt has been made to establish the chronological sequence of these sets.　　　　　　　　　　　　　　　　　　　　　　　　*[Z10/93]*

— — — — —. See also nos. 34-35, 679, 1024.

34.　**Ashhurst, John,** 1839-1900. Memoranda booklets. *Philadelphia, 1875-98.*

24 v., 1 envelope. 16 cm (box, 26.5 cm). Chronological record of visits to patients, meetings, and hospitals, including Episcopal and Children's. Also notes on nurses, books, medical students, subscriptions. Laid in: business cards, advertisements, correspondence, two summons to appear as a witness in court (1891, 1897). Most of the volumes have signature of John Ashhurst and A.P.C. Ashhurst.　　　　　　　　　　　　　　　　　　*[10b/44]*

35.　— — — — —. Papers, incl. childhood journal, essays and addresses while an undergraduate at the University of Pennsylvania, medical essay, lecture notes, student grades, correspondence, etc., catalogue of his library and bio-bibliographical items by his son A.P.C. Ashhurst. *Philadelphia, 1845-1901.*

4 boxes. 39.5 cm. Largely autograph; some photocopies. Contents: Box 1. Journal 1848-49 (bound); papers and addresses (2 vols., incl. 1 on Anaxagoras, 6 ff.); some addresses in Greek and English translation (bound); photocopies of biography and bibliography of John Ashhurst by his son (2 envelopes). — Box 2. Notes for lectures on inflammation, abscesses, ulcers, erysipelas, etc. (2 env.); students' examinations and final grades in course on surgery (1890-96; 4 env.); index to 1st edition of his *The Principle and Practice of Surgery* (1871; 1 env.); medical essays and addresses (2 folders), incl. Contribution to surgical literature; Surgery before the days of anaesthesia; Surgery of the larger bloodvessels; The ethics of nursing (carbon, 3 ff.); Valedictory address, Univ. of Penna. 1879; letters to J.A. during his illness, and condolences upon his death (1 folder). — Box 3. Bibliotheca medica; Catalogue of a collection of books on medicine and the allied sciences (1866-93?; bound), and smaller catalogue (1856-63?; bound); Table of cases treated (1877-82; 1 fold.). — Box 4. Letters to John Ashhurst (originals and photocopies, 1874-93; partial[?] calendar); misc. (notes on lectures; booklist; cash book; exercise book, 1850; Univ. of Penna. reports, notices, etc.; *International Encyclopedia of Surgery* controversy [5 folders]); U.S.A. General Hospital, Chester, Penna. Ward D. Case book (1862-98; broken binding).
　　　　　　　　　　　　　　　　　　　　　　　　　　　[Z10/81]

36.　[— — — — —]. Letters and notes to John Ashhurst. *V.p., 1863-1900.*

1 box (11 folders). 32 cm. Extensive collection of letters, a considerable number concerned with Ashhurst's activity for the Committee on Publication of the International Medical Congress, the Committee of Publication of the College of Physicians of Philadelphia, and as editor of various editions of the *International Encyclopedia of Surgery.* A list of correspondents is filed with the

collection; some major writers of letters are: William Allen, J.S. Billings, J.H. Hutchinson, William MacCormac, W.F. Norris, C.B.G. de Nancrède, G.A. Otis, L.A. Sayre, J.C. Warren and J.C. White.   *[n.c.]*

————. See also nos. *185.13*, 361, 675, 804, 846, 1079-80.

37. **Ashmead, Albert Sydney,** 1851-1911. Correspondence (original letters to, and copies of letters, by A.S. Ashmead, hand- and typewritten articles primarily by Ashmead, printed items, etc., a large part concerned with leprosy). *V.p., 1894-1910.*

3 boxes (in excess of 700 items); illus. 32 cm. Boxes 1-2 contain primarily letters to Ashmead; several deal with the International Leprosy Conference, Berlin, 1897. Well represented among correspondents are Juan de Díos Carasquilla (21 items), David G. Brinton (18 items), Jules Goldschmidt (27 items), H. Polakowsky (19 items), Alfred Stillé, and a few others. — Box 3 contains besides copies of letters by Ashmead (incl. one to R. Virchow) some addressed to him, articles and notes by Ashmead and others, a few photographs, printed items, etc. — Alphabetical index of correspondents (complete?) and partial analysis of contents filed with the collection. Contents of Box 3 unsorted and in need of further study (some items torn and/or fragile).   *[n.c.]*

————. See also no. 65.

38. **Association of the Out-door Physicians of the Guardians of the Poor of the City of Philadelphia.** Constitution, list of members, and minutes. *Philadelphia, 1872-74.*

24 pp. 34.5 cm. Misc. letters and printed materials laid in. Presented by Edwin L. Evans.   *[Z10/59]*

39. **Atmospheric Air, its Physical and Chemical Properties.** *Philadelphia?, 1806-07.*

[1 blank], 16, [1 blank] ff. 20 cm. Paper submitted "to your inspection," (cf. f. 16); the "inspector" not identified. With reference to a Count Morozzo (f. 9) and Joseph Priestley (f. 12).   *[n.c.]*

40. **B., H.** Compendium medicum, das ist, ein kurtzes, aber doch nützliches Artzneybüchlein, wie man alle Gebrästen unnd Kranckheiten des menschlichen Leibs, von dem Haupt bis auff die Füszsolen, mit gewissen und approbirten Experimenten curiren soll. Jetzunder wider auffs newe sehr verbessert, vermehrt, auch mit einem nützlichen Register gezieret. Durch.*HB* von Ruchheim Anno. 1724. *Germany (or Pennsylvania?), 1724.*

3 ff., 1004 pp. (irregularly numbered, e.g. 878 omitted; pp. 319-20, 665-66, 789-94 removed; 2 or more ff. after p. 1004 missing), 8 ff. 21 cm. Folio 2 of the introduction with caption title Oeconomiae hiatricus genannt zu Deutsch, ein Artzney Buch oder Hausartzney. — The title page (p. 1) resembles the style of a

printed book; this ms. may have been copied from a published text. The author has not been identified. Several prescriptions and some passages in Latin. Authorities cited belong largely to earlier periods. — Bookplate of Carl Bensel, son of Georg Bensel, dated 1763.   *[10a/299]*

41. **Babcock, William Wayne,** 1872-1963. Babcock's notes on pathology. *Philadelphia, ca. 1920?*

[1], 15, 49, [3] ff. 33 cm. Typescript (carbon). "Copied for students at Temple College" on title page.   *[10a/493]*

—————. See also no. 622.

42. **Bache, Franklin,** 1792-1864. Papers and correspondence. *Philadelphia, etc., 1814-59.*

2 boxes (30 envelopes, nos. 1-28). 39 cm. Contents: I. Lectures, essays, reviews, etc. Envelope 1. Essay on emphysema; inaugural thesis (34 ff., 1814); 2. Lecture before the Medical Society on the Brunonian theory of life and disease (25 ff., 1820); 3. Notice of his chemistry textbook; outline for medical students (10 pp., 1820); 4. Elucidation furnished by chemistry; lecture before the Medical Society (18 ff., 1821); 5. Review of the *U.S. Pharmacopoeia* 1820, publ. in *Medical Recorder*, July 1821 (31 instead of 32 ff., 1821); 6. Review of nosological arrangements of Drs. Cullen, Hosack, and Rush (22 ff., 1823); 7. Account . . . of the atomic theory; lecture at the Academy of Natural Sciences (27 pp., 1823); 8. Lecture on the theory of volumes of Gay-Lussac, *ibid.* (20 pp., 1823); 9. Small pox and vaccination; clipping from *National Gazette*, signed A.B.C., with added notation "by Fr.B." (1 f., 1823); 10. Lecture on the application of chemistry to the science of medicine before the Medical Society (1 f., 22 pp., 1824); 11. Remarks on the action of hydrogen on spongy platinum (3 ff., ca. 1830); 12. Draft of regulations on conferring the M.D. at the Philadelphia Medical College (6 ff., 1836); 13. New method of chess notation (5 ff., 1855); 14. Corrections to 1859 Amer. ed. of Fownes' *Manual of Chemistry*, with acknowledgment by Robert Bridges (9 ff., n.d.); 15. Memorial of the physicians of the Southern Dispensary for the Medical Relief of the Poor; draft by F. Bache (6 ff., n.d.).

II. Letters primarily by F. Bache. 16. Printed form, on inquiry from the Committee on Commerce of the Pennsylvania House of Representatives on prevention of spasmodic cholera (2 ff.) with copy of B.'s answer (7 pp., 1832); 17. Letter of Andrew Boardman on address on political economics and currency in New York, with F.B.'s answer (2 + 4 ff., 1841); 18. Letter to Robley Dunglison on errors in D.'s 4th ed. of *New Remedies* (14 pp., 2 ff., 1846); 19. Letter to Benjamin Gerhard on questions of hygiene and environment (4 pp., 1 f., 1849); 20. Letter to John Churchill with list of corrections (1, 3 ff., 1858).

III. Letters primarily to F. Bache. 21a-b. Letter of T. Sewall introducing Wm. Beaumont, and from Beaumont, concerning analysis of gastric juices of A. St. Martin (4 ff., 1833); Beaumont soliciting testimonial on same matter (2 ff., 1834); 22. Letter of Nicholas Chervin and draft of answer, on yellow fever (2 ff., 6 pp., 1821); 23. Letter of Robert Hare on the heating of prison cells, with notes (incl. drawings) by B. (7 ff., 1830); 24. Letter of Joseph Lovell referring to Beaumont's account (2 ff., 1833); 25a-b. Fourteen letters of Benjamin Silliman on Edward Turner's *Elements of Chemistry*, etc. (together 24 ff., 1829-33, 1836, 1855); 26. Correspondence between Edward Turner and F. Bache on various editions of the *Elements of Chemistry* (22 ff., 1831-34); 27. Six letters of J.C. Warren on anesthesia (13 ff., 1826, 1851-54); 28. Four letters by J.W. Webster on need for an inexpensive textbook of chemistry at Harvard, etc. (8 ff., 1836-43). — Partial contents filed at end of box 2, with letter of transmittal by the donor, Franklin Bache (1931).   *[10a/292]*

————. See also nos. 112, 169, 787-8, 980, 1103, 1112, 1115-6.

43. **Baker, George Fales,** 1864-1929. Manuscript notes in syllabus of the Department of Medicine, University of Pennsylvania. *Philadelphia, 1884-85.*

2 v. 23 cm. Printed interleaved text with extensive notes on James Tyson's "General Pathological Anatomy" (v. 1, pp. 189-249), followed by 23 pp. ms. additions, and on R.A.F. Penrose's "Obstetrics and Diseases of Children," D.H. Agnew's "Surgery" (v. 2, pp. [251]-450), followed by 38 pp. ms. additions.
[10b/62]

44. **Baltz, Theodor Friedrich,** 1785-1859. Les suites nuisibles de la circoncision: lettre missive au concile des rabbins à Frankfort. *Berlin, 1845.*

[10] ff. (last blank). 28 cm. "Imprimée comme manuscrit et distribuée particulièrement." Two leaves with dedications: Aux hauts ministères du culte de tous les états, and À l'Institut de France, à l'Académie royale des sciences . . . . — Manuscript inscription: Mr. Dieffenbach à Mons. Vanier (f. 2). Presented by Alfred Stillé to the Lewis Library. Bookplates of Samuel Lewis and Stillé.   *[10b/41]*

45. **Barton, Benjamin Smith,** 1766-1815. Lectures on materia medica . . . in the University of Pennsylvania. *Philadelphia, 1802-03.*

2 v. ([2], 764, 21 ff.). 21 cm. Signatures of Robert Patterson on front fly-leaf of v. 1, of John S. Mitchell in v. 2. "Index of the classes" on final 21 leaves of v. 2. Pencilled prose and poetry on versos of ff., in reverse, by earlier relatives of E.B. Krumbhaar, acc. to note in back of v. 1. Letter to Jasper Yeates by William Barton dated July 15, 1774 pasted in v. 2. — Gift of E.B. Krumbhaar.
[10a/394]

46. ————   ————. *Philadelphia, 1806-07.*

246 ff. 22.5 cm. Student unidentified.   *[10a/6]*

47. ————   ————. *Philadelphia, ca. 1812.*

481 pp. 26 cm. Inscription on flyleaf: "Wm. Elmer, April 20th 1812."
[10a/377]

48. ————   ————. *Philadelphia, 181—?*

4 v. (268, 190, 190, 262 ff.). 21 cm. Presented by Hugh Lenox Hodge; with his bookplates.   *[10a/10]*

49.   — — — — —. Notes from a course of lectures on the institutes and practice of medicine . . . . *Philadelphia, 1814-15.*

284 pp. 20.5 cm. Notes taken by Henry Vander Veer, Somerville, N.J., according to the donor, Fred B. Rogers.   *[10a/402]*

50.   — — — — —. Notes from Dr. Barton's lectures on natural history or zoology. *Philadelphia, 1809-10.*

56 pp. 21 cm. Student not identified.   *[10a/8]*

51.   — — — — —. Notes on lectures of B.S. Barton. *Philadelphia, 1815.*

[24] ff. 21 cm. Notes on "Barton's practice," taken by Robert Alison.
[10a/178]

52.   — — — — —. Notes on the lectures of Dr. Benj. S. Barton . . . taken by Thos. D. Mitchell. *Philadelphia, 1809-10.*

447 pp. 25 cm. Includes index. — Bound with Thomas Duché Mitchell's *Notes on the lectures on surgery delivered by Drs. Physick and Dorsey in the University of Pennsylvania*, 1809-10; 371 pp., with partial index. — Presented by W.W. Keen.   *[10a/11]*

53.   — — — — —. Notes on the materia medica from the lectures of B.S. Barton. *Philadelphia, 1808-09.*

2 v. (250, 272 ff.). 24.5 cm. Title pages mutilated to delete a name. — Presented by the heirs of Joseph Carson.   *[10a/7]*

54.   — — — — —. Notes taken from the lectures of Doctor Barton on the practice of physick as delivered in the University of Pennsylvania, by James P. Freeman. *Philadelphia, 181—.*

229 pp. (title on fly-leaf; blank leaves at end). 20 cm. It is doubtful that James P. Freeman attended the lectures of Barton; Freeman received his A.B. in 1816, i.e. the year after Barton's death, and his M.D. in 1819. He may have copied the notes from somebody else's manuscript or he may have been the owner.   *[10a/9]*

55.   — — — — —. Samuel Betton's notes on Dr. Barton's lectures. *Philadelphia, 1803-04.*

[512] pp. 26 cm. Bookplate of Thomas Forrest Betton.   *[10a/5]*

— — — — —. See also nos. 114, 150, 805h, 816.

56.   **Barton, William Paul Crillon,** 1785-1856. Manuscript relating to Jefferson Medical College. *N.p.d.*

47 ff. 33 cm. Presented by Geo. M[?]. Abbot, June 9, 1893: "This paper by my grandfather Wm. P.C. Barton has something to do with the early history of the Jefferson College . . . ." — An account of a "fantastic vision of the imagination,"

evidently representing in allegory the early rivalry between the medical schools of Jefferson and the University of Pennsylvania. Typewritten transcript (15 pp.) included.   *[Z 10/2]*

—————. See also nos. 114, 364.

57.   **Bayle, Antoine Laurent Jessé,** 1799-1858.   Notice sur Laënnec. *Paris, 1826?*

18, 20 pp. 27.5 cm. Manuscript of article which appeared in *Revue médicale* (1826). With typescript copy (20 pp.). — Note accompanying manuscript states that it was presented to Francis R. Packard by Flammarion, Paris, 1933.   *[10c/71]*

58.   **Bechet, Paul Esnard,** 1881-1962.   Papers. *V.p., 1911-57.*

2 boxes. 31.5 cm. Manuscript, typescript, and reprints. Consists chiefly of correspondence from dermatologists and of materials relating to the history of American dermatology. Partial content: 40 letters, etc., concerning the 6th Int'l. Dermatological Congress, N.Y., Sept., 1907; G. Nobl, Fifty years of Vienna dermatology, from *De dermatologia,...* Budapest, 1936, tr. by G. Riehl; correspondence on Bechet's *Hist. Amer. Derm. Assoc., 1876-1951.* — Gift of Mrs. Bechet.   *[Z 10c/21]*

Beck, David de, *see* **De Beck, David.**

59.   **Bedell, Arthur Joseph,** b. 1879.   The macula in the elderly. *Albany, N.Y., 1949.*

117 pp. 29 cm. Typescript; photographs. This was the 1949 George E. de Schweinitz Lecture of the College of Physicians' Section on Ophthalmology.
                    [ZZ 10d/13]

60.   **[Beerman, Herman,** b. 1901].   The publications of Dr. Herman Beerman. *Philadelphia, ca. 1947.*

1 folder (4 ff.). 28 cm. Typescript (carbon copy).
                    [Z 10/180]

61.   **Beers, John B.**   Description and patent of a new instrument, called the wife's protector . . . to prevent conception. *Rochester, N.Y. and Washington, 1846-47.*

[2] ff., 2 printed forms, 1 f. engr. illus. 23-32.5 cm. Patent no. 4729. Bookplate of Samuel Lewis.   *[Z 10/107]*

62.   **Behrend, Moses,** 1877-1969.   Security against illness and injury in the State of Pennsylvania today. *Philadelphia, 1939.*

2, 15 ff. 33 cm. Typewritten. Read before the Section on Public Health, Preventive and Industrial Medicine of College of Physicians, Feb. 6, 1939. Published (without summary, 2 ff. at beginning) in *Pennsylvania Med. Jour.,* v. 43: 18-20 (1939).   *[ZZ 10d/5]*

63. **Bellott, M.?** Lecture notes on silver, platina, palladium, etc., galvanism (ff. 7v-13v), fluids, in particular water and vegetable nature, April 6-17, 1810. *Edinburgh?, 1810.*

[24] ff.; illus. 16 cm (in envelope). Pencilled. "M. Bellott Esq. care of T. Thorburn Esq. Writer George Square Edin." (f. 24v). [n.c.]

Benneville, George de, *see* **De Benneville, George.**

64. **Berens, Conrad,** 1889-1963. Evaluation of certain glaucoma operations with especial reference to cycloelectrolysis, cyclodiathermy and iridocorneosclerectomy. *New York, 1954.*

69 pp. 29 cm. Typescript; photographs. 1954 George E. de Schweinitz Lecture of the College of Physicians' Section on Ophthalmology.

[ZZ 10d/12]

65. **[Beri-Beri].** Collection of some foreign opinions on pathological matters peculiar to Japan [etc.], collected by A.S. Ashmead. *N.p.d. (ca. 189—?).*

3 folders in 2 boxes (39 cm.). Translations (or versions) of studies on beri-beri (kakke) from the pens of a great variety of authors. Not analyzed. [n.c.]

66. **Bernardus de Gordonio.** Lilium medicinae. *England (Oxford?), 1348.*

xxiv, 256 ff. (ff. 1, 30-1, 71, 88, 122, 135, 148, 172-4, 201, 203-6, 218-9, 239, 241, 243 missing, f. 242 repaired with loss of text). Few illuminated initials. Restored, near-contemp. Oxford binding. 18.5 cm (in box). Listed under title *Practica dicta Lilium medicine* in L.E. Demaitre, *Doctor Bernard de Gordon* (Toronto, 1980), no. 58 (pp. 185-8). Sixteenth-century title page on preliminary first leaf, followed by early 16th-cent. alphabetical index (incomplete, begins with letter E). Purchase note, unsigned, in a 15th-cent. hand "Istum librum emi a doctore Kokkes" (Cokes, Coxe?; f. 2r); W. Patten. 1555 (f. 1r). With marginal and interlinear contemporary corrections. — Various descriptions, correspondence, etc., relating to the ms. are enclosed. — Gift of Sir William Osler.

[10a/249]

— — — —. See also no. 643.

67. **Betton, Thomas Forrest,** 1809-75. Lectures on surgery. *Philadelphia, 184-?*

238 ff. 26 cm. "Presented to Dr. H.E. Goodman by the author . . . upwards of 25 years ago; . . . presented to College of Physicians by H. Earnest [sic] Goodman . . . 6/28/1895." Lectures chiefly concern inflammation. [10b/2]

— — — —. See also nos. 55, 141, *185.613*, 412, 914.

68. **[Bilious Remitting Fever].** *N.p., first half 19th cent.*

   9 ff. 25.5 cm (in envelope). Without indication of authorship. Slight, contemporary editorial corrections. Blind-stamped "Ames" (name of stationer?) on front leaf.   *[10a/413]*

69. **Bines, D. A.** A dissertation on phlegmasia dolens . . . to be read in the 22nd district, Medical Society of Ohio, May 26th, 1829. *N.p., 1829.*

   Title page, pp. 1-4, blank f., 39 ff. 26.5 cm. Presented by Robert L. Pitfield.
                                                                          [Z 10/123]

70. **Bisbé y Perez, José.** Report of two hundred and eighteen anomalies found in the anatomical rooms of the University of Pennsylvania with eighty-four illustrations and a general statement of their average frequency.   Presented to the demonstrator of anatomy, Dr. Lenox Hodge. *Philadelphia, 1875-76.*

   1 v. (84 drawings on 21 pp.). 25 cm. Offered in competition for a student prize awarded by Hodge.   *[10a/52]*

71. **Bishop, William,** b. 1818. An inaugural essay on Asiatic cholera, presented to the faculty of the Philadelphia College of Medicine, for the degree of doctor in medicine. *Philadelphia, 1859.*

   [20] ff. 25 cm.   *[n.c.]*

72. **Bitner, Abraham,** d. 1854.   Note's [sic] taken from the Philadelphia Alms House. *Philadelphia, 1824-25.*

   1 v. only. 19.5 cm. Added: Notes on lectures of Nathaniel Chapman, dated 1825.   *[10a/397]*

73. **Black, Joseph,** 1728-99.   Lectures on chemistry (notes taken[?] by Caspar Wistar, 1784). *Edinburgh, 1784.*

   4 v. 19 cm. Consists of notes on 118 lectures. Inscribed inside front cover of each volume: "1784. From Dr. Caspar Wistar's Medical Library; presented to the College of Physicians in the name of Dr. Mifflin Wistar, 1887." Inscribed on p. [1] of v. 1: "C. Wistar junr."   *[10a/12]*

74. — — — — —. Notes from Dr. Blacks lectures on chemistry. *Edinburgh, ca. 1792-93.*

   1 v. 19.5 cm. "Tho C James" (presumably Thomas Chalkley James, the notetaker) on t.-p., and "Supposed to be about 1792 or 3" on following p. Case notes on few pp. at end of volume. — With bookplate of Hugh Lenox Hodge.   *[10a/14]*

75. —————. Syllabus of a course of chemistry by Dr. Black. *Edinburgh, 1792-93.*

1 v. 18 cm. A note on earlier catalogue card states "Taken by Thom. C. James." — Bookplate of Hugh Lenox Hodge.   *[10a/13]*

—————. See also no. 111.

76. **Blayney, Arthur,** 1762?-1814. Accounts for visits to, and medicines for, patients. *Philadelphia, 1802-14.*

262, [30] pp. 38.5 cm. Inscribed inside front cover: "Dr. Blayney." Brief ms. notes *re* travels of Richard Stone Blayney in 1809 on p. 1. — Presented by his descendant, Willis H. Blayney, through the generosity of Herbert A. Greene, March, 1972.   *[Z 10c/20]*

Blockley, Philadelphia, *see* **Philadelphia. General Hospital.**

77. **Bodenhamer, William,** 1808-1905. Fissure of the os uteri as a cause of sterility; its symptomatology, aetiology, pathology, diagnosis and treatment. *New Rochelle, N.Y., 1905.*

[3], 11 ff. 17.5-39 cm. Autograph. Letter of transmittal to L.H. Adler (1/24/1905) and letter from Lewis H. Adler, Jr., to A.B. Cooke, *re* publication (article remained unpublished). — Gift of L.H. Adler.   *[Z 10/134]*

78. **Bogen, Emil,** 1896-1962. Drunkenness; a quantitative study of acute alcoholic intoxication. *Cincinnati, 1927.*

36, [7] ff.; charts, tables, 5 plates. 28 cm. Typewritten. Alvarenga Prize Essay no. 25, 1927. Published in altered or abbreviated form as "Diagnosis of Drunkenness; Quantitative Study of Acute Alcoholic Intoxication," in *Calif. & West. Med.,* v. 26: 778-83 (1927), and as "Drunkenness; Quantitative Study of Acute Alcoholic Intoxication," in *JAMA,* v. 89: 1508-11 (1927).   *[10d/18]*

79. **Boggs, Thomas Richmond,** 1875-1938. Notes on clinical microscopy taken by B.B. Vincent Lyon, Johns Hopkins University. *Baltimore, 1905-06.*

144 ff. 20 cm.   *[10a/398]*

80. **[Bohemia. Laws, statutes, etc.]** Königliche Böhmische Stadt Rechte, welche von ... Pawl Christian von Rostina zusammen getragen, nachgehents aber in ... Druck auzgangen vnd ... Anno 1579 ... Rudolpho [II, emperor of the Holy Roman Empire and king of Bohemia] ... praesentirt worden. *Prague?, 1579?*

154 ff. (ff. 149-54 blank). 32 cm., boxed. Alphabetical index on ff. 134-48. Manuscript copy.   *[Z 10/33]*

81. **Bókay, János,** 1858-1937. The history of pediatrics: ... In celebration of the 80th year of the Budapest Stefanie Children's

Hospital, formerly the Contagious Hospital for Poor Children; and of the 100th birthday anniversary of Johann Bokai, Sr. Translated by S.X Radbill. *Philadelphia, 1933.*

70, 15 pp. 29 cm. Typescript. Presented by the translator, March 29, 1933. Originally published in Berlin in 1922 as *Geschichte der Kinderheilkunde.*

[10d/149]

82. **Bond, Henry,** 1790-1859. Prescriptions collected by Henry Bond. *Philadelphia?, 1815-23?*

169 pp. 18 cm. References to Drs. Borrows, Samuel Jackson, Physick, Ferriar, etc. Entry on p. 73 dated Nov. 20, 1823. Includes household formulae. − Presented by Miss S.C. Dewey.   [10a/48]

−−−−−. See also no. *185.12.*

83. **Bond, Thomas,** 1713-84. Introductory lecture to a course of clinical observations in the Pennsylvania Hospital delivered there December 3rd, 1766. *Philadelphia, n.d. (1827?).*

1 f., 13 pp. 33.5 cm. Published in *North American Medical & Surgical Journal*, v. 4: 264-75 (1827) where it is noted that a manuscript copy was made for the purpose by "Mr. Paul Eve, student of medicine" (i.e., Paul Fitzsimmons Eve), which may be this copy; if so, it was extensively edited as to spelling and punctuation before publication; publ. also in T.G. Morton and Frank Woodbury, *The History of the Pennsylvania Hospital, 1791-1895,* rev. ed. (Phila., 1897; pp. 462-67), where it is noted (p. 461) that a copy was deposited in the Library of the Hospital; also in *Jour. Hist. Med. and Allied Sci.*, v. 2: [10]-19 (1947) with commentary by Carl Bridenbaugh, who used as his text a transcription from the minutes of the Managers of the Pennsylvania Hospital.   [Z 10/3]

84. −−−−−. Ledgers of Thomas and Phineas Bond. *Philadelphia, 1751-70.*

6 v. 38.5-43 cm. Volume 1, 1751-4; 2, 1754-6; 3, 1756-9; 4, 1763-7; 5, 1764-70; 6, 1765-7. All except v. 4 and 6 contain accounts, arranged by names of patients, including many well-known individuals (e.g., Benjamin Franklin, Isaac Norris, Thomas Wharton, several Wistars [Caspar, John and Richard], members of the families Mifflin, Pemberton, Penrose, Rhoads, etc.). − Bookplate of Samuel Taylor, bookbinder in v. 4. − Presented by Henry Chapman and v. 2 by Charles Cadwalader.   [Z 10/1]

−−−−−. See also no. 285.

85. **Bowditch, Henry Pickering,** 1840-1911. Physiology lectures. Transcribed by H.A. Anderson. *Boston, 1892-93.*

349 pp. 29 cm. Typewritten. Inscribed on front flyleaf: "'97, Harry P. [i.e., T.] Handy, Harvard Medical School, from H.A. Anderson, Jan. '93."   [10d/9]

−−−−−. See also no. 486.

86. **Bradbury, Samuel,** 1883-1947. Note on influenza at 16 (Phila. U.S.) Gen. Hosp., Oct. 12 to Nov. 12, 1918 by S. Bradbury and E.B. Krumbhaar . . . *Philadelphia, 1918.*

4, [3] ff. text, [4] ff. addenda. 20-35 cm. 4 numbered ff., the main text, are in Krumbhaar's hand, the 3 following, meant as inserts, in Bradbury's. Letters and memos to Influenza Committee and the Surgeon General included.
[10a/422]

87. **Bradley, William Nathaniel,** 1871-1962. Florence Nightingale, 1820-1910; Dr. William Smith Forbes, 1831-1905. *Philadelphia, 1951.*

36 ff., incl. photographs and photostats. 31 cm. Typewritten (carbon copy).
[Z 10c/37]

88. —————. William Ellery Hughes. *Philadelphia, 1944.*

5, 4, [4] ff. 28.5 cm (in envelope). Typescript (carbon), etc. Text of biography in carbon and mimeographed copies, with few items of correspondence and obituary notice from *N.Y. Times.*   *[10d/91]*

—————. See also no. 289.

89. **Bram, Israel,** 1883-1955. Sleeping habits; questionnaire and replies. *V.p., 1927-37, [ca. 1950].*

1 box. 31 cm. File of some 150 replies to questionnaire sent to distinguished men and women (see *Fugitive Leaves*, n.s., no. 16 [1957]), in preparation of a book on the relationship of sleep and dream phenomena to the ductless or endocrine glands and the involuntary nervous system; the book remained unpublished. Some replies were extensive, among them B.A. De Voto, Ernest Hemingway, H.L. Mencken, and R.P. Scripps. Beyond the questionnaires further material on sleep, e.g., reprints of articles, notes, preface and two chapters of projected book by Dr. Bram, also material (illustrated) on goiters, and typed copies of reviews of the author's *Exophthalmic Goiter and Its Medical Treatment* (1936) are included. List of replies received enclosed.   *[10c/152]*

90. **Brandner, Georg Heinrich.** Verschiedene medizinische Vorschriften. *Pottsville, Pa., 1840.*

1 v. 19.5 cm. Contains "Namen der Mitglieder des Teutschen Lyceums zu Pottsville, 19ten August A.D. 1839." — Prov.: "Albert H. Brandner Pottsville Nov. 18/55."   *[10a/395]*

91. **Brinton, John Hill,** 1832-1907. Papers and documents. *V.p., 1854-96.*

2 boxes (3 bundles, 2 v.). 39 cm. Manuscript, incl. printed forms and notes, and typewritten items. Contents: 1. Fee book, 1854-58. — 2. Requisitions, receipts and few letters while with the army during the Civil War, 1864-65. — 3. Orders and letters, U.S.A. Medical Department, 1864-65. — 4. Record of 2 wounded soldiers, n.d. — 5. (Printed) Monthly return of clothing, camp and

garrison equipage, received . . . at (in manuscript:) Army Medical Museum Washington . . . by . . . J.H. Brinton, 1864. — 6. Correspondence, incl. business and legal items, reports on and letters by patients, their relatives and doctors, few relating to Jefferson Medical College, letter from Mrs. W.T.G. Morton with reference to her husband's contribution to anesthesia, etc., 1889-96. — 7. Two small booklets and pamphlets: physicians visiting lists, 1856 and 1873, diary, 1878.   *[10a/482]*

92. **[Broca, Benjamin Auguste,** 1849-1924.] Tirages à part du professeur A. [Benjamin Auguste] Broca et André Broca. *N.p., ca. 1930.*

[2] ff. 27 cm (in envelope). 77 entries for B.A. Broca (non-consecutively numbered 1-168) and 21 for André Broca (numbered 1-43), 1882-1923. Compiled by Mrs. B.A. Broca? (cf. enclosed typed note).   *[n.c.]*

93. **Bromer, Ralph Shepherd,** 1886-1957. Roentgen ray studies of the ankle joint. *Philadelphia?, 1921.*

14, [5] ff. 32 cm. Read before the American Surgical Association, June 14, 1921. Published in *Archives of Surgery*, v. 4 (1922). Accompanies an article by Bromer and Ashhurst, "Classification and mechanism of fractures of the leg bones . . ."   *[10a/322]*

— — — — —. See also no. 32.

94. **Brooks, Henry Harlow,** 1871-1936. Clinical record of William Bedner, February 8, 1918. *Camp Upton, N.Y., 1918.*

[9] ff. 32 cm (in envelope). Typescript (carbon copy) and manuscript. 3 pp. polygraphs and pencil sketch by Herbert S. Kates. Diagnosis is of aneurism of right auricle.   *[n.c.]*

— — — — —. See also no. 483.

95. **Brothers, Abram,** 1864-1910. Infantile mortality during childbirth, and its prevention: "Vive l'enfant." *New York, 1895.*

[12], 246 ff.; tables. 27 cm. Typescript. — "This essay received the prize . . . from the trustees of the William F. Jenks Memorial Fund . . . Jan. 1895." Published separately and as part of *Trans. & Stud.*, ser. 3, v. 17 (1895).   *[10a/15]*

96. **Brown, Alexander.** A family book. *Ireland, 1717-46.*

[8], 232 ff. (many missing or omitted, some unnumb. ff. interspersed). 32 cm. 2nd prel. f. torn, 3rd on the "oeconomy of human life" in cipher, followed by extensive table of contents (referring to "pages" instead of leaves). Recipes and remedies, some general medical observations, ff. 1-166; followed by a miscellany incl. poetry, preparation of ink powder, explosives, genealogical information, financial tables, etc. Presented to Lewis Library by Arthur V. Meigs.   *[Z 10/104]*

97.   **Brown, Frederick,** 1837-94.   Prescription ledgers.   *Philadelphia,*
       ca. 1860-90.

       14 v.   46 cm.   Firm founded in 1822 by Frederick Brown (1796-1864), a great-
       nephew of Charles Brockden Brown. — Presented by Free Library of
       Philadelphia; bindings removed; paper in poor condition.   *[Z 10a/2]*

98.   —————.   Private memorandum book belonging to Frederick
       Brown, chemist & druggist . . . .   *Philadelphia, 1860-69, 1889.*

       1 v.   25 cm.   Presented by Mrs. M. Henry Wells (granddaughter); correspond-
       ence, including family relationships, with the volume.   Consists chiefly of
       recipes and formulae.   Addresses of various physicians and agents or suppliers
       in distant places at beginning.   Includes copy of letter to Surgeon Robert
       Crooke Wood, U.S.A., Washington, August 30, 1861 (p. 30), recommending
       the firm's essence of ginger for use in the field; (at end) copy of list given to
       police showing articles stolen from 1018 Spruce Street, Sept. 30, 1861;
       newspaper clippings advertising the store or its products; printed list of
       imports, dated April, 1874, laid in.   *[ZZ 10c/18]*

99.   —————.   Private prescriptions.   *Philadelphia, 1860.*

       1 v.   29.5 cm.   Formulary, showing originator of formula in most cases;
       alphabetical index. — Presented by Mrs. M. Henry Wells.   *[ZZ 10c/19]*

100.   **Bryn Mawr Hospital.**   Admissions — Discharges, October 10,
       1893 - July 2, 1905.   *Bryn Mawr, Pa., 1893-1905.*

       50 ff. (ff. 1-2, with title?, removed; ff. 46-50 blank).   51 cm.   2461 admissions
       with name, date, diagnosis, free or paid status, address, ward, initials of
       resident physician, place of birth, age, sex, occupation.   The discharge records
       show revised diagnoses, outcome ("cured," "relieved," "died"), discharge date
       and length of hospital stay.   Note concerning patient 151, under care of S.
       Weir Mitchell, on p. 3.   Gift of Samuel B. Sturgis.   *[Z 10c/33]*

101.   **Burr, Charles Walts,** 1861-1944.   Notes on lectures on mental
       diseases.   *Philadelphia, 1907-08.*

       20 ff.   22 cm (in envelope).   Notes taken by E.B. Krumbhaar, University of
       Pennsylvania.   *[10a/423]*

102.   —————.   Personality and physiognomy.   *Philadelphia, 1935?*

       10 ff. (with 1 f. inserted as 1a).   28 cm (in envelope).   Typewritten, with
       pencilled corrections and some additions: "Read Febr. 15 at meeting of Phila.
       Co. Medical [Society] and district dental societies."   *[n.c.]*

       —————.   See also nos. 356, 519, 529.

103.   **[Butler, Charles St. John,** 1875-1944].   Bibliography of Charles
       S. Butler . . . to July 1, 1937.   *N.p., 1937.*

       5 ff.   26.5 cm (in envelope).   Mimeographed.   Lists 65 items.   *[Z 10/156]*

104. **Butler, Samuel Worcester,** 1823-74. Journal of cases treated, beginning June 29th 1849 and diary, May 1, 1852 - June 1, 1855. *Philadelphia and Burlington, N.J., 1849-55.*

1 v.   30.5 cm.   Acquired 1975 in part through donations by F.B. Rogers, J.F. Huber, S.J. Peitzman, Clara Manson in memory of W.B. McDaniel, II, and Mrs. S. Hoffman, Mr. and Mrs. B. Hoffman, and Dr. and Mrs. S. Make, to mark 50th wedding anniversary of Dr. and Mrs. S.X Radbill.   Correspondence included. — Contents: pp. [1]-6, cases seen in Philadelphia, in joint practice with Joseph Parrish; pp. 9-119 combine diary entries with some case reports. — At end, 7 pp. of clippings from *The Weekly Picayune*, New Orleans, July 31 to August 20, 1853, on that city's yellow fever epidemic.   *[ZZ 10c/25]*

105. **Cadwalader, Thomas,** 1708-79. Essay on the West India dry gripes; original manuscript notes. *Philadelphia, 1740?*

[50] pp.   19 cm.   Autograph of printed version published in Philadelphia by B. Franklin in 1745. — Presented by S. Weir Mitchell.   *[10a/197]*

106. **Caldwell, Charles,** 1772-1853. Accounts with patients. *Philadelphia, 1815-19.*

[xii], 213 ff.   41.5 cm.   Pasted inside front cover: sworn affidavits, dated July 14, 1820 and June 14, 1822 (attesting to correctness of entries for William Cummings), in proceedings Caldwell against Cummings, in Philadelphia Court of Common Pleas, 1820. — Inscribed on front cover: "Vol. IX"; on flyleaf, "A. [i.e., Exhibit A?] Charles Caldwell." — Presented by the Free Library of Philadelphia.   *[Z 10c/29]*

107. **Cameron, Sir Gordon Roy,** 1899-1966. Pancreatic anomalies; their morphology, pathology, and clinical history. *Victoria, 1924.*

24 pp.; 4 plates.   33 cm.   Typewritten.   Alvarenga Prize Essay, no. 22, 1924.   Published in *Trans & Stud.,* ser. 3, v. 46: 781-820 (1924).   *[10d/11]*

108. **Cameron, John Allan Munro.** The physiological sphincters of the alimentary canal and their affections. *Glasgow, 1929.*

31, 57, 12 ff.; 26 photographs on 12 ff. at end.   26 cm.   Typescript (carbon copy).   Inscribed on flyleaf "J.A. Munro Cameron, Assistant Pathologist, Victoria Infirmary, Glasgow, Scotland."   *[10d/45]*

109. **Cancer cure.** *N.p., 19th cent.*

1 f.   27 cm.   Manuscript (primitive style and handwriting).   Torn in pieces, reassembled, and then mounted.   Presented by Robert Bookhammer.
[ZZ 10a/1]

110. **Carbonell, Louis Philip.** Record of anomalies. *Philadelphia, 1879.*

2 v.; illus.   16.5 cm.; 28.5 × 38 cm (oblong).   Vol. 1 (text).   Anomalies of session 1878-79 (and) 1877-78 ([2], 40, [1] and blank ff.). — 2. Colored

drawings of anomalies (mounted, 35 ff.). "Prof. Leidy's subject" on f. 1 (marked page 1) of vol. 1. — Offered in competition at the University of Pennsylvania Medical Department for a student prize awarded by Hugh Lenox Hodge. With Hodge's bookplate. *[Z 10/14]*

111. **Carson, Joseph,** 1808-76, comp. Collection of engraved portraits of faculty, autograph certificates of attendance, and cards of admission relating to two students attending the University of Edinburgh Medical School, and the "Extra-Academical School of Medicine and Surgery," i.e., Donald McIntyre, attending 1767-69, and Samuel Lewis, 1835-40. *Philadelphia, etc., various dates (1761-1840?).*

1 v. 19.5 cm. Among contents Announcement, dated 1797, in Latin, of the Medical School, listing graduates to 1750, with inscription "Henry U. Onderdonk, Glasgow, 1809;" ornamented certificate, Latin, dated Dec. 15, 1761, and signed by Alexander Russell, for "Aberdonia Academia," specifically for William Chancellor, "Philadelphiensis;" among professors signing cards of admission or certificates of attendance are Thomas Young, Sir Charles Bell, Alexander Munro, Thomas Charles Hope, James Home, Robert Jameson, Wm. Pulteney Alison, Alexander Russell, Alexander Jardine Lizars. Also a prescription of (John Coakley?) Lettsom, and a holograph note of Sir William Fordyce. Among engraved portraits are those of William Cullen, Joseph Black, John Gregory, William Cuming, Patrick Russell, John Johnstone, Andrew Duncan, John Lorimer, John Armstrong, George Cheyne, etc. — Presented by the heirs of J. Carson. *[10c/7]*

112. —————, comp. Collection of letters, a few poems, memoranda, invitations, announcements, prescriptions, obituaries, death certificates, estate notices (manuscript and printed), portraits, illus., etc. *V.p. and various dates.*

5 v. 33 cm. The extensive collection, brought together by Dr. Carson, includes besides correspondence addressed to him, a great variety of materials documenting the medical scene of his approximate period, primarily in the United States, but including foreign correspondents. The number of persons involved is too large to be listed in its entirety, but the following is a fair sampling: David H. Agnew (vol. V), Franklin Bache (I), Elisha Bartlett (I), John Bell (II), Ralph M. Bird (II), Daniel Drake (I), Charles Frick (II), Addinell Hewson (I), Oliver Wendell Holmes (incl. poem; I), David Hosack (I), Samuel Jackson (V), Edward Jenner (III), Daniel C. Macreight (III), Charles D. Meigs (I), Edward Miller (V), Valentine Mott (I), Thomas D. Mütter (I), Florence Nightingale (III), Josiah C. Nott (II), Henry U. Onderdonk (many letters to him; V), Joseph Pancoast (I), Robert M. Patterson (II), Jonathan Pereira (III), Edward F. Rivinus (II), William S.W. Ruschenberger (II), Alexander Somervail (II), Edward Stanley (III), William Tilghman (many letters to him; V), Gaetano Valeri (III). Volume IV is primarily a collection of portraits (from antiquity to 19th cent.). An unedited index of 86 pages is available; copies may be obtained at cost (estimated at $5.00). *[Z 10c/10]*

113. $-----$, comp.   Collection of letters, notes, lists of specimens, portraits (incl. photographs), clippings, etc., principally of botanists. *V.p., 1786, 1821-72.*

> 1 v.; illus. 31 cm. Scrapbook. Among persons represented are William Darlington, Thomas Nuttall, Henry Muhlenberg, Asa Gray, Joseph Henry, Amos Eaton, Elias Durand, Charles L. Bonaparte, Alymer Bourke Lambert and F.G. Cuvier. The collection includes 3 clippings on, and engraving of J. J. L. Audubon, 2 autograph letters of James D. Dana, clippings and a note on the invention of the telegraph by S.F.B. Morse, a letter on Indian language by Theodore Schulz, obituaries of J.L.R. Agassiz, etc.   *[10c/6]*

114. $-----$, comp.   Scrap book, consisting of portraits, letters, clippings, documents, admission cards, etc.; illustrating and supplementing Carson's *History of the Medical Department of the University of Pennsylvania* (Philadelphia, Lindsay and Blakiston, 1869). *V.p., 1706-ca. 1875.*

> 6 v.; illus. (incl. 89 portraits). 31 cm. Manuscript and printed. Besides material relevant to the history of the Medical Department, and more generally to the history of the University, the scrap book contains items relating to the University of Edinburgh and other medical institutions (primarily in Philadelphia), learned societies (incl. the American Philosophical Society); the letters contain information beyond medicine, e.g. on chemistry, botany and occasionally on historical and social topics. Among the large number of letter writers are William Hall (described as a surgeon, Philadelphia, 1706), Benjamin Franklin, Cadwallader Coldon, John Morgan (10 or more letters), Wm. Hewson, John Redman, Benjamin Rush (six letters), Joseph Priestley, Benjamin Smith Barton, Caspar Wistar (4), P.S. Physick (4), John Redman Coxe, William P.C. Barton (3), J.G. Dorsey (6), Samuel L. Mitchell, Benjamin Silliman, Robert Hare (4), N. Chapman (4), George B. Wood (many), Samuel Jackson (4), William Pepper (3), J.K. Mitchell, plus various letters to Joseph Carson (incl. several from Joseph Leidy, Henry H. Smith and Alfred Stillé). Furthermore included are printed book and book auction announcements, and clippings dealing with a variety of topics. One letter in v. VI by M. Leib briefly describes the yellow fever in Philadelphia, 1797.
>
> *[ZZ 10c/4]*

115. $-----$.   Division III.   General consideration [in connection with] therapeutics.   Chapter I.   Effects of medicines.   *Philadelphia, 186—?*

> [61] ff. 25 cm. Autograph, with paste-ins, corrections, emendations. Unidentified; begins: The end proposed in cultivating medical science is the cure. — Gift of the heirs of Dr. Carson.   *[n.c.]*

116. $-----$.   A history of the Medical Department of the University of Pennsylvania from its foundation in 1765. *Philadelphia, 1869.*

> 1 v. 25 cm. A draft of Carson's published *History* (Philadelphia, Lindsay and Blakiston, 1869) with many corrections and additions tipped in. — Gift of Mrs. Hampton L. Carson.   *[10a/241]*

117.   —————. Introductory lecture on therapeutics. *Philadelphia,*
       ca. 1845.

       18 ff.   26 cm.   Not listed in Carson's bibliography by Ruschenberger, *Trans. &*
       Stud., ser. 3, v. 4: lxi-lxvii (1879).   *[10a/21]*

118.   —————. Lectures by Joseph Carson. *Philadelphia, ca. 1848.*

       35, [3] ff.   20 cm.   Notes confined to the subject of emetics.   Student not
       identified.   *[10a/18]*

119.   —————. Lectures on pharmacy delivered in the Philadelphia
       College of Pharmacy. *Philadelphia, 1848?*

       1 v.   25.5 cm.   Lectures 1 through 5 only.   *[10a/17]*

120.   —————. Notes for a medical history of the revolutionary
       army. *Philadelphia, ca. 1840?*

       1 v.   26 cm.   Not listed in Carson's bibliography (for citation see no.
       117).   Transcriptions and digests of documents written between June 1775
       and Dec. 31, 1776.   *[10a/20].*

121.   —————. Notes for his lectures on materia medica and phar-
       macy, delivered at the University of Pennsylvania, Department
       of Medicine. *Philadelphia, 1850-73.*

       4 boxes (1 envelope, 77 notebooks [in 8 binders], few loose ff.).   32
       cm.   *[10a/291]*

122.   —————. Notes made with reference to the University of
       Pennsylvania. *Philadelphia, ca. 1840-50.*

       1 v.   21 cm.   Chiefly odd ff. of notes cut and pasted over the blank leaves of
       ruled exercise-book.   *[10a/22]*

123.   —————. Notes on copaiba. *Philadelphia, ca. 1861.*

       [48] ff. (misnumbered).   25 cm.   Autograph.   Not listed among Dr. Carson's
       books and articles (*op. cit.*, see no. 117). — Gift of the heirs of Dr. Carson.   *[n.c.]*

124.   —————. Notes on topics connected with materia medica and
       therapeutics. *Philadelphia, 1849-53?*

       2 v.   25 cm.   Autograph?   *[10a/16]*

125.   —————. Notes taken [by H.M. Howe] upon lectures . . . on
       materia medica, Oct.14.63. *Philadelphia, 1863.*

       1 v.   17.5 cm.   *[10a/384]*

126.   —————. On puerperal eclampsia. *Philadelphia?, 1870?*

       157 ff.   26 cm.   Published (with some revisions) in the *American Journal of the*
       Medical Sciences, n.s., v. 61: 433-66 (1871).   *[10a/19]*

127.   —————. On the operation of medicines by introduction into the circulation. *Philadelphia, ca. 1864-67.*

Ff. 118-63.   25 cm.   Autograph with corrections and additions, but incomplete. Constitutes lectures III and IV of his *Synopsis of the Course of Lectures on Materia Medica.* With this are filed some misc. letters.   Gift of the heirs of Dr. Carson.   *[n.c.]*

128.   —————. Printed *Synopsis of the Course of Lectures on Materia Medica and Pharmacy,* 3rd rev. ed. (Philadelphia, 1863), interleaved with handwritten lecture notes and marginalia entered by William Furness Jenks, medical student at the University of Pennsylvania. *Philadelphia, 1863[-64?]*

vii, [17]-244 pp.   23 cm.   Inscribed on front flyleaf "W.F. Jenks, Sept. 1863, Philadelphia."   He received his degree in 1866. — Gift of Warren Weiss.
                                                                                   [10a/484]

129.   —————. Secretion of bile. — Notes on the American Revolution. *Philadelphia, ca. 1870-75.*

21, 4 pp.   25.5-28 cm.   Secretion of bile (autograph) written on backs of old letters, advertisements and notices; among letter writers are Norris Cadwalader Shallcross and Alfred Bower Taylor. — The notes on the American Revolution are extracted from various primary and secondary sources.   *[10a/503]*

130.   [—————]. Letters to J. Carson. *V.p., 1854-75.*

1 envelope.   21-28 cm.   Introductions of persons beginning at the University of Pennsylvania Department of Medicine, exchange of laboratory specimens, matters of meetings, etc., as well as 2 letters by J. Carson.   Mostly brief items.   List of correspondents enclosed.   *[n.c.]*

—————. See also nos. 201, 416, 476, 765, 1032, 1119.

131.   **Carter, John T.,** 1850-1936.   Narcotic drug distribution. *Tridelphia, W. Va., March 10, 1920 - July 1, 1933.*

39 pp. (2 loose prescriptions laid in, 1 blank leaf).   15.5 × 10.5 cm.   Pocket notebook containing chronological list of doses, with names of patients.   Gift of Richard W. Foster.   *[10a/508]*

132.   **Carter, William Spencer,** 1869-1944.   The relation of the parathyroids to the thyroid gland by "Parathyroids". *Galveston, Texas, 1903.*

200 pp. (partly blank).   36 cm.   Alvarenga Prize Essay, 1903.   Description of sections (5 ff.) inserted at end.   With box of 24 slides and explanatory text.   *[Z 10/13]*

133.   **Catanensis, Joannes Panormitanus,** 1690-1753.   Ars medica.
       Italy, 1738?

    [23] ff., 573 pp. (incl. blank ff. and pp.).   21 cm.   Partial contents: 1. Physiologia
    [Dissertatio I] (pp. 20-93). — 2. De temperamentis (pp. 94-120). — 3. De
    humani corporis fluidis (pp. 121-217). — 4. De humani corporis partibus, seu
    de anatomia corporis humani (pp. 225-426). — 5. De spiritibus et calido
    innato veterum (pp. 439-87). — Pars secunda. Semiotica, De pulsibus, De
    urinis (pp. 493-550). — Pars tertia. Hygiene (pp. 559-73).   *[10a/297]*

134.   —————. Repertorium omnium medicaminum morbis om-
       nibus specificorum curandis, tam propria experientia, tam
       celebriorum medicinę luminum auctore comprobatum, ab . . .
       Joanne Catanese Panormitano, magno cum studio elaboratum
       in suorum discipulorum emolumento, et amore . . . *Italy, first
       half 18th cent.*

    20 ff. (index)., 227 ff. (irregularly paged; ff. 220-27 blank).   21 cm.   16 ff. at
    end entitled De signaturis plantarum humana membra similitudine reprae-
    sentantium ex Osualdo Crollio. Alternate title on f. 1 (following index):
    Practicae animadversiones . . . alphabetico ordine digestae.   *[10a/298]*

135.   **Chambers, George Hamilton,** 1865-1938.   Book of prescrip-
       tions for various patients. *Philadelphia, 1887-98.*

    1 v.   21 cm.   One hundred fifty prescriptions. Incomplete (leaves removed
    for period between Jan. and late March 1892). Presented by Samuel X
    Radbill.   *[10a/468]*

136.   **Chance, Burton,** 1868-1965.   John Cooke Hirst, M.D.; a sketch
       of his life. *Philadelphia, 1925.*

    4 ff.   27.5 cm.   Typewritten.   *[ZZ 10d/2]*

137.   —————. Miscellaneous prescriptions. *Philadelphia, ca. 1890.*

    18 ff.   13 cm.   Notebook with pencilled inscription: ". . . from Woods Course."
    [n.c.]

138.   [—————]. Extensive collection of letters to Dr. Chance. *V.p.,
       1901-59.*

    1 box.   39.5 cm.   Includes letters from a large number of prominent
    physicians (among them several ophthalmologists). List of writers filed with
    the collection. Special mention is made of 50 letters by Fielding H. Garrison,
    30 by D'Arcy Power, and (more or less at random) those by Harry Friedenwald,
    William W. Keen, Robert R. James, William R. LeFanu, Francis R. Packard
    and Casey A. Wood. One of the recurrent topics is the history of medicine. —
    With a few notes concerning the Library of the College of Physicians, 5
    addressed to W.B. McDaniel.   *[n.c.]*

139.   [— — — — —]. Record of the writings of Burton Chance, M.D.
        Philadelphia, 1952.

> v, 45 pp. 21.5 cm. Compiler not indicated. — Typescript, with manuscript
> additions. A catalogue of the scientific and literary works of Burton Chance
> (published and unpublished). — Principal topic of the former is ophthalmolo-
> gy.   *[10a/362]*

        — — — — —. See also nos. 209, 1015, 1139.

140.   **Chapman, Nathaniel,** 1780-1853. Apoplexia, or apoplexy.
        Philadelphia?, after 1837?

> 114 ff. 25.5 cm. Incomplete. — References to "the late Dr. Physick" imply a
> date 1837 or later. — Presented by Henry Cadwalader Chapman. — Unpublish-
> ed?   *[10a/123]*

141.   — — — — —. Copy of a course of medical lectures .... *Philadelphia,*
        1833?

> 2 v. 33 cm. With bookplate of Thos. Forrest Betton. Catalogue of the Betton
> Collection lists this manuscript under G.H. Wikoff as "Manuscript notes
> delivered by Prof. N. Chapman." From internal evidence it appears that it was
> transcribed by G.H. Wikoff. End flyleaf of v. 2 with inscriptions "John Mark
> Smith, 131 S. 3rd St., Phila." and "J.K. Mitchell, M.D. Lecturer on Chemistry,
> Philadelphia Medical Institute and Franklin Institute." Contains list of
> faculty of the Medical Institute for 1833.   *[Z 10/5]*

142.   — — — — —. Epidemic[s] of America. *Philadelphia, ca. 1822.*

> 1 v. 25.5 cm. Lectures, including one on Diseases of the alimentary canal. —
> Formerly attributed to John Marshall Paul.   *[10a/410]*

143.   — — — — —. Examinations on Dr. Chapman's lectures by John
        K. Mitchell. *Philadelphia, 1816-17?*

> 300 pp. 34.5 cm. Interleaved with blank sheets. Begins with lecture on
> physiology and concludes with smallpox. Described (with some errors) by
> Richman, pp. 71-72. — Presented by S. Weir Mitchell.   *[Z 10/4]*

144.   — — — — —. Hydrophobia. *Philadelphia, after 1828.*

> 1 v. 25 cm. Section on hydrophobia (66 ff.) shows close correspondence
> (sometimes word-for-word), often with new material added, to Chapman's
> thesis, *An Essay on Canine Fever,* 1801. With annotations in Chapman's hand,
> referring to material dated 1828. Contains sections on tetanus (49 ff.);
> diseases of the medulla spinalis or spinal cord (18 ff.); chronic myelitis (15 ff.);
> spinalgia, spine ache or spinal irritations (22 ff.). — Unpublished? Gift of
> Henry Cadwalader Chapman.   *[10a/122]*

145.   — — — — —. Lectures on materia medica. *Philadelphia, Nov. 1814 -March 1815.*

    2 v. (246, [9] ff.). 20.5 cm. Inscribed on flyleaves: "Edward Barton, Philadelphia, April 1815." — Some notes laid in.   *[10a/26]*

146.   — — — — —. Lectures on pathology, medical physiognomy and the practice of physic. *Philadelphia, 181—?*

    2 v. (383, 377 ff.). 21 cm. The work of a trained copyist? Each v. with separate index. — Former owner's name removed in both volumes.   *[10a/25]*

147.   — — — — —. Lectures on physiology. *Philadelphia, 1822.*

    211 pp. 25.5 cm. Inscribed inside front cover: J.K. Mitchell. — Presented by S. Weir Mitchell.   *[10a/31]*

148.   — — — — —   — — — — — and the practice of medicine. *Philadelphia, 1817-18.*

    v. 1, 3, 5-8, 10, 12-15. 20 cm. Volume 1 entitled "Chapmans Lectures. Supplement. Vol. 1st, 1817." Name on flyleaf of v. 3 "G.B. Wood." — Gift of Hugh Lenox Hodge.   *[10a/29]*

149.   — — — — —. Manuscript notes of the medical lectures of Dr. Chapman from the library of Dr. Wilmer Worthington. *Philadelphia, 182—?*

    2 v. (464, 380 pp.). 25 cm. Inscribed on flyleaves "John B. Roberts, 1874," and on flyleaf of vol. 2 "W. Worthington"; both volumes include Worthington's bookplates, numbered 58 and 59.   *[10a/33]*

150.   — — — — —, comp. Notes from Dr. Barton's lectures on materia medica, etc., taken by Nathaniel Chapman Jr. during the Winter 1798-9. *Philadelphia, 1798-99 and after?*

    1 v. 19 cm. Contrary to the title (on cover and title-page), this contains only 2 pp. on Barton's lectures. Much more extensive notes follow: 1. Lectures on natural philosophy, by James Cooke (magnetism, gravitation, hydrogen); 2. Hydrophobia, from [Thomas] Percival's *Essays*, v. 2; and, 3. Cullen's *Practice*, v. 3 and 4. — Mentioned as commonplace book by Richman, p. 29.   *[10a/4]*

151.   — — — — —. Notes from Dr. Chapman's lectures on the materia medica, as delivered in the Pennsylvania University. *Philadelphia, 1814-15?*

    221, [11, 1] pp. 20.5 cm. Aphorisms, receipts, etc. dated 1856-63, at end of volume. — Notes by Henry Vander Veer, according to the donor, Fred B. Rogers.   *[10a/403]*

152.   ——————. Notes from the lectures of Nat. Chapman . . .
        Philadelphia, 1815-16.

> 285, [12] pp. 20 cm. "An abridged view of the whole materia medica . . . .,"
> 12 pp. at end.   *[10a/27]*

153.   ——————. Notes on his lectures on clinical medicine. *Philadel-*
        phia, 181— or 182—.

> 498, [3] pp. 26 cm. Leather binding stamped "L. Lemer." Begins with
> medical physiognomy and continues with practice of medicine, incl. diseases
> of circulatory, digestive, glandular, muscular, etc. systems, ending with
> pathology.   *[10a/441]*

154.   ——————. Notes on lectures on physiology, pathology and
        materia medica. *Philadelphia, ca. 1817-20.*

> 3 bound, 1 unbound v. 20 cm (in envelope). Notes with corrections,
> additions and few inserts. Text not consecutive; the unbound volume, in a
> different hand, parallels to some extent parts of the bound volumes. In two or
> more hands, owned by, prepared for, or written by R. La Roche (cf. pencilled
> entry on back cover of volume marked 3). Bound volumes within illustrated
> children's exercise book covers.   *[10a/313]*

155.   ——————. Notes on the lectures of Nathaniel Chapman . . .
        recorded by R.E. Griffith, jr. *Philadelphia, 1818-20.*

> v. 1 (42 ff.). 19 cm. Incomplete; contains only part of fevers, in section on the
> circulatory system (first part of Chapman's course on practice). — Gift of
> Francis Fisher Kane.   *[10a/271]*

Note: *Items 156-162, which follow, are various presentations of Nathaniel*
Chapman's Practice of Medicine.

156.   ——————. Lectures on the practice of medicine. *Philadelphia,*
        185—.

> 1 v. (pp. 495-663). 24.5 cm. Apparently the second volume of a set of
> Chapman's lectures, incl. only the diseases of the respiratory system. Inscribed
> "Isaac Norris Jr. 2.3.[18]53" and with paste-in of newspaper clipping
> "Transfusion of the blood," with inscription "*Evg. Bulletin,* Feb. 8, 1851, G.P.
> Norris."   *[10a/32]*

157.   ———— ————. *Philadelphia, after 1813.*

> 1 v. 20 cm. Incomplete; begins with part 1 of Chapman's course, Diseases of
> the circulatory system, chiefly treating of fevers and hemorrhages, cf.
> Chapman's Lectures on the more important eruptive fevers, haemorrhages
> and dropsies . . . ., Philadelphia, 1844. — Student not identified.   *[10a/24]*

158.   ———— ————. Notes on Chapman's Practice of medi-
        cine, with classification of Cullen. *Philadelphia, 184—?*

1 v. only. 24.5 cm. Inscribed on title-page and throughout George Douglass. This is vol. 2 of Chapman's lectures. Includes part of the section on digestive diseases, and diseases of the absorbent and respiratory systems. — Table of contents included for this and missing volumes.   *[10a/459]*

159.   — — — —   — — — —. Notes on the lectures . . . on the practice of medicine . . . . *Philadelphia, 1821-22.*

2 v. 15.5 cm. Signature of Jacob Jeanes on end flyleaf of v. 1. Pencil sketch of Isaac Hays on end paper of the same volume. — Gift of Hahnemann Medical College.   *[10a/365]*

160.   — — — —   — — — —. Notes taken [by John Kearsley Mitchell the Elder] from the lectures . . . on the practice of medicine . . . *Philadelphia, 1816-17.*

v. 2 & 8 only. 21.5 cm. The latter v. with inscription "Index to & abstract of my notes on the lectures of Professor N. Chapman year 1816-1817 in seven volumes lost by being loaned, J.K. Mitchell . . . ." — Gift of S. Weir Mitchell.   *[10a/28]*

161.   — — — —   — — — —. Notes taken from the lectures of N. Chapman on the practice of medicine. *Philadelphia, ca. 1838-40.*

[2] ff., 162 pp. (vol. I only; pp. 163[-64?] missing). 19 cm. Inscribed in pencil on title-page "Jno. Neill" (University of Pennsylvania, M.D. 1840). Table of contents on f. 2. — Presented by H.R. Wharton.   *[10a/138]*

162.   — — — —   — — — —. Practice of medicine. *Philadelphia, 1818.*

314 (incl. blank) pp. 19 cm. Attributed to Robert Alison. — Consists of sections on diseases of the circulatory, alimentary, respiratory, and perspiratory system.   *[10a/181]*

163.   — — — — —. Tic douloureux, neuralgia, nerve ache, &c. *Philadelphia, ca. 1834.*

56 (and many blank) ff. Not autograph, but with some corrections in Chapman's hand. Printed version in *Amer. Jour. Med. Sci.*, v. 14: 289-320 (1834).   *[10a/124]*

164.   — — — — —. Valedictory, as delivered Feby. 1818, taken by G.B. Wood. *Philadelphia, 1818.*

[12] pp. 26.5 cm. Incomplete; page [12] begins in the middle of a word and ends in the middle of a sentence.   *[10a/34]*

— — — — —. See also nos. 4, 72, 114, 260, 329, 382, 384, 459, 631, 636, 707, 765, 806, 836, 925.

165.   **[Charles II, King of England].** The state of his late Majesty's body when opened February 7th 1684, read to the Councell the same evening (2 ff., text on recto of f. 1, title on verso of f. 2). — A

short character of Charles ye Second, King of England, setting forth his untimely death (2 ff., verso of f. 2 with title "my Lord's Mulgraves character of King Charles ye 2nd"). *England, ca. 1684.*

29.5 cm. Autopsy report, translated from the original Latin, attributed to John Sheffield. Gift of E.B. Krumbhaar and described by him in *Trans. & Stud.*, ser. 4, v. 6: 51-9 (1938/39).   *[Z 10/111]*

166.   **Charles, Steven Tudor.** John Jones, American surgeon and conservative patriot. *N.p., 1964.*

1 envelope (30 ff., genealog. table); plate. 31 cm. Typescript (carbon). Published in *Bull. Hist. Med.* v. 39: 435-49 (1965), with plate, but without genealogical table. — Gift of author, letter of transmittal enclosed.   *[10c/144]*

167.   **Charlton, John.** An essay on the reciprocity of mind and body . . . Preceptor F. Julius Le Moyne. *Philadelphia, 1842.*

53 pp. 25.5 cm (in envelope). Title printed, text handwritten. Submitted as dissertation at University of Pennsylvania (but degree apparently not granted). Letter of transmittal by R.W. Mays and acknowledgement enclosed. Gift of Thomas S. Martin.   *[10a/411]*

168.   **Cheek, Stephen H.,** b. 1829. An inaugural essay on yellow fever, presented to the faculty of the Philadelphia College of Medicine, for the degree of doctor in medicine, by Stephen H. Cheek of New Orleans. *Philadelphia, 1857.*

[1], 17 ff. 25 cm.   *[n.c.]*

169.   **[Chemistry].** Lecture 33rd. Notes and demonstration for a lecture in chemistry. *Philadelphia?, ca. 1818-20.*

16 ff. 16 cm. References to selenium, "last and latest discov^{d}" element, suggests composition shortly after 1817. Comparison with printed and manuscript lectures of Franklin Bache, Jacob Green and Robert Hare indicate some similarity with Hare in organization and with Bache in contents.   *[n.c.]*

170.   **Chirac, Pierre,** 1650-1732. Reports on the treatment of various ailments, recorded by Cuthbert Constable. *Montpellier?, ca. 1700-18.*

407 pp. (2 unnumb. blank pp. between pp. 99 and 100, p. 132 omitted in contemp. numbering), 26 ff. (1-13 and 24-6 blank). 16 cm. French and some Latin. The reports are irregularly dated 1699 (p. 334), 1700-01, 1703 and 1706 (p. 361), the period during which Chirac treated his patients. — The attribution to Chirac is based on statement by Dr. Cuthbert Constable (p. 274), in the same hand as the text. Since Constable changed his name from Tunstall to Constable in 1718 it is assumed that the manuscript was finished, or possibly even written, in, or soon after, 1718. — Bookplate of William Constable.
                                                            [10a/183]

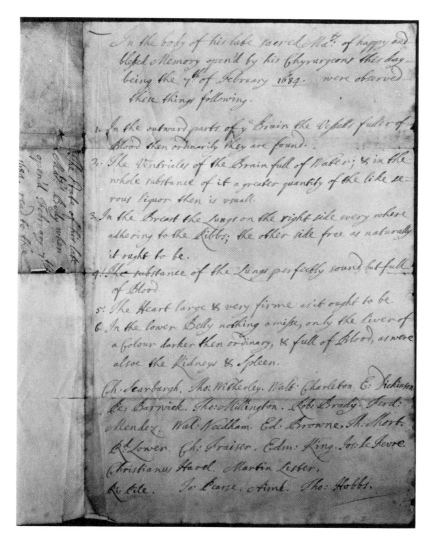

Plate 2.   165.   Autopsy report of Charles II, 1684.

171. **[Cholera].** Lecture on cholera, etc. *Philadelphia, ca. 1821-25?*

    65 ff. 32 cm. Notes from lectures of an unnamed Philadelphia physician, by unnamed notetaker. Topics, besides cholera, include dysentery, diabetes, hepatitis, heart diseases, dyspepsia, etc., with cases cited. A number of Philadelphia doctors are mentioned, e.g. Wood, Hewson, Wistar, Physick, Griffitts, etc. Several dates between 1818 and 1821 are mentioned (e.g. ff. 14, 26, 30). — Presented by William Ashmead Schaeffer.   *[10a/167]*

172. **Chomel, Auguste François,** 1788-1858. Remarques sur la clinique de Mr Chomel; notes de M. Lacaze. *Paris, 1832.*

    193 ff. 23 cm. Ff. 1-169 contain paragraphs 1-1029; ff. 169-93 paragraphs 1-162. The first series consists chiefly of remarques or aphorisms of Chomel, with other items interpolated: "Maladies des enfans par M. Guersant" (paragraphs 235-67); "Aphorismes de Louis" (483-593); "Cayol" (594-605); "Andral" (669-77); "Louis (1830)" (816-993); "Louis - 1830" (994-1029). The second series is headed "Professor Fouquier" (paragraphs 1-103); and "Louis" (104-62). — Prov.: C. Wistar Pennock. Gift of W.W. Gerhard.   *[10a/35]*

173. **Church, Benjamin,** 1734-76. Doctor Churches[!] defence. *N.p., Oct. 27, 1775.*

    [11, 3, 3] pp. 32.5 cm. The "Defence," 11 unnumbered pp. with corrections and revisions, recounts in the first person Church's removal from prison at the summons of the Massachusetts Provincial Congress, to explain before it his cipher letter of June 17th, conveying to the British information on American forces and intentions. Two copies of the cipher letter, translated into English, are included. — On p. [11] of the "Defence" is inscribed (in a different hand) "This defence of Dr. Church was found among the papers of Dr. Jonathan Potts at Pottstown by Robert E. Hobart & given to me by him in 1868. Isabella James." Correspondence included with W.F. Norwood, 1973, and also photocopy of his article, "The Enigma of Dr. Benjamin Church", *Medical Arts and Sciences,* 2d quarter, 1956, and of other biographical materials on Benjamin Church.   *[ZZ 10c/2]*

174. **Churchman, John Woolman,** 1877-1937. Selective bacteriostasis of gentian violet. *New York, 1921.*

    2 boxes (206 ff., 11 plates; plates 12-60). 28 cm (in box). Typescript. Alvarenga Prize Essay, 1921.   *[10d/5]*

175. **[Civil War].** Return of the southern medical students home in 1859. *Philadelphia, etc.?, 1859.*

    12 ff. 26 cm (in envelope). Collection of newspaper clippings pasted on sheets. The students came from the University of Pennsylvania, Department of Medicine.   *[10d/154]*

176. **Clarke, Mary A.** Correspondence on a proposed memorial statue for Jacob Mendez Da Costa on the island of St. Thomas (Virgin Islands). *Philadelphia, 1934-35.*

    1 envelope. 31 cm. Presented by Mary Clarke.   *[10c/149]*

177. **Cline, Henry,** 1750-1827. Lecture on surgery. *London, 4th quarter 18th cent.*

[2] ff., 300 pp., [5] ff. 22 cm. Lecture notes taken by John Wallis Brooks. Contents: Of sutures; Operations about the head and neck; Fistula lachrymalis; On hernia; Of the paracenthesis; Lythotomy; Phymosis; Amputation; Index. References in the text to St. Thomas Hospital (London), William Cheselden, Benjamin Cowell, Richard Mead, etc. Similar lecture notes exist in the St. Thomas Hospital Medical School Library (information kindly supplied by D.T. Bird). Signature and contemporary stamp "I.W.Brooks" on f. 2v, ms. entry of his birth and signature of his grandson Albert C. Morrison (b. 1862) *ibid.* Genealogical account begins with statement that Brooks died during a yellow fever epidemic in New York at the beginning of the 19th century (fragile early 20th-century insert inside front cover).   *[n.c.]*

178. **Cloud, Joseph Howard,** 1872-1968. Acute meningococċic endocarditis and septicemia, by J.H. Cloud and E.B. Krumbhaar. *Le Treport (France), 1917?-18.*

9, [1] ff. 27 cm. Pencilled autograph; with additions and some corrections by Dr. Krumbhaar, in ink. From Base Hospital no. 10, A.E.F., and Gen. Hosp. no. 16, B.E.F., both in Le Treport. Published in *JAMA*, v. 71: 2144-46 (1918).
          [ZZ 10b/1]

179. **Coates, Samuel,** 1748-1830. Letter to Joseph Paschall with report on victims of the yellow fever. *Philadelphia?, 1793.*

2 ff. 34 cm (binding 35 cm.). Gift of William Pepper.   *[Z 10/46]*

180. **Cole, Harold Newton,** b. 1918. A history of dermatology in Cleveland, and the first fifty years of the Cleveland Dermatological Society, 1923-1973. *Cleveland, 1973?*

24 ff. 28 cm. Reproduced from typewritten copy; presented by the author.
          [10c/133]

181. **Colhoun, John,** 1740-82, supposed author. Miscellaneous notes, accounts, cures and prescriptions, with diary of a journey from Fredericksburg, Va. *Chambersburg (Pa.), 1764-77.*

2 v. in 1. 17 cm. Presented by Historical Society of Pennsylvania, with note indicating a connection with Dr. Cahoon of Chambersburg, Pa. John Colhoun (or Colhoon, as he signs himself on some occasions) married Rhuhammah Chambers (cf. A.W. Thrush, *Medical Men of Franklin Co.*, p. 56). Most entries not dated. The only internal indication of a connection with Colhoun is a partly illegible entry mentioning both "Mrs. Chambers" and "Colhoun."   *[10a/145]*

182. **Collectanea** zu Beantwortung der mir vorgelegten Fragen, begins: Ich Apotheker sagte. *N.p., late 18th cent.*

4 ff. (f. 3-4 blank). 22 cm. Examination paper, German and Latin, without indication of examiner, examinee or institution, but with references to authorities, incl. Boerhave.   *[n.c.]*

183. **Collection of Autographs**, portraits, caricatures, printed forms and advertisements, etc. *V.p., 1668-1885.*

1 v. (79 items); illus. 29.5 cm. The collection contains 27 letters and notes (incl. a prescription), among them items by William Heberden (1765), James Currie (1804), J.C. Lavater (n.d.), Matthias Baillie (1820), A.P. Cooper (1837), J.C. Spurzheim (1829), B.C. Brodie (1838), J.A. Paris (n.d.), Charles Hastings (1841) and T.H. Huxley (1875). Besides portraits (among these a water-color portrait of Joseph Priestley) are included several broadsides, few watercolors and sketches. Later acquisitions were entered towards the end by the donor (E.B. Krumbhaar), i.e. letter of gynaecological interest by Giovanni Apostolis (1668), 2 printed appointments as military surgeons in the British army (1794) and 4 fragmentary prescriptions (France, 17th cent.). — Detailed analysis of contents available.   *[Z 10/121]*

184. **Collection of Letters** in Honor of W.B. McDaniel, II, on his retirement as Curator, Historical Collections of the Library, College of Physicians of Philadelphia, October 30, 1973. *V.p., 1973.*

2 boxes. 25-27 cm. Solicited by the President of the College, Katharine R. Sturgis, from former associates, friends and fellows; bound for presentation to him (volume in Box 2); additional letters in folder (Box 1). Also included (in Box 1): photocopies of the letters, list of persons solicited, and related material; 1 vol. of similar letters from the staff; 1 folder of letters on his death (1975). — Excerpts from the letters publ. in *Trans. & Stud.*, ser. 4, v. 43: 45-54 (1976).

[ZZ 10c/21]

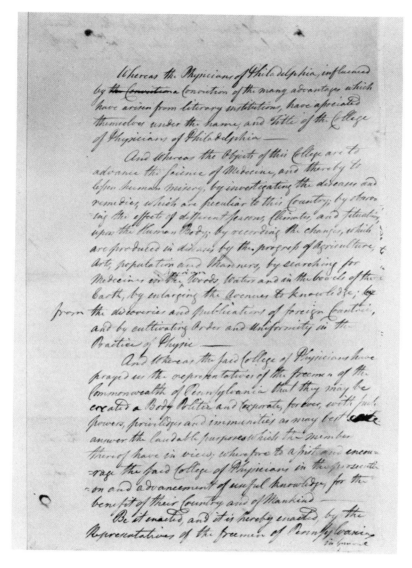

Plate 3. 185.11 College of Physicians of Philadelphia *Charter.* Draft by Benjamin Rush, 1788.

185.   **COLLEGE OF PHYSICIANS OF PHILADELPHIA. ARCHIVES.**
        Philadelphia, 1787ff.

ARRANGEMENT

.1   Government (8 entries)
.2   Committees (54 entries)
        .23 Lectures and Orations (9 entries)
.3   Fellows (5 entries)
.4   Sections (10 entries)
.5   Special Meetings & Celebrations (11 entries)
.6   Major Operating Units (10 entries)
        .61 Library
        .62 Historical Collections
        .63 Mütter Museum
        .64 Office of Continuing Education

.1   **GOVERNMENT OF THE COLLEGE OF PHYSICIANS.**

.11   **Charter and By-Laws,** 1788-1972.
      First draft of charter by *Benjamin Rush* and by-laws, the latter
      with several revisions. Also includes related materials.
      1 v., 2 boxes, 2 envelopes; 23 printed pamphlets (1790-1972).
      [Vault; Z 10/17; 1h/557; n.c.]

.12   **Minutes,** 1787-1974.
      Minutes recording monthly meetings, 1787-1974 (some with
      index). Minutes of annual meetings, 1974-78, with notes and
      correspondence. Rough drafts of minutes, 1854-1909. — Index
      to papers presented at meetings, 1787-1833. — Brief calendar of
      activities, 1787-90, incl. note by *Henry Bond*. — List of dates, time,
      and rooms for meetings, 1899-1901.
      This part contains furthermore miscellaneous correspondence,
      1793-1950, among these, letters about *yellow fever* epidemic of
      1769; resignation of *Benjamin Rush*, 1793.
      16 v., 4 boxes, 2 envelopes.   *[Z 10/227; Z 10/17; n.c.]*

.13   **Office of the President,** 1833-1978.
      Miscellaneous correspondence, speeches, newsletters, announce-
      ments and clippings of presidents, ranging from extensive to
      very limited files and even complete absence of College-related
      documents.
      6 v., 12 boxes, 3 envelopes, 1 carton.   *[Z 10/57; 10c/123, 153; ZZ 10d/8; n.c.]*
      Note: Specific information on the extent of each president's file can be

supplied; see also under the names of presidents in the alphabetical sequence: *John Redman* (1787-1805); *William Shippen* (1805-08); *Adam Kuhn* (1808-18); *Thomas Parke* (1818-35); *Thomas C. James* (1835); *Thomas T. Hewson* (1835-48); *George B. Wood* (1848-79); *William S.W. Ruschenberger* (1879-82); *Alfred Stillé* (1883-84); *Samuel Lewis* (1884); *Jacob Mendez da Costa* (1884-86; 1895-97); *S. Weir Mitchell* (1886-88; 1892-94); *David H. Agnew* (1889-91); *John Ashhurst, Jr.* (1898-99); *William W. Keen* (1900-01); *Horatio C. Wood* (1902-04); *Arthur V. Meigs* (1904-06); *James Tyson* (1907-09); *George E. de Schweinitz* (1910-12); *James C. Wilson* (1913-15); *Richard H. Harte* (1916-18); *William J. Taylor* (1919-21); *Thomas R. Neilson* (1922-24); *Hobart A. Hare* (1925-27); *John H. Gibbon* (1928-30); *Francis R. Packard* (1931-33); *Alfred Stengel* (1934-36); *George P. Muller* (1937-39); *Edward B. Krumbhaar* (1940-42); *O.H. Perry Pepper* (1943-45); *Jacob P. Schaeffer* (1946-49); *T. Grier Miller* (1949-52); *Richard A. Kern* (1952-55); *Lewis C. Scheffey* (1955-58); *Jonathan E. Rhoads* (1958-60); *Thomas M. Durant* (1961-63); *John H. Gibbon, Jr.* (1964-66); *Francis C. Wood* (1967-69); *George I. Blumstein* (1970-72); *Katharine R. Sturgis* (1972-73); *John P. Hubbard* (1974-78); *George P. Rosemond* (1978-80).

.14   Office of the Secretary (Executive Secretary, 1940-52), 1840-1952.

Annual reports and correspondence (mainly concerning election and resignation of fellows, procedures and duties of the office), 1840-1940. — Papers of the executive secretary *James Harold Austin*, 1940-52, incl. correspondence concerning pension plans, congressional legislation about *experimentation on animals,* library of the College of Physicians, *building fund, Therapeutic Trials Committee of the Council on Pharmacy and Chemistry* of the *American Medical Association, statistics.* — Minutes of the Medical Board of the *University of Pennsylvania,* and various activities at the same institution. — Surveys evaluating hospitals and laboratories in Pennsylvania, New Jersey and New York, 1946-51.

3 v., 7 boxes, 6 envelopes.   *[Z 10c/5; Z 10/131; n.c., partly Vault]*

.15   Office of the Treasurer, 1787-1961.

Annual reports, 1841-1911, 1933, and monthly reports, 1883-1908. — Two sets of correspondence, 1810-1905, and 1877-1904, 1941. — Accounts and account books, 1787-1961, incl. dues and contributions from fellows (1834-1959).

34 v., 17 boxes, 5 envelopes.   *[10c/116-7, 119, 122; 10d/33; n.c.]*

.16   Council, 1864-1979.

Minutes, 1864-1979, incl. drafts and correspondence (1868-1979). — Reports, pamphlets and clippings from representatives from the Council to the *Pennsylvania State Quarantine Board,* 1893-1911. — Correspondence, reports and memoranda on plans to establish a medical school at the *University of Ghana at Accra* with assistance by Philadelphia medical schools, 1961-3.

5 v., 8 boxes, 3 envelopes, 1 folder.   *[Z 10/226; n.c.]*

.17   **Censors,** 1836-1941.
Minutes, notes and correspondence, 1887-91. — Reports and testimony concerning fellows of the College of Physicians, 1836-1911, and death notices of fellows, 1934-41. — Reports to the secretary, 1902-10, 1920-31.
1 v., 3 boxes, 1 envelope.   *[10c/121]*

.18   **Office of the Executive Director,** 1967-80.
Reports, financial papers, grant administration, fund raising, correspondence, etc. of directors *W. Wallace Dyer*, 1967-70; *Charles E. Ingersoll*, 1970-72 (including material of the *Greater Philadelphia Committee for Medical-Pharmaceutical Sciences*); *F. Robert Michael*, 1972-74; *William F. Chaveas*, 1975— (including the *"Third Century Program"*). Also material relating to personnel, visitors registration and miscellaneous administrative details.
2 boxes.   *[n.c.]*

.2   **COMMITTEES.**

.21   **Standing Committees** (in chronological order).

.211   Committee on the *Pharmacopoeia,* 1790-1950.
Minutes, 1877-99, incl. lists of accepted and rejected drugs. — Correspondence (incl. letter from the physicians of New Haven to College of Physicians president *John Redman* [1790], approving his call for a pharmacopoeia), circulars and reports on the U.S. Pharmacopoeia, 1790-1950.
1 v., 2 boxes, 2 envelopes.   *[n.c.]*

.212   Committee on *Public Hygiene*, 1834-38, 1851.
Correspondence and reports concerned with the purity of water from the Schuylkill River and with filling stagnant ponds and lots in and near Philadelphia.
2 envelopes.   *[n.c.]*

.213   *Library* Committee, 1836-1978.
Annual reports, 1836-1939; minutes, 1865-1978; correspondence and reports, 1864-1978. — Alphabetical listing of portraits, statues and other items displayed in the College of Physicians, 1898-1915. — Financial records (reports, account books, ledgers), 1839-1953. — Correspondence, reports and accounts of a sub-committee appointed for the collection of funds for the revision of the catalogue, 1901, 1910.
25 v., 10 boxes, 3 envelopes.   *[10a/285, 309; 10c/8, 21, 29, 46-7, 118; 10d/88]*

.214   Committee on the *Theory and Practice of Medicine,* 1837.
Papers on the treatment of *scarlatina* with belladonna, *bloodletting*, new treatment of *cholera*, and counterirritants.
1 envelope.   *[n.c.]*

15   *Building* Committees, 1840-1979.
      Committee on the Erection of a Hall, 1840. Report of a joint
      committee of the College of Physicians, the *Philadelphia Medical
      Society* and the *Philadelphia Medical College*, 1840. — Building
      Committee of 1850ff. Minutes, 1860-2; correspondence, 1906-
      11, 1915; two files of reports, 1906-12 and from the Subcommit-
      tee on Furniture, 1909-10; specifications, 1907-9; blueprints and
      plans, 1907-13. — Committee of Seven, 1859-60. Minutes of a
      committee to solicit additional contributions. — Building Com-
      mittee, 1904-15. Minutes, 1904-12; reports, 1906-12; correspond-
      ence, 1906-11, 1915 concerning general activities, the Wood and
      Gross rooms; specifications, blueprints and plans, 1907-13;
      reports of the Subcommittee on Furniture, 1909-10. — Building
      Committee, 1948-56. Minutes, reports, financial records and
      correspondence concerning fundraising and construction of the
      new stacks; blueprints of alterations and additions to the
      building, 1955-56. — Building Committee, 1967-68, 1979. Min-
      utes, reports and correspondence, mostly on library construction
      and in 1979 for additions to the Medical Documentation Service
      facilities.
      5 v., 4 boxes, 6 envelopes.   *[Z 10/6, 139; Z1h/5; ZZ 10d/19; n.c.]*

6   Committee on *Surgery*, 1840.
      Resignation of the chairman *Joseph Pancoast.*
      1 envelope.   *[n.c.]*

7   *Publications* Committee, 1840-1976.
      Reports, 1840-1976 and annual reports, 1874-1956. — Correspond-
      ence and misc. papers concerning the *Transactions & Studies.* —
      Financial records, 1885-86, incl. bills, receipts and treasurer's
      statements.
      5 boxes, 2 envelopes.   *[10c/94; Z 10c/7; n.c.]*

8   Committee on a *Pathological Museum*, 1849 and *Mütter Museum*
      and *College Collections Committees*, 1863-1981.
      Minutes with report by *John Neill* about efforts to establish the
      pathological museum, with partial listing of the collection,
      consisting largely of specimens presented by *Isaac Parrish*, 1849.
      — Mütter Museum Committee. Annual and semi-annual
      reports, 1863-1978; minutes, 1973-77, of the committee of the
      Museum and College collections; correspondence, 1901-35;
      financial records, 1863-1966, incl. account books, tax statements
      and auditors' reports; scrapbooks containing essays, resolutions,
      proposals, etc. (concerning lectureship and misc. affairs of the
      committee), 1866-1912. — Committee on the College collections,
      1935-81. Annual reports, 1935-72. — Minutes, 1935-81. —

Correspondence, 1935-66, mainly dealing with acquisitions and acknowledgements of gifts. — Catalog, 1940. — Notebooks, 1938-69, with information on accessions.
27 v., 26 boxes, 25 envelopes.   *[n.c.]*

.219   *Hall* Committee, 1863-1977.
Annual reports, 1863-1970. — Minutes, 1884-1977. — Misc. correspondence and reports, 1880-1977, concerning construction, design, purchase, sales, repair, rental, etc., of the building of the College of Physicians. — Financial records, 1867-1908, largely on rental charges.
15 v., 6 boxes, 3 envelopes, 1 binder.   *[10a/308; n.c.]*

.2110   Committee on *Entertainment*, 1886-1941.
Minutes, 1885 and 1909. — Reports, 1886-1941. — Address by *Horace Howard Furness*, 1886, presenting a silver loving cup (gift of *Mary Cadwalader Mitchell* and *Sophia Stevens Conover*). — Miscellany, 1886-1941 (vouchers, invitations and responses).
2 v., 5 envelopes.   *[10c/16; Z 10/56, 224]*

.2111   *Finance* Committee, 1887-1978.
Annual reports, 1935-78. — Minutes, 1887-1978. — Appraisal of the contents of the building of the College of Physicians (except books and archives), 1936. — Misc. correspondence.
2 v., 2 boxes, 1 envelope.   *[10c/11, 120; n.c.]*

.2112   *Directory of Nurses* Committee, 1881-1936.
Annual reports, 1925, 1933-36. — Correspondence, 1881-1913 (15 vols., incl. index) dealing with evaluations and recommendations by physicians and patients. — Financial accounts, 1881-1909. — Scrapbook, 1882-1932. — Miscellany.
18 v., 1 box.   *[Z 10c/23, 25, 27; n.c.]*
Note: The directory provided information on private-duty nurses.

.2113   Committee on *Scientific Business*, 1911-1981.
Annual reports, 1911-40. — Minutes, 1938-40, 1974-75, of the committee responsible for evening lectures. — Calendars, 1936-81, listing speakers and their lectures. — Some texts of lectures and correspondence, 1972-76.
3 boxes.   *[n.c.]*

.2114   Committee on *Public Health and Preventive Medicine*, 1913-1980.
Annual reports, 1913-48. — Minutes, 1914-24, 1967-80. — Correspondence on the practice of the *New York Life Extension Institute* (1922), the investigation into the *Philadelphia Hospital for Mental Illness* at *Byberry* (1938-40) and committee business.
1 v., 3 boxes, 2 envelopes.   *[10d/134; n.c.]*

15   Committee on *Nominations* for the College *Elections*, 1935-1978.
       Reports, 1935-40, with lists of nominees. — Proposed slates of
       officers, election returns, etc., 1970-78.
       1 box.   [n.c.]

16   *Joseph N. Pew, Jr.* Memorial Loan Fund Committee, 1961-1979.
       Minutes, reports, correspondence, accounts, memoranda, 1961-
       74, including results of a survey (1962) evaluating the financial
       needs of interns and residents and letters of appreciation from
       grantees. — Financial records, 1962-75. — Correspondence with
       rejected applicants, 1965-73. — Files of applications with
       supporting documents, 1963-75. — Clippings and articles, 1963-
       78.
       11 boxes.   [n.c.]

17   Committee on *Ordinances and By-Laws*, 1967-1977.
       Minutes, 1973-76. — Reports, correspondence and proposals,
       1967-77.
       1 box.   [n.c.]

18   *Women's* Committee, 1971-1978.
       Draft of by-laws, 1972. — Minutes, 1971-78. — Correspondence,
       1972-78. — Financial report, 1973. — Guest list of party given for
       descendents of founders of the College of Physicians, 1976.
       1 box.   [Z 10c/30]

19   *Fellowship* Committee, 1974-1978.
       Reports, correspondence, etc.
       1 box.   [n.c.]

20   Long-range *Planning* Committee, 1975-1978.
       Minutes, reports, memoranda, etc. on *Forward-Looking Program. . .,
       Third Century Program,* fund-raising campaigns, and cooperation
       with other medical institutions in the Philadelphia area.
       1 box.   [n.c.]

Pro-Tem Committees (in chronological order).

Committee on the Use of *Tobacco*, 1833.
Report in response to petition from the *Young Men's Association* of
Philadelphia.
1 envelope.   [n.c.]

Committee on the Inventory of the *Kappa Lambda* Archives,
1836.
Material on the presentation of the society's archives to the
College of Physicians.
1 envelope.   [n.c.]

.223   Committee on the *Fee Bill*, 1836.
        Report including "Table of Charges for Professional Services."
        1 envelope.   *[n.c.]*

.224   Committee on the State of the *Medical Profession*, 1839.
        Report outlining reforms for the improvement of the medical
        profession in Philadelphia.
        1 envelope.   *[n.c.]*

.225   Committee on *Standing Committees*, 1840.
        Report suggesting revision of the by-laws.
        1 envelope.   *[n.c.]*

.226   Committee on the *Right to the Floor*, ca. 1840.
        Report suggesting further revision of the by-laws.
        1 envelope.   *[n.c.]*

.227   Committee to Examine the Protective Powers of *Revaccination*,
        1845.
        Records with names of, and observation on, children who had
        been vaccinated against *smallpox*.
        1 v.   *[Z 10/8]*

.228   Committee on the circular from the *New York Medical Society*,
        1845.
        Report opposing participation in organizing a *national medical
        convention*.
        1 envelope.   *[n.c.]*

.229   Committee on *Anatomy Act*, 1867.
        Report in support of an act passed by the Pennsylvania Legisla-
        ture "For the Promotion of Medical Science, and to Prevent the
        Traffic in Human Bodies in the City of Philadelphia and County
        of Allegheny."
        1 folder.   *[n.c.]*

.2210   Committee to Confer with Committees from the *Philadelphia
        Obstetrical Society* and the *Philadelphia County Medical Society*, 1878.
        Report supporting a law assuring *privileged communication* between
        patient and physician.
        1 folder.   *[n.c.]*

.2211   Committee to Address Select and Common Councils with
        regard to the threatened invasion of *cholera*, 1885.
        Report and recommendations.
        1 folder.   *[n.c.]*

212   Committee on Tablets, 1885.
Report of the committee established to honor fellows of the
College of Physicians who died during the *epidemic*, with brief
history of the College of Physicians.
1 folder.   *[n.c.]*

213   Committee to Collect and Distribute Funds for the Relief of the
Profession following the *Johnstown Disaster*, 1889.
Report with account of letters received from Johnstown (Pa.)
practitioners.
1 folder.   *[n.c.]*

214   Committee on *Cholera*, 1893.
Report on efforts to promote cooperation among physicians to
prevent a cholera epidemic in Philadelphia.
1 folder.   *[n.c.]*

215   Delegates to the Union Committee on *Water Supply*, 1893.
Report on efforts to establish committees on a permanent water
supply and general *sanitation.*
1 folder.   *[n.c.]*

216   Committee on Trolley Car Gong and Bell, 1894.
Report on meeting with Mayor *Edwin S. Stuart* on the necessity
for continuously ringing bells.
1 folder.   *[n.c.]*

217   Committee on National Board of *Public Health*, 1895.
Letter to the College of Physicians requesting continuation of the
committee.
1 folder.   *[n.c.]*

218   Committee on *Professional Confidence*, 1895.
Report, memoranda and clippings on *privileged communications.*
1 envelope.   *[n.c.]*

219   Committee in Regard to Duties on Books, 1895; 1910.
Reports on efforts to prevent imposition of duties on *importation
of medical books and equipment.*
1 folder.   *[n.c.]*

220   Committee to City Council on Proposed Site for *Municipal
Hospital* (Philadelphia), 1897.
Report.
1 folder.   *[n.c.]*

221   Committee on Placarding Houses for *Contagious Diseases*, 1898;
1900-01.
Reports.
1 envelope.   *[n.c.]*

.2222   Committee on Proposed Act of Assembly of the *Law Reform* Committee, 1900.
Report on expert testimony.
1 folder.   *[n.c.]*

.2223   Committee on Prevention of *Contagious Diseases*, 1904.
Report with resolutions to be adopted by the *Board of Health* (Philadelphia) regulating and preventing such diseases.
1 folder.   *[n.c.]*

.2224   Committee on the Desirability of Free Distribution of *tetanus antitoxin*, 1910-11.
Reports, including proposal to restrain the use of explosives on Fourth of July celebrations.
1 folder.   *[n.c.]*

.2225   Committee on the Wearing of Gowns by the Officers at Meetings, 1910.
Report.
1 folder.   *[n.c.]*

.2226   Committee on Combined Meeting with the *American Academy of Political and Social Science*, 1934.
Report.
1 envelope.   *[n.c.]*

.2227   Committee on Special *Library Privileges*, 1935; 1938.
Reports.
1 envelope.   *[n.c.]*

.2228   Committee on *Air Hygiene*, 1937.
Report on air pollution, etc.
1 envelope.   *[n.c.]*

.2229   Committee on *Internship* and *Residency*, 1962.
Compilation of responses to inquiry on financial condition and needs.
1 v.   *[n.c.]*

.2230   Committee to Consider the Proposal to Combine the *Mütter Museum, College Collections* and *Historical Collections*, 1970-77.
Minutes, reports, correspondence and notes.
1 envelope.   *[n.c.]*

.2231   Committee for the Division of *Medical History*, 1973-78.
Minutes, reports, memoranda and correspondence on the establishment and purpose for the Institute for the History of Medicine, incl. transcript of a symposium (1974) and applications for the position of director of the institute.
1 binder, 1 box.   *[n.c.]*

232   Search Committee, 1974-75.
Minutes and correspondence concerning the selection of the
executive director of the *College of Physicians.*
1 box.   *[n.c.]*

233   *Continuing Education* Committee, 1976-78.
Correspondence.
1 envelope.   *[n.c.]*

234   Steering Committee for *Fund Raising* and Public Affairs, 1976-78.
Minutes, reports and correspondence.
1 box.   *[n.c.]*

3   **Lectures and Orations** (Committees), 1864-1976.

31   *Thomas Dent Mütter* Lectureship, 1864-82.
Proceedings, 1864-82, including appointment of lecturers, announcements and reports to the secretary of the College of
Physicians. Subject of lectures: *surgical pathology.*
1 envelope.   *[10a/400]*

32   *Alvarenga Prize* Committee, 1887-1941.
Minutes and notes, 1887-92. — Correspondence, 1890-1941. —
List of candidates, including titles of essays submitted, 1897-
1939. — Essays, 1897-1933, having failed to receive prizes.
1 v., 5 boxes.   *[10a/375; Z 10/150]*

————. See also Alvarenga Prize in subject index.

3   *William F. Jenks* Prize Committee, 1890-95.
Correspondence, 1890-95, including announcements and rules.
Subject of essays: *obstetrics.*
1 envelope.   *[n.c.]*

4   *Nathan Lewis Hatfield* Prize and Lectureship, 1900-35.
Reports and correspondence, 1900-35. Subject: original *research*
in medicine.
1 box.   *[n.c.]*

5   Committee on the *Silas Weir Mitchell* Oration, 1922-40.
Reports and correspondence.
1 envelope.   *[n.c.]*

6   *Mary Scott Newbold* Lectures, 1923-34; 1968.
Reports and correspondence, 1923-34. — Transcript of Symposium
(1968) on legal and ethical implications of the non-medical use
of *drugs.*
1 box, 1 envelope. Fund established by *Clement B. Newbold* as a tribute to Mrs.
Newbold, *William J. Taylor,* et al.   *[n.c.]*

.237   *George E. de Schweinitz* Lectures, 1949, 1954.
Typescript of lectures by *Arthur J. Bedell* (1949) and *Conrad Berens* (1954).
3 v., 1 envelope.   *[ZZ 10d/12-13; Kc 402]*

.238   *Ralph Pemberton* Lectureship, 1972-73.
Reports, correspondence, copy of will, etc. (established by R. Pemberton in the field of *arthritic and metabolic conditions*).
1 envelope.   *[n.c.]*

.239   *Kate Hurd Mead* Lectures, 1973; 1975-76.
Correspondence, 1973-76. — Copies of lectures sponsored jointly by *Medical College of Pennsylvania* and the *College of Physicians*.
1 envelope.   *[n.c.]*

.3   **FELLOWS** (Membership).

.31   *Biographical Material:* Lists of fellows, 1793-1979. — Rollbook, including proposals for membership, 1935-69. — Biographical sketches and memoirs, 1918-68. — Biographical files of fellows, most with miscellaneous correspondence, applications for membership and some printed items. — Correspondence and responses, 1937-79, concerning bequests and gifts given by and in honor of fellows.
8 v., 2 boxes, 5 envelopes.   *[10c/19; Z 10/135; n.c.]*

.32   Announcements, programs, brochures, pamphlets, and other printed material, 1848-1980. *With* Calendars of officers and committees, 1869 to present. — Meeting announcements, 1848 to present. — Announcement of lectures, etc., 1895 to present. — *Fellows Forum*, a review of College news and activities, 1974-77, 1980.
4 v., 8 boxes, 1 envelope.   *[1h/14; n.c.]*

.33   Scrapbooks and clippings, 1888-1956.
12 v.   *[Z1b/31]*

.34   Memorials: *James Harold Austin*, 1952-53. Correspondence and accounts of fund raising for addition to library as a memorial. — *Samuel Lewis*, 1873; 1892.   List of subscribers to raise money for a portrait of Dr. Lewis. — *Wharton Sinkler*, 1911-69. Correspondence, reports and blueprints concerning the herb garden of the College of Physicians.
5 envelopes, 1 folder, 1 cylinder.   *[n.c.]*

.35   Special Fellows' Associations: *Journal Association*, 1871-75. Constitution, annual reports, minutes, letter-book and correspondence of fellows concerned with subscriptions to journals, etc. for

the *library.* — *S. Weir Mitchell* Associates, 1972-74. Reports and correspondence, mainly concerned with support for the *library.*
2 v., 2 envelopes. *[10c/40; Z 10/131; n.c.]*

SECTIONS.

1   *Ophthalmology,* 1890-1947.
Annual reports, 1934-40. — Minutes, etc., 1890-1913; 1947.
4 v. *[Z 10/147]*

2   *Otolaryngology, Otology* and *Laryngology,* 1893-1939.
Annual reports, 1894-1939. — Minutes, etc., 1893-1927; 1937-38.
3 v., 2 boxes. *[Z 10/148; n.c.]*

3   General *Surgery,* 1894-98.
Annual reports.
1 folder. *[n.c.]*

4   *Orthopedic Surgery,* 1894-95.
Annual reports.
1 folder. *[n.c.]*

5   *General Medicine,* 1897-1966.
Annual reports, 1897-1957. — Minutes, 1897-1927. — Correspondence, 1927-64. — Lectures (texts and abstracts), 1948-61. — Financial records, 1911-66. — Announcements, etc., 1927-65.
2 v., 13 boxes. *[10a/193; Z 10/179]*

6   *Gynecology,* 1897-1907.
Annual reports.
1 folder. *[n.c.]*

7   *Medical History,* 1905-79.
Annual reports, 1905-57. — Minutes, 1950-53. — Correspondence, 1948-57. — Financial records (including reports, dues, etc.), 1936-57. — Lectures and related material, 1948-57. — Announcements, etc., 1948-56; 1979.
8 boxes, 1 envelope. *[Z 10/218; n.c.]*

8   *Public Health, Preventive and Industrial Medicine,* 1920-28; 1974.
Annual reports, 1920-28; 1974. — Minutes, 1923-74. — Correspondence, etc., 1923-74.
2 boxes, 1 envelope. *[ZZ 10c/3; n.c.]*

9   *Internal Medicine,* 1976-77.
Correspondence; section failed to be established.
1 envelope. *[n.c.]*

.410   *Basic Sciences,* 1977.
Correspondence concerning formation of this section.
1 envelope.   *[n.c.]*

.5   **SPECIAL MEETINGS AND CELEBRATIONS**

.51   *Centennial* Celebration, 1886-87.
Report (1887) of the Committee for the Centennial Celebration.
— Scrapbook, including program, with poetry by *S. Weir Mitchell*
and *Henry Hartshorne*, correspondence, notes, clippings, printed
materials, proceedings. — Catalogue of portraits lent, listing
subject, date, name of artist and owner.
1 v., 1 box, 1 binder, 1 envelope.   *[10c/12; Mütter Museum]*

.52   *Silas Weir Mitchell* Memorial, March 31, 1914.
Program and invitations.
1 envelope.   *[n.c.]*

.53   *Marie Curie* special meeting honoring Madame Curie during her
visit to the College of Physicians, May 23, 1921. Correspondence, clippings, sketch of quartz-piezo electrometer given to the
College of Physicians by *Pierre Curie.*
1 envelope.   *[Z 10/140]*

.54   *Lister* Centenary, April 6, 1927.
Correspondence and misc. records of the Committee organizing
the celebration.
1 box.   *[Z 10/151]*

.55   *Harvey* Celebration, March 22, 1928.
Reports, 1927.
1 envelope.   *[10d/86]*

.56   *Sesqui-Centennial* Celebration of the *College of Physicians of Philadelphia*, May 14-15, 1937.
Reports, correspondence (incl. letters of acceptance and regrets),
invitations and lists of invited guests, miscellaneous accounts,
draft of program.
1 box.   *[10c/33]*

.57   *Alfonso Corti* Commemoration, November 21, 1951.
Reports, correspondence, photographs from Corti's works.
1 box.   *[10c/135]*

.58   Fiftieth Anniversary of the Dedication of the Hall of the *College of
Physicians*, December 14, 1959.
Presidential newsletter, program and memorabilia.
1 envelope.   *[10c/60]*

59   *Bicentennial* Committee, 1972-73. Minutes, reports and correspondence concerning the plans for medical exhibits in connection with the U.S. Bicentennial of 1976.
1 envelope.   *[n.c.]*

510   Scientific Program Committee for the *Bicentennial*, 1973-76.
Minutes, correspondence, etc. to arrange lectures, including *"World Health* in Human Perspective" (1976), also series of taped lectures by distinguished scholars. — List of persons attending.
1 box, 11 tape cassettes.   *[ZZ 7c/1; n.c.]*

511   *John Heysham Gibbon, Jr.* Memorial, February 13 and May 5, 1973.
Correspondence, memorials, photographs, clippings and symposium (May 5) celebrating the 20th anniversary of *open-heart surgery*.
1 box.   *[n.c.]*

6   **MAJOR OPERATING UNITS.**

61   **Library,** 1792; 1864-1981.
By-Laws (1792) regulating the use of the library. — Reports, 1864-1981: annual reports, 1864-1931, monthly reports, 1883-1981.
5 v., 8 boxes, 1 envelope.   *[10c/21, 36; Librarian's Office]*

611   Office of the Librarian, 1882-1981.
Correspondence and a great variety of documents of the librarians *Charles Perry Fisher*, 1882-1932; *Walton Brooks McDaniel II*, 1931-52; *Elliott H. Morse*, 1953-81.
144 v., 151 boxes; 29 envelopes, 19 folders (some of them in boxes); 5 posters. *[10a/128, 170-1, 237, 310; 10c/23, 24e, 28, 36, 39, 41, 49-50, 55, 61, 95-6; 10d/58; Z 10/35, 77, 110, 113-4, 133, 138, 142, 162, 167, 225; Z 10c/41; ZZ 10d/14; n.c.]*
Note: For details send inquiries to the office of the librarian, College of Physicians of Philadelphia. — Included are: Rules of the staff, 1912, 1940-48. — Records of department head meetings, 1970-73. — Items relating to cataloguing and classification, 1818-1911 and later. — Book catalogues, 1818-1911; journal catalogues, 1885-1900; dissertation catalogue, 1895. — Shelf lists and inventories, 1887-1934. — Annual reports and documents of the reference and the circulation departments, 1792-1960; visitors' registers, 1880-1956, binders' list, 1868-1935 (of the circulation department) and bibliographies on special topics (of the reference department). — Financial records, 1869-1978. — Grant proposals, 1964-79 (including "Philadelphia and the *Pharmacopoeia*," [1964-67]; bio-bibliography of *aging* to 1900 [1965-68]; reorganization of journals [1971]; "Medical Library Resource Project" [1972]; strengthening of research library resources [1978]; improvement of cataloguing and distribution to advance medical knowledge [1978]; restoration of water-damaged library collection [1978-79]. — Proposed cooperation with Philadelphia area medical libraries, 1971). — *Mid-Eastern Regional Medical Library Service*, 1966-79. — *Medical Documentation Service*, 1968-73.

.612   Institute for the Advancement of *Medical Communications*, 1968-73.
Reports, correspondence, etc. (discontinued in 1972).
1 box.   *[n.c.]*

.613   Gifts of collections, 1857-1913.
Catalogues, accession books, shelf lists of donors *Thomas Betton*, 1857; *Samuel Lewis*, 1860, 1880-1912; *George Ord*, 1865-66, 1882; *Samuel David Gross*, 1889-1905, 1913.
13 v., 2 boxes, 2 envelopes.
                              [10a/304; 10c/37; Z 10/109, 133; Z 10c/34; (G)Za/184-5]

.614   Purchase of Hough Collection, ca. 1901.
Catalogue of the *John Stockton Hough* Library (duplicates and non-medical items sold to the *University of Pennsylvania*).
2 boxes.   *[Z 10c/19]*

.62   **Historical Collections,** 1953-78.
Correspondence, reports, list of duplicates for sale, record of reference questions, users' records, purchase orders, accounts, grant proposals (for the cataloguing of the collection, one supported by the *American Philosophical Society*), etc., under the curators *Walton Brooks McDaniel II* (1953-75) with material on his involvement with the *Medical Library Association*, the *History of Science Society* and the *American Association for the History of Medicine*; *Lisabeth Marie Feind Holloway* (1969-76), again including material on the *Medical Library Association* and the *American Association for the History of Medicine* as well as assistance to the *Pennsylvania Hospital* with its cataloguing project and the preparation of a guide to their collection; *Ellen Gartrell*, 1976-78 (acting curator and curator).
1 v., 32 boxes, 1 folder, 2 envelopes.   *[ZZ 10c/21; n.c.]*

.63   **Mütter Museum,** 1856-1980 (currently under the *Institute for the History of Medicine*).
Papers, 1856-71, 1901, including articles of agreement, deed and insurance policy, correspondence. — Annual reports, 1909-29, and curators' reports to the *Mütter Museum Committee*, monthly reports, 1920, 1925-26, correspondence and resolutions on the purchase and release of museum objects, 1835-82. — Correspondence, information on acquisitions and generally on museum objects, and financial records issued by curators *Thomas Hewson Bache* (1865-81), *Guy Hinsdale* (1884-99), *Ward Brinton* (1900-09), *Clarence Hoffman* (1910-22), *Henry Morris* (1908-11; 1926) with correspondence on the *Robert Morris* family; curators *Harry P. Schenck* (1927-36), *Joseph McFarland* (1937-45), *Ella N. Wade* (1945-63), *Elizabeth Moyer* (1973-80).
32 boxes, 1 envelope, 3 packets.   *[Mütter Museum; n.c.]*

31   Museum *catalogues*, 1856-1941, with descriptions, accession record and name of donor. — Accession of donations, 1866-1950. — Deeds of gifts, 1935-50. — Inventories, ca. 1903. — Financial records, 1926-67. — Articles, 1944-78 (many by *E.N. Wade* and citations of publications referring to objects in the museum, 1929-41). — Scrapbook, and miscellaneous items, 1931-66, largely gathered by *H.P. Schenck, J. McFarland* and *E.N. Wade*.
        22 v., 5 boxes, 1 envelope, 2 binders.   *[Mütter Museum; n.c.]*

32   Special collections: *Hyrtl* collection, accession book of skulls and hearts, ca. 1874; *Robert Abbe*, 1923-35; *G.B. Fraser*, 1923 (lantern slides); *Addinell Hewson*, 1924 (lantern slides); *R. Tait McKenzie*, 1934 (photographs); *Charles K. Mills*, 1921 (lantern slides); *Alexander B. Randall*, 1923 (lantern slides with notebook); *Joseph McFarland* collection of materials, 1934-66, compiled in preparation of his article on the "Mütter American Giant."
        6 v., 1 box.   *[Mütter Museum; n.c.]*

4   **Office of Continuing Education,** 1974-81. Programs: *Practice related educational programs* (PREP) with correspondence, reports, etc., mostly on the establishment and management of the program; monthly reports, 1977-79; statistical analysis and evaluation of participants; files of applicants, 1976-80; financial records, 1974-78, etc. *Training program in emergency medicine*, 1975-79. — Reports, correspondence (1977-79). — General and financial records, educational material, and evaluations. — Grant proposal, 1975. Proposal and correspondence for the creation of an institute for continuing *mental health education*.
        12 boxes, 1 folder.   *[n.c.]*

————. For related College entries, see also nos. 1, 3, 36, 59, 62, 64, 78, 95, 107, 138, 184, 231, 254, 322, 366, 368, 370, 374, 376, 398, 432-3, 456-7, 466, 486-7, 524, 557, 600, 617, 619-20, 626, 642, 678-9, 686, 696, 718, 752, 755, 766, 780, 788, 800, 854, 878, 883, 941, 1003, 1007, 1034, 1036, 1074, 1077, 1104-5, 1115, 1127.

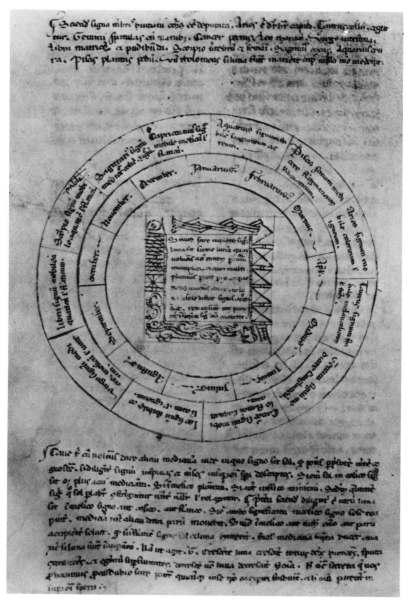

Plate 4. 190. Astrological Calendar appended to *Viaticum, Libri I-VII* by Constantinus Africanus, first half 13th century.

186. **Collins, Joseph,** 1866-1950. Aphasia; a contribution and a critical study. *New York, 1897.*

[1], 350, 33, 7, [64] ff.; 14 plates. 28.5 cm. Typewritten. Published as *The Genesis and Dissolution of the Faculty of Speech; a Clinical and Psychological Study of Aphasia* (New York, 1898). Alvarenga Prize Essay no. 6, 1897.   *[10a/172]*

187. ——————. Bibliography on aphasia. *N.p., ca. 1897.*

64 ff. 28 cm. Photocopy.   *[Pam F 1022]*

188. **Commonplace Book.** *Pennsylvania?, after 1913.*

1 v. 20 cm. Presented by Edward Blanchard Hodge; in his handwriting? — Includes notes on Richard Clarke Cabot, clippings from journals, etc.

[10a/242]

189. **La Connoissance des urines** par leur couleurs avec cel que chacune marque & signifie, tirée des bons autheurs modernes, principalement du R.P. De Mombreloz (Secondary title on p. 1, La Science de la connoissance des maladies par la couleur des urines). *France, ca. 1700.*

Title, 38 pp., 1 f., "Table des chapitres." 16 cm. Prov.: Debruas; Mellet; E.B. Krumbhaar.   *[10a/399]*

190. **Constantinus Africanus.** Viaticum, libri I-VII, *inc.:* Quoniam quidem ut in rethoricis [ait] tullius (ff. 2r-81r). — *With* **Nicolaus Salernitanus.** Antidotarium, *inc.:* Ego nicolaus rogatus a quibus (ff. 82r-105r). *Italy, first half 13th cent. (1244 or earlier).*

105 ff. (f. 1 lacking). 28.5 cm. Neither part contains the name of author or the title. For the Constantinus Africanus see Thorndike & Kibre, col. 604; the *incipit* of Nicolaus Salernitanus (Ibn al-Jazzar? See article by W.B. McDaniel) agrees with that of the incunable edition of 1471 (Hain-Reichling 11764). On the verso of f. 81 is an illustration of the zodiac with indication of its medical implications, and text beginning: Sciendum signa membri humani. Following the explicit of the Nicolaus Salernitanus (Laus Christo detur operis quod finis habetur) is a 23-line verse (*inc.:* Prima etas ab adam usque noe/...) which includes the presumable date of writing, i.e. March 1244 (see W.B. McDaniel, "Notes from the Library," *Trans. & Stud.*, ser. 4, v. 9: 125-6 [1941-42]). Additions by the same scribe on bottom margins of f. 104v and 105r; further notes on f. 105v.   *[Z 10/76]*

191. **Cook, Floyd Harrison,** 1881-1949. Case reports on eye diseases. *N.p., 1911-19.*

Folder (29 ff.), boxed. 32.5 cm.   *[n.c.]*

192. **Cooper, Astley Paston,** 1768-1841. Surgery. Clinical lectures. Midwifery; lecture notes. *London, 1817.*

2 v. (incl. many blank leaves). 21 cm. Comparison with "Notes taken [by Henry U. Onderdonk] from the course of surgery delivered by Mr. Astley Cooper in St. Thomas Hospital London," 1809-10 makes it almost certain that at least the extensive lectures on surgery are by A.P. Cooper; his name does not appear in the ms., but is entered with a question mark at the head of title in both volumes (20th-cent. hand). Volume 2 begins with an introduction to clinical lectures, stressing the importance of observation of actual cases. Beginning at the end of the volume are 2 lectures on midwifery. — Presented by Mrs. A.P.C. Ashhurst.   *[10b/39]*

————. See also nos. 183, 484, 587, 605, 743.

193. **Cooper, Thomas,** 1759-1839. Chemical notes, being the substance of a course of lectures . . . in Philad[a] during the spring of 1817. *Philadelphia, 1817.*

2 v. ([6, incl. 5 blank], 153, [1], 154-319 and few blank ff.). 20 cm. "Taken by Hugh L. Hodge," signatures and bookplate of Hodge in each volume. — Caption titles: "Lectures on chymistry by Judge Cooper" (v. 1); "Lectures on chemistry . . ." (v. 2). — Pencilled corrections.   *[10a/36]*

194. **Corson, Edward Foulke,** 1834-64. Case book kept by Edwd. F. Corson, M.D., U.S. sloop of war "Hartford," commenced June 15th/59 [ended Oct. 5/59]. *N.p., 1859.*

37 pp. 35 cm.   *[Z 10/228]*

195. ————. Register of patients for U.S.S. Mohican, cruise beginning October 17th/62. *N.p., 1862-64.*

1 v. 20.5 cm.   *[10a/396]*

196. **Cowles, Edward,** 1837-1919. Psychiatry. *Boston, 1903.*

1 v. 26.5 cm (in envelope). Mimeographed? "Abstracts of lectures in part, and tabulated statements of symptoms, etc., used in the courses on psychiatry at Harvard Medical School and Dartmouth Medical School . . . Papers revised for the course of 1903." — With reprints of published papers. — Lecture 1 lacks pp. 1-2.   *[10d/29]*

197. ————. A study of the principles of hospital organization and methods of management. *Boston, 1903.*

1 v.; tables. 27 cm (in envelope). Mimeographed?, with manuscript additions. Discusses expenses and policies, 1881-1903, for diet, laundry, grounds, staff, etc. "Chapters from the appendix illustrating the subject from the accounts of the McLean Hospital. Other chapters required to complete the 'Study'."   *[10d/28]*

198. **Coxe, Edward Jenner,** 1801-82. Materia medica; notebook. *Philadelphia, middle 19th cent.?*

[iv], 212, [2] pp. 24.5 cm. Lists drugs and remedies, chiefly of vegetable origin, with their applications. — Gift of Mrs. T. Wistar Brown.   *[10a/360]*

199.   — — — — —. Notebook. *Philadelphia, ca. 1831?*

> 1 v. 24 cm. An alphabetical arrangement of medical terms, especially those
> relating to vegetable materia medica, with definitions and citations to journal
> articles, all, or nearly all, before 1831. — Gift of Mrs. T. Wistar Brown.
>
> *[10a/361]*

200.   **Coxe, John Redman,** 1773-1864, comp.   Collection of letters,
etc., on yellow fever recorded by John Redman Coxe. *Philadelphia, 1794-95.*

> [2] ff., 171 (vero 172) pp., [9] blank ff. 22 cm. Contents: John Mitchell's
> letter to B. Franklin on yellow fever in Virginia, 1741/2 (pp. 1-80). — John
> Kearsley on the same outbreak (pp. 82-3). — John Redman on the yellow fever
> in Philadelphia, 1762 (pp. 86-130). — John Redman Coxe on bilious remitting
> yellow fever in Philadelphia in 1793 (pp. 132-58). — Extract from letters by
> Benjamin Rush, Ashton Alexander, Thomas Drysdale, and John R. Coxe (pp.
> 162-71). "J.R. Coxe 1794" inside front cover. — Gift of S. Weir Mitchell.
>
> *[10a/175]*

201.   — — — — —. Notes from the lectures ... on materia medica. *Philadelphia, 1827-29?*

> [40] ff. 18 cm. Title-page with two dates, 1827 and 1829. — Inscribed on
> verso of title-page: "Joseph Carson, Philadelphia." His autograph?   *[10a/39]*

202.   — — — — —. Notes from the lectures ... taken by Wm. S. Wallace.
Philadelphia, 1821-22.

> 143 pp. 27 cm. Text on recto of each leaf, the verso contains occasional
> addenda or comments.   *[10a/37]*

203.   — — — — —. Notes on Dr. Coxe's lectures on materia medica and
pharmacy ... by WWG [William Wood Gerhard]. *Philadelphia,
1826-27.*

> 82, [4] ff. 17.5 cm. Drawing of Passaick Falls at Paterson [N.J.] on
> frontispiece.   *[10a/38]*

204.   — — — — —. Phlegmasiae — Exanthemata. *Philadelphia, ca. 1818-
19.*

> [iv] ff., 173 (vero 174), 38 pp. 20 cm. Shorthand notes taken by Robert Alison
> (M.D. 1819, University of Pennsylvania)? Table of contents on prel. ff. The
> arrangement is that of Cullen's Nosology.   *[10a/179]*

205.   — — — — —. Will (copy); miscellaneous family letters and papers
relating to his estate. *Philadelphia, 1857 and later.*

> 1 envelope. 37 cm. List of contents filed with the collection.   *[10c/83]*

— — — — —. See also nos. 114, 200, 339, 384, 459, 805t.

206. **Craig, Frank Ardary,** 1876-1959. Golden jubilee, Henry Phipps Institute, 1903-1953. *Philadelphia, 1953.*

    3 ff. 28 cm (in envelope). Mimeographed. Added autograph letter by Dr. Craig addressed to "Dear George" (G. William Norris) and printed one-page article by Hugh Scott, entitled 50 Years at Phipps. *[n.c.]*

207. —————. The story of White Haven Sanatorium, 1901 to 1956; a tribute to Lawrence F. Flick. *Philadelphia?, 1956?*

    1 box; illus., ports. 27.5 cm. Manuscript and typescript; pencil sketches on manuscript t.-p. — Circular of the sanatorium, published in Philadelphia (1959) included. *[10c/80]*

208. **Creighton, Charles,** 1847-1927. Commonplace book on vaccination. *London, 1912.*

    2 v. in 1. 18 cm. Label on cover: "No. 1 Given to Porter F. Cope, 1 Nov. 1912. C. Creighton." Autograph at end of first volume. *[10a/426]*

209. **Crichton-Brown, James,** 1840-1938. Nine letters from C.-B., and one from his widow, to Burton Chance. *Crindau (Scotland), and London, 1926-38.*

    1 envelope. 30.5 cm. Incl. some letters concerned with Chance's work in the history of ophthalmology. *[n.c.]*

210. **Crile, George Washington,** 1864-1943. An experimental and clinical research into certain problems relating to surgical operations. *Cleveland, 1901.*

    179, [5] ff.; graphs. 27 cm. Alvarenga Prize Essay, 1901; published with minor revisions in *Trans. & Stud.*, ser. 3, v. 23: 59-82 (1901). Contents: On the effect of severing and mechanically irritating the vagi; Research into the effects of intra-venous infusion of saline solution; On the physiologic action of cocain and eucain; On the effect of temporary closing of carotid arteries. *[10b/22]*

211. **Croskey, John Welsh,** 1858-1951, comp. Biographical data of medical men (and women) who are, or have been, members of the staff of the Philadelphia General Hospital. *Philadelphia, 1918-19.*

    6 boxes. 26.5 cm. Typewritten and manuscript. Close to 1,000 records (printed forms with typed and some handwritten entries) giving the basic biographical data, incl. early education, medical degrees, positions at Philadelphia General Hospital, memberships. Most, if not all, persons were included in Dr. Croskey's *History of Old Blockley* (Philadelphia, 1929). Name index filed with the collection. *[Z 10c/9]*

    —————. See also no. 752.

212. **Crowell, Bowman Corning,** 1879-1951. Notes on pathology lectures. *Philadelphia, 1924-26.*

1 v.; illus. 29 cm. Notes taken during sophomore and junior year by unidentified student at Jefferson Medical College. Includes notes on neuropathology of M.A. Burns. *[ZZ 10a/27]*

213. **Cruice, John Joseph,** d. 1863. Papers. *V.p., 1856-63.*

1 envelope. 37.5 cm. Contents: Folder 1. Puerperal convulsions (1861). 17 ff. (Thesis, M.D., University of Pennsylvania, Department of Medicine). – 2. Civil War papers, relating to appointment and service as medical officer in the Union army (Philadelphia and St. Louis) and death, including photocopies of letters of recommendation by W.F. Atlee, James J. Levick, S. Weir Mitchell, John F. Randolph; photocopy of letter by W.B. Slaughter concerning Cruice's loyalty to the U.S.; photocopy of letter by Robert Blake Cruice, resigning his commission because of J. J. Cruice's death. – 3. Financial and legal papers, chiefly relating to the purchase of real estate in Philadelphia. *[10c/102]*

214. **Cruice, John Mulchinock,** 1873-1956. Lecture notes, etc. *Philadelphia, 1898-1914.*

1 box. 32 cm. Contents: 1. Notes on W.F. Norris' lecture on ophthalmology (typed with extensive ms. notes and pencilled additions; 138 ff.). – 2. History of St. Joseph's Hospital, Philadelphia (ms., 12 ff.). – 3. Lecture on nurses' training (ms., 9 ff.). – 4. Lecture notes on materia medica (ms., 61 ff.). *[10a/485]*

215. ————. Records and Manual on nursing. *N.p., 1899-1914.*

1 box. 39 cm. Contents: Casebook and ledger, 1899-1914, containing records of cases and prescriptions; also record of daily expenditures, 1911-14. – Inscribed on flyleaf: "John M. Cruice, Oct., 1899." Manual on nursing, typewritten, ff. 1-10 and 63-102 only. *[Z 10a/5]*

216. **Cruice, Robert Blake,** 1838-99. Account books. *Philadelphia, 1891-98.*

2 v. 36 cm. Manuscript records of visits to patients, with fees. *[Z 10c/8]*

217. ————. Papers. *V.p., 1861-99.*

2 boxes. 31.5-39.5 cm. Contents: Box 1. Civil War papers, relating to his enlistment, service, injury, resignation, pension, etc. – Box 2, Folder 1. Biographical sketch; folder 2. Certificates of memberships, appointment as U.S.A. pension examining surgeon, etc.; folder 3. Miscellaneous letters to Cruice, some in photocopy, etc.; folder 4. Letters to Wm. Welsh, Dec. 23, 1872, applying for post of attending physician at Girard College. With photocopies of letters of recommendation. *[10c/103]*

————. See also no. 1118.

218.   **Cruice, William Robert,** 1842-86. Account book. *N.p., 1863-71.*

> 1 v. 24 cm. Includes records of prescriptions for patients. — In front of books are poems copied by Ellen J. Cruice.   *[10c/100]*

219.   **Cruice family.** Papers. *Ireland and Philadelphia, 1832-98?*

> 1 envelope. 37.5 cm. Includes legal papers relating to the family's affairs in Ireland; correspondence with Sir Bernard Burke, Ulster-king-at-arms, about the family coat-of-arms, with a painting of it; certificate of American citizenship of James P. Cruice, 1855; letters signed John Hopkins, Sarah Cruise; miscellaneous photographs, mostly not identified. Calendar filed with the collection.   *[10c/104]*

220.   **Cruikshank, William Cumberland,** 1745-1800? Notes from Cruikshank's lectures on surgery, etc. *England, ca. 1790.*

> 72 ff. (ff. 36-72 blank). 20 cm. Author of the Notes unnamed. The assignment to William Cumberland C. is not entirely certain, but likely, in part because of the reference to Dr. Hunter (f. 3), with whom W.C. Cruikshank was associated. "L.2" on the first leaf seems to indicate that this is the text of a second series of lectures.   *[10b/4]*

221.   — — — — —. Rough notes from Mr. Cruikshank's lectures on surgery: *London, 1791.*

> [1] f., 133 (irregularly numbered) pp., [4] ff. 21 cm. Notes taken by Thomas Chalkley James. — Bookplate of H. Lenox Hodge.   *[10b/3]*

222.   **Cullen, William,** 1710-90. Clinical lectures. *Edinburgh, 1770?*

> 3 v. 20 cm. Imperfect. 1371 paragraphs; sections 294-99 of v. 3 out of order; one or more pp. missing in v. 1. — Inscribed on flyleaf: "Dr. Rhodes, James Evans." — Gift of Jane B. Evans.   *[10a/247]*

223.   — — — —   — — — — —. *Edinburgh, 1772-73?*

> [vi], 791, [1] pp. 23 cm. Inscribed on flyleaf: "Wm.Ashmead's 1823" and on p. [vi] "D.Stuart" and "Wm.Ashmead, April 2nd, 1823." — Total of 40 lectures. — Gift of Wm. Ashmead Schaeffer.   *[10a/166]*

224.   — — — — —. Notes on the clinical lectures of Wm. Cullen by Adam Kuhn. *Edinburgh, 1767?*

> [85] pp. (20.5 cm.); 92 ff. (25 cm.).   *[10a/78]*

— — — — —. See also nos. 42, 111, 150, 204, 354, 573, 805a, 931, 1091.

Curatio morborum, *see* **Sixteenth-Century Lecture Notes.**

225. **Curci, Beniamino.** Breve memoria sull' emostatico Curci . . . *Bari, 1869.*

> 8 ff. (last blank). 35 cm. The text of the Breve occupies 3 ff. Prefaced by letter addressed to Egregio Signor Presidente dell' Academia Americana delle Scienze Mediche-Cerusiche, Filadelfia and synopsis in English signed A.S. (Alfred Stillé?) — Presented by William R. Nicholson. *[Z 10/122]*

226. **Curtin, Roland Gideon,** 1839-1913. Notes on lectures in obstetrics and gynecology. *Philadelphia, 1863-66.*

> [73] ff. (ff. 28-35 blank). 10×17 cm (in envelope). Contents: R.A.F. Penrose, Obstetrics, Dec. 2, 1863 - Oct. 27, 1864 (ff. 1-13r). — J.G. Allen, Didactic lecture on the diseases of females, 4/16 to 6/15, 1866 at the Nurses Home (Lying-in Charity Hospital), ff. 13v-27v). — A.H. Smith. Obstetric lecture, 9/22 to 10/20, 1864; 4/12 to 6/27, 1866, at the Nurses Home (from back of volume, ff. 73-36). — Signed by R.G. Curtin in several places. *[10a/342]*

227. **Da Costa, Jacob Mendez,** 1833-1900. Address delivered before the Association of Military Surgeons of the United States, at Philadelphia, Pa., May 12th, 1896. *Philadelphia, 1896.*

> 9 ff. 26 cm. Typewritten. Published in the Association's *Transactions*, v. 6: 14-16 (1896). *[10d/8]*

228. —————. Notes of lectures on the practice of medicine. *Philadelphia, 1887-91.*

> 2 v. (279, [5]; 221, [4] ff.). 34 cm. Reproduced from typewritten copy. "Taken in shorthand by Thomas G. Ashton" (M.D., 1888, Jefferson Medical College). *[Z 10/80]*

229. —————. Professional aspirations; valedictory address to the graduating class of the Jefferson Medical College of Philadelphia. Delivered April 15th 1891 . . . . *Philadelphia, 1891.*

> 36 ff. 25 cm. Enclosed holograph letter, 1891 Sept 29: "My dear Charlie, you asked me to give you the manuscript of something I have written. I give you this, — my valedictory, and the last thing I wrote before resigning my professorship. Ever affectionately, your father, J.M. Da Costa." — Published Philadelphia, Lippincott, 1891. *[10a/284]*

—————. See also nos. 176, *185.13,* 444, 675, 765, 993, 1105.

230. **Daland, Judson,** 1860-1937. Cardio-vascular sclerosis in soldiers. Read at the ninth annual meeting of the U.S. Pension Examining Surgeons, held in Washington, D.C., May 2, 1910. *N.p., ca. 1910.*

> 6 ff. 25 cm. Typewritten, with pencilled notes. *[10a/432]*

231.   — — — — —. Trephining of the skull by the Incas of Peru. *Phila-delphia, 1934.*

18 ff.; table. 29 cm. Typescript (carbon copy). Case histories from the Medico-Chirurgical Hospital on the verso of most leaves. Read before the Section on Medical History, College of Physicians of Philadelphia, Dec. 10, 1934. Published, with modifications and 8 illustrations, as "Depressed Fracture and Trephining of Skull by Incas of Peru," *Ann. Med. Hist.*, v. 7: 550-58 (1935). — Presented by the author.   *[10d/52]*

232.   **David,** anatomist. Two lectures on dissection, from the labora-tory of Dr. Gregory, performed by Dr. David, August 13, 1761. *London?, 1761.* — With **Gregory, John.** Two lectures on materia medica, Nov. 17 and 22, 1762. *London?, 1762.*

Fragment of [8], 14 pp. 21 cm.; with reproduction in envelope (37 cm). Frag-ile and damaged.   *[n.c.]*

233.   **Davison, Wilburt Cornell,** 1892-1972. The superiority of inoculation with mixed triple vaccine (B. Typhosus, B. Paraty-phosus A, and B. Paratyphosus B) over successive inoculations with the single vaccines, as shown by agglutinin curves in men and rabbits. *Baltimore, 1917.*

[2], 99 ff.; unnumb. tables, charts. 27 cm (in envelope). Typescript (carbon), copyedited. Alvarenga Prize Essay no. 19, 1917. With reprint of published paper from *Arch. of Int. Med.*, v. 21: 437-509 (1918).   *[10d/31]*

234.   **Davison, Willis T.,** 1858-1928. Separation of the lower epiph-ysis of the femur. *Philadelphia, 1881-82.*

15, [1] ff. 29 cm. Inaugural dissertation "entered with specimen for prize number 4," Jefferson Medical College.   *[Z 10/129]*

235.   **Deatherage, George E.** Letters to Frederick L. Hoffman and Willy Meyer, on the causes of cancer. *South Charleston, W. Va., 1931.*

25 ff. (together 9 letters) in envelope (30 cm). Carbon copies. Interspersed between the 5 letters to Hoffman and 3 to Meyer by Deatherage, is one letter from Dr. Stafford L. Warren to Hoffman.   *[10a/440]*

— — — — —. See also no. 952.

236.   **Deaver, John Blair,** 1855-1931. Gastric and duodenal ulcer. *Peoria, Ill.?, 1922.*

30 ff. 28 cm. Typescript. Read before Tri-State District Medical Association, October 30th, 1922.   *[10b/58]*

237.   — — — — —. Progress of medical science during the 19th century. *Philadelphia?, ca. 1910?*

15 ff. 20.5 cm. Address, without indication of audience, place or date. Beginning on f. 9 a lengthy characterization of "my friend Dr. Ziegler" (Jacob Lindemuth Z., 1822-1906?). *[10c/85]*

238. **[— — — — —].** Forty-seven letters to J.B. Deaver. *V.p., 1886-1926.*

1 envelope. 37.5 cm. Among the letters are note from President Coolidge (thanking for care of his son), 2 letters by S.W. Mitchell, 6 by J.B. Murphy and 3 by M.H. Richardson. Typed list of correspondents enclosed. — Added 1 letter by J.B. Deaver to Dr. Anthony Ambrose. *[n.c.]*

239. **Deaver, Joshua Montgomery,** 1901-78. Acute and chronic appendicitis. *Philadelphia, ca. 1951?*

[1], 12 ff. 31.5 cm (in envelope). May be identical with the 1951 Annual Oration of the Philadelphia Academy of Surgery by Dr. Deaver on the same subject. Unpublished. *[n.c.]*

240. **— — — — —.** Examination in surgery, University of Pennsylvania, Medical School. *Philadelphia, ca. 1927-28.*

[1], 3 ff. 35.5 cm (in envelope). Dr. Deaver received his M.D. in 1928. *[n.c.]*

241. **De Beck, David,** 1857-1929. A monograph on the diseases of the eye due to malaria. *Seattle, 1900.*

353, 35 ff.; 2 plates, 41 illus. 33 cm (in box). Typescript. With extensive bibliography. — Alvarenga Prize Essay no. 9, 1900. *[10d/6]*

242. **De Benneville, George,** 1703-93. Medicina Pensylvania; Or The Pensylvania physician, containing I. The theory and practice of pharmacy. II. A distribution of medicinal simples, according to their virtues and sensible qualities, the description, use, and dose of each article. III. Directions for extemporaneous prescription, with a select number of elegant forms, with the astralis, and other diseases in general. IV. With a instruction, how to judge the diseases by the urine, and the knowledge of the pulse beating, for the use of mankind. By a French author, G. De B., Senior. *Philadelphia, etc., ca. 176- — 79, with later additions, to 1841 (lower margin f. 39v).*

[20], 149, [19] ff. (=188 ff., incl. a few blank ff.). 23.5 cm. Spelling reproduced as found in the manuscript. Title-page and most of the text in English and German, on opposite pages. Contents (from caption headings): Ad lectorem benevolum (German text, prel. ff. 3r-7r). — Matteria medicament-[or]um, oder die zu der Medecin gehörige[n] Simplicia (prel. ff. 8r-20r, incl. trilingual vocabulary of "simplicia" (Latin, German, English, ff. 10v-19r). — Preparationes simpliciores; simple preparations; einfache Zubereytungen (ff. 1-65). — Table of diseases . . . with the principal remedies . . . (followed by German title on facing p., ff. 66-117). — Appendix or guide for womans and

childrens diseases . . . and the principal remedies (with German title, ff. 122-36). — Instruction how to judge the diseases of the urine and the knowledge of the beating of the pulse (with German title, ff. 137-47). — Remedies . . . (incl. prescriptions of Rush [f. 148r], Louis Martinet [f. 7r at end] and George Parkman [f. 15r, *ibid.*]); description of epidemics of 1821-23 (ff. 149r-1r); horse medicines (ff. 3v-4r) and Observations on the medical treatment of General Washington in his last illness, addressed to his physicians Messrs. Craik & Dick, by John Brickell, Savannah, 23 Jan. 1800 (ff. 12v-13v). Inscribed "George De Benneville student in physic" (ff. 54r, 60r, 67r), "George De Benneville junior student in physic February 13 1779" (f. 76r), "Harriett de B. Keim January 13. 1841. from her Father" [i.e. the younger G. De B.] (flyleaf and similar but faint, on cover). — Photocopy of paper by Douglas Macfarlan, with information on the watermarks of Sauer (Sower) and Rittenhouse in this ms., filed with the volume, together with early newspaper clippings and notes (in the hand of the younger G. De B.).   See also A.D. Bell, *The Life and Times of Dr. George de Benneville* (Boston, 1953). — Gift of Leonard S. Myers.   *[Z 10/44]*

—————. See also no. 620.

243.   **Delaware Township, Northhampton County, Pennsylvania.** Document of certification for Abraham Howell, "practitioner in the art and theory as a skillful physician," 1787, 1794, here in a copy dated 20 November 1811, witnessed by Ezekiel Schoonover, justice of the peace, and on the recto by the Board of Health of Philadelphia, dated 18 October 1811; sworn and subscribed by Joseph Hemphill, with seal, and countersigned John Allison. With 17 testimonials of patients, 1802-11, purporting to have been cured from various ailments (sores and rheumatism) by Howell. *Philadelphia, 1811.*

1 sheet; vellum. 86 x 71 cm.   *[Z 10/190]*

244.   **Dermatological Research Laboratories, Inc., Philadelphia.** Documents, reports, correspondence, etc. (incl. mimeographed and printed material) on the manufacture, testing and distribution of salvarsan and salvarsan-related (arsphenamine and neoarsphenamine) products. *V.p., 1915-53.*

3 boxes. 31 cm. Contents: Box 1. Involves primarily J.F. Schamberg (Dermatological Research Laboratories), G.W. McCoy (Public Health Service), J.O. Stieglitz (Univ. of Chicago), U.S. Congress (abrogation of German patent) and the Scientific Chemical Co., N.Y. (Herradora's arsenic, mercury and iodine compounds), 1915-22. — Box 2. H.A. Metz (Farbwerke-Hoechst Co.) and J.F. Schamberg before the Committee on Judiciary of the U.S. Senate on alleged dye monopoly (1922); the same and legal counsel I.L. Bamberger on supply and manufacture of salvarsan, etc. (1915-18, and 1916-22). — Box 3. Dermatological Research Institute (successor to the Laboratories) and the Abbott Laboratories, Trustees and Finance Committee minutes (1917-40); Research Institute of Cutaneous Medicine (history, board membership, extensive list of publications [456 items]), Trustees and Finance Committee minutes (1938-

49); J.A. Kolmer and the Institute of Public Health and Preventive Medicine at Temple University (1950-53), incl. copy of 1923 paper on mechanism of non-specific protein.   *[ZZ 10c/26]*

De Schweinitz, George Edmund, *see* **Schweinitz, George Edmund de.**

245. **De Wecker, Louis,** 1832-1906.   Iridotomy . . . translated by S.L. Ziegler.   *Philadelphia, 1890.*

[1], 27, 68 ff.   20 cm.   Contains besides the translation of pp. 392-97 of L. De Wecker's and E. Landolf 's *Traité complet d'ophthalmologie* (v. 2, Paris, 1886) the section iridotomy (pp. 383 ff.) of X. Galezowski's *Maladies des yeux* (Paris, 1888) and L. De Wecker's *De l'iridotomie* from *Annales d'oculistique,* v. 70 (= ser. 10, v. 10): 123 ff. (Paris, 1873). — Gift of the translator.   *[10b/38]*

246. **Dickens, Paul Frederick,** b. 1885.   Benign lymphocytic chorio-meningitis, a new disease entity (acute aseptic meningitis) by Paul F. Dickens . . . and Charles Armstrong.   *N.p., ca. 1934-35.*

11 ff.   26 cm.   Typescript (carbon copy).   Published in *U.S. Naval Med. Bull.* v. 33: 427-34 (1935).   *[10d/140]*

247. **Diem, Oscar,** b. 1875.   Notes and remarks on Professor Ernest Fuchs' lectures on histology and pathology of the eye, by Oscar Diem and Henry J. Minsky.   Revised by Prof. Fuchs.   *New York, 1921.*

66 ff.   27 cm.   Mimeographed.   *[10d/39]*

248. **Dinwoodie, William,** 1854?-1938.   Report of surgical clinic of Dr. R.J. Levis at the Pennsylvania Hospital from Wednesday Oct. 18th 1876 to Wednesday Jan. 31st, 1877 inclusive . . . .   *Philadelphia, 1876-77.*

135 pp.   21 cm.   Inscribed on cover "For Dr. Levis' Prize."   *[10b/7]*

249. **Doane, Joseph Chapman,** 1884-1973.   Scrapbooks, chiefly on Philadelphia General Hospital.   *Philadelphia, ca. 1919-29.*

2 v., 3 envelopes in box.   26.5 cm.   Photographs, clippings, and correspondence.   Detailed table of contents laid in. — Gift of Jesse F. McClendon.   *[Z 10c/36]*

250. **Dock, George,** 1823-75.   Records of events from the commencement of my medical studies in Philadelphia, Oct. 10th, 1840 . . . . With a record of the principal surgical cases & operations that I have had during my professional life, up to the date of July 1856.   *Philadelphia, 1840-56.*

1 v.   19 cm.   Some of W.E. Horner's cases are briefly described.   Dock served a year as one of the resident physicians at Blockley.   Pasted in at end "List of operations and remarkable cases in the Blockley Hospital during my residence therein from May 1842 until May 1843." – Gift of Wm. L. Holt.   *[10a/344]*

251.   **Dodd, Robert J.,** 1809-76.   Papers.   *V.p., 1826-92.*

1 box.   39 cm.   Contents: Envelope 1.   Personal papers (marriage certificate, certificate of church membership; audit of estate, 1891-92, etc.). – Envelope 2.   Family papers (copies of wills, etc.).   Papers concerning his medical inventions (a patented catheter-bougie, with copy of endorsement by George W. McClellan, Sept. 20, 1843, and a patented cupping apparatus, with copy of endorsement by Geo. C. Shattuck, March 28, 1844). – Env. 3.   Naval orders, 1826-78. – Env. 4.   Business papers *re* railroad investments; also naval miscellany; copy of memorial of W.N.B. Waters, USN, 1852; postmortem examination of C.U. Alden, chaplain, USN; copy of circular (USN, 1850) *re* suspension of corporal punishment; instructions on bezique.   *[Z 10/155]*

Donnelly (F.W.) Memorial Hospital, Trenton, *see* **Trenton Municipal Colony Hospital.**

252.   **Dorland, William Alexander Newman,** 1864-1956.   The evolution of man.   *Chicago?, post 1939.*

18 ff.; 26 charts (illus.; all but one printed).   28-56 cm.   *[ZZ 10c/1]*

253.   – – – – –.   Papers, memorabilia, clippings, reprints, etc.   *V.p., 1886-195–.*

8 v.; illus., photogrs., portrs.   46 cm.   Contains in v. I material illustrating Dr. Dorland's activities in World War I (memorabilia, incl. decorations) and in v. III record of his role in the Medical Reserve; in v. II-V articles on longevity, poem by unnamed student at Medical College, Loyola Univ. (Chicago) on Dorland; among institutions represented (besides Loyola Univ.) are Chicago Medical Society, AMA, Amer. College of Surgeons, Medical School of the Univ. of Pennsylvania, among correspondents D.H. Agnew, Grover Cleveland, H.W. Cushing, J.C. Da Costa, M.W. Ireland, W.W. Keen, Joseph Leidy, C.H. Mayo, S.W. Mitchell, William Osler, F.R. Packard, David Riesman, Theodore Roosevelt, G.E. de Schweinitz, Alfred Stillé (alphabetical index of correspondents inside front cover in v. II-V); v. VI-VIII mainly printed miscellanea and photographs (Univ. of Pennsylvania Med. Class of 1886, Christmas cards, etc.).   *[Z 10/69]*

254.   **Dorrance, George Morris,** 1877-1949.   Congenital insufficiency of the palate.   *Philadelphia, 1929.*

70 typewritten ff., 72 plates, in loose-leaf notebook.   30 cm.   Drawings by Erwin Frank Faber.   Alvarenga Prize Essay, 1929.   Published in *Arch. of Surg.* v. 21: 185-248 (1930).   *[10d/25]*

255. **Dorsey, John Syng,** 1783-1818.   Daybooks. *Philadelphia, 1805-17, 1833.*

    3 v. 19.5-39.5 cm. Volume 1 contains notes, partly in shorthand, on cases of women patients, evidently intended for eventual publication; a note on receipt of militia fines Dec. 2, 1805; and a list of receipts from patients, Jan. 1805-Jan. 1806. — V. 2 contains at end some notes by the executor (not named) of the estate of E. Dorsey, in 1833; some unused sketches, etc., for JSD's bookplate, with a landscape sketch. — V. 3 contains a list of JSD's private pupils and their fees; and a collection of surgical case reports (44 pp.). — Gift of Mrs. B. G. du Pont.   *[Z 10/60]*

256. —————. Fee book. *Philadelphia, 1805-17.*

    [42] pp. 38.5 cm. Summarizes Dorsey's total annual income from practice, without listing fees for individual visits or services; JSD's biographical notice in Kelly & Burrage cites some of these figures. — Gift of Mrs. B.G. Du Pont.   *[Z 10/62]*

257. —————. Lectures on materia medica. *Philadelphia?, ca. 1816.*

    2 v. 20 cm. Inscribed on flyleaf of v. 2: "Presented to Isaac Hays by his friend Dr. G.B. Wood." — Gift of I. Minis Hays.   *[10a/40]*

258. —————. Ledger. *Philadelphia, 1804-18.*

    2 v. 39 cm. Entries show both services and fees. — Gift of Mrs. B.G. Du Pont.   *[Z 10/63]*

259. —————. Notes from cases of surgery which have occurr'd in the practice of Dr. P.S. Physick. *Philadelphia, 1798-1811.*

    2 v. 31 cm. Sketches, drawings and watercolors of cases occur throughout both volumes. Vol. 2 (1801-11) contains some case reports revised from v. 1; also (pp. 105 ff.) a draft of Dorsey's famous ligation of the external iliac artery (G.-M. no. 2930), with a different drawing from that in the report published in *Eclectic Repertory*, v. 2: 111-15 (1811). — Gift of Mrs. B.G. Du Pont.   *[Z 10/65]*

260. —————. Notes on lectures on materia medica, taken by Thomas Shivers. *Philadelphia, 1817.*

    2 v. ([5], 119, [3 blank] ff., pp. 128-270 [misnumbered]; 255 ff.). 20.5 cm. Title on spines: Dorsey's Notes, with date 1817. Labels of student "T. Shivers" on front covers; Shivers received his M.D. at the University of Pennsylvania in 1820. Volume 2 contains partial or summary notes on Nathaniel Chapman's lectures on the practice of medicine. — Gift of Mrs. H.L. Huston.   *[n.c.]*

261. —————. Notes on the lectures of John Syng Dorsey . . . by John Y. Clark. *Philadelphia, 1816-17.*

    131, 250, 11 ff. 26 cm. Gift of Alfred Stengel.   *[10a/306]*

262.   — — — — —. Notes on the lectures of John Syng Dorsey. *Philadel-phia, 1817.*

[64] pp. 19 cm. Inscribed inside front cover: R.P. Richardson, Philadelphia. On cover: "Notes on Dorsey, Volume I." Inside, below caption title: "Vol. II[?] Nov. 7th 1817. 2nd lecture." Continued through 8th lecture (undated). — Gift of Montgomery Harris.   *[10a/198]*

— — — — —. See also nos. 52, 114, 255, 329, 817, 821, 928.

263.   **Dover, Levi.** Levi Dover's book of remedies of vegetable origin. *Philadelphia?, 19th cent.*

1 v. 16 cm. Label on cover: "Levi Dover's Book"; printed at bottom, "Sold by Benjamin Johnson, no. 249, Market Street," Philadelphia. Remedies are grouped according to their purpose, e.g., "Remedies to stay bleeding"; "Remedies for the head and brain." Each entry followed by a number (page reference to another work?).   *[10a/343]*

264.   **Drayton, Joseph,** illus. Nine numbered and two unnumbered colored drawings of sections of stomach or intestines. *Philadel-phia, 1827.*

9 plates. 17-21 cm. Prepared for William E. Horner in connection with Horner's "On the Anatomical Characters of Asiatic Cholera, with Remarks on the Structure of the Mucous Coat of the Alimentary Canal," published in *American Journal of Med. Sciences,* v. 16: 58-81 (1835).   *[10c/148]*

265.   **Duhring, Louis Adolphus,** 1845-1913. Notes on the lectures on dermatology delivered to the medical class of the University of Pennsylvania. *Philadelphia, 1892-93.*

1 v. 21 cm. Notes taken by John M. Swan; dated 7 Oct. 1892 - 17 Dec. 1892 (47 pp.) and notes on lectures on genito-urinary diseases by Edward Martin, 6 Jan. - 24 Feb. 1893 (23 pp.).   *[10a/329]*

266.   **Dulles, Charles Winslow,** 1850-1921. Fractures of cranium. *Philadelphia, ca. 1880-84, 1894.*

Slips mounted on 44 pp. and inserts; illus. 17 cm. Except for an insert dated 1894 probably notes in preparation of the "Historical Study," part of his "The Mechanism of Indirect Fractures of the Skull," *Trans. & Stud.,* ser. 3, v. 8: 273-96 (1886) and separately under the same title. — Gift of the author.   *[10b/33]*

267.   — — — — —. Hydrophobia notes, book A. *Philadelphia, 1882.*

60, [10] ff. 22 cm. Pencilled notes from various publications and history of hydrophobia (in ink, final leaves), preliminary to his published articles on the topic. — Fragile.   *[10a/489]*

268.   **Duncan, Andrew,** 1744-1828.   Extracts of lectures. *Edinburgh, 1793-94?*

> 178 pp. 19 cm. Signatures on title page of John Brown and James McHenry. Notes taken by McHenry? Main divisions "Fluids" (1-154) and "Solids" (156-74). — Bookplate of George McHenry.   *[10a/346]*

269.   — — — — —.   Institutions of medicine ... delivered in 1799 & 1800 (title page and contents only). — Lectures on animal heat and respiration *(Edinburgh?, 1802 or later* [cf. f. 34], ff. 19-29, 33-40*)*. — Lectures on therapeutics... *(Edinburgh, 1800,* vol. 1; f. 41, pp. 1-31, followed by quote in French on p. [33]*)*. — **Physick, Philip Syng,** 1768-1837. Notes on lectures entitled Inflammation *(Philadelphia, 180-;* 135 ff.*)*.

> [8] ff. (3-8 blank), ff. 19-29, 3 blank ff., [ff. 33-41], 33 pp., [140] ff., (136-40 blank). 21 cm. Title page poorly repaired, measures 18 cm., the table of contents with initials *"MS"* in upper left corner 19.8 cm; they belong to a lecture not included in this composite volume. The lectures on animal heat and respiration have the headings "Is respiration essential to the evolution of animal heat" (f. 19v) and "On the respiration of oxymunale (?, i.e. oxygenote?) acid gas" (f. 33r). — The notes on lectures by Dr. Physick contain references to many medical authorities, among them John Hunter, Anton de Haen, Richard Mead, Pierre Joseph Desault, Alexis Boyer, Caspar Wistar, Percival Pott, and Benjamin Rush.   *[10a/41]*

   — — — — —.   See also no. 111.

270.   **Dunglison, Robley,** 1798-1869.   Autobiographical ana. *Philadelphia, ca. 1852-55.*

> 8 v., 4 env., in 2 boxes; portr., etching. 26 cm. Autograph. Volume 1 begins with table of contents to all 8 volumes. The numbering of pages and leaves of this volume is highly irregular, omitting pp. 42-99 and 106-136, but it seems complete. His "earliest letters" (p. 109 in table of contents) are found in envelope 1, and some unnumbered ff. belonging to the "ana" are in envelope 4. An alphabetical index is at end of v. 7. Includes a large number of letters, e.g. some by W.C. Rives, S.A. Allibone, J.K. Kane, J.P. Kennedy, etc. Considerable extracts appear in S.X. Radbill, "The Autobiographical Ana of Robley Dunglison," *Trans. of the Amer. Philos. Soc.*, n.s., v. 53, part 8 (1963). — Volume 1 gift of Charles Perry Fisher, others of Mrs. Violette Fisher Dunglison.
>
>   *[10c/14]*

271.   — — — — —.   Correspondence (largely letters addressed to Dr. Dunglison), items relating to the Society of Apothecaries, London, etc. *V.p., 1830-69.*

> 1 env. (3 folders). 37.5 cm. Contents: Folder 1. Letters to Dunglison, among them Bowen, and Gray and Bowen, London publishers; Sir Henry Holland about his *Medical Notes*, his election to the American Philosophical Society and a letter with information on Michael Faraday; Charles Folsom on editorial matters concerning the printing of Dunglison's *Dictionary of Medical*

Science; John Forbes on the *Cyclopaedia of Practical Medicine*; Joseph Pancoast, statement "Examination of thorax"; Rev. William Taylor on Dunglison's concern with the blind; G.S. Pattison on various appointments. – 2. Miscellaneous items, incl. 7 letters of R. Dunglison, 1840-66, with lengthy letter to Mr. Nussey of the Society of Apothecaries; statements of the Board of Jefferson Medical College, accepting with regret the resignation of R.D., and making him professor emeritus (1868); financial statements. – 3. R.D. and the Society of Apothecaries, London.   *[n.c.]*

272.   – – – – –. Introductory lecture, session 1853-4 (crossed out, begins: Although Gentlemen, the subject of the human biology . . .). *Philadelphia, 1853-54.*

ff. [3]-30, [12] ff. 20 cm (in envelope). Autograph, corrections throughout. Pencilled on upper left margin: "Oct. 11, 1858," possibly the date of subsequent use of the text at Jefferson Medical College.   *[n.c.]*

273.   – – – – –. Introductory lecture to the course of institutes of medicine, etc., delivered (at Jefferson Medical College) 13th of October 1856. *Philadelphia, 1856.*

57 ff. (last 2 loose). 20 cm (in envelope). Autograph with corrections throughout. Presumably covering more than one lecture. Deals primarily with historical development and with qualifications.   *[n.c.]*

274.   – – – – –. Introductory observations to medical jurisprudence. *Philadelphia, 1832.*

Cover, [8] ff. (f. [7] blank), 1 f. inserted. 21 cm (in envelope). Autograph, corrections throughout 7 ff. Unquestionably an introductory lecture.   *[n.c.]*

– – – – –. See also nos. 42, 338, 386, 427, 507, 980.

275.   – – – – –, **and Richard James Dunglison,** 1834-1901, comp. Diplomas, certificates of appointments, citizenship document, lecture invitations, etc. of Robley Dunglison . . . compiled by Dr. Richard J. Dunglison. *V.p., 1816-62.*

92 ff. (ff. 66, 68, 74-92 blank). 39 × 52 cm (oblong). Handwritten, printed and engraved. Record of regular, corresponding and honorary memberships (see S.X Radbill, "The Autobiographical Ana of Robley Dunglison," *Trans. of the Amer. Philos. Soc.* n.s., v. 53, pt. 8 [1963], "List of institutions to which he belonged," pp. 194-96); appointment to positions (Royal College of Physicians, London, Univ. of Virginia, Univ. of Maryland, Jefferson Medical College, etc.); degrees (Edinburgh, Erlangen, Yale Univ., LLD Jefferson Medical College); record of activities on behalf of medical, scientific, religious, social, and public organizations. With signatures of many well-known persons, incl. Thomas Jefferson (f. 17). 2 items on f. 51, now blank, removed. Some items on vellum, several have seals. – Gift of R.J. Dunglison.   *[Z 10/29]*

276. **Dunton, William Rush,** 1831-1911.   List of patients.   *Philadelphia, 1859-69.*

> 1 v.   29 cm.   Case records, 1859-69, and List of prescriptions given to patients from the Union Benevolent, 1859-60.   *[Z 10/149]*

277. **Duvernoy, Georges Louis,** 1777-1855.   Mémoire sur l'hymen, ou l'on démontre, que la membrane, qui porte ce nom, chez la femme, existe dans plusieurs mammifères, lu à l'Institut national [= Institut de France?] le 3 thermidor an XIII.   *Paris, 1805.*

> 20 pp.   24 cm.   Autograph, signed, with corrections.   Bound with printed "Extrait d'un mémoire sur l'hymen" (pp. 186-91) of *Bulletin de l'Ecole et de la Société de Médicine de Paris* (v. 1, 1812).   At head of title: ...A imprimer Savant étranger.   Rapport du 8 fructidor an 13. — Adopté pour le 2ᵉ vol. du Savant étranger. — Prov.: J. Stockton Hough Library.   *[10a/161]*

278. **Eagle, Harry,** b. 1905.   The present status of the blood coagulation problem.   *Philadelphia, 1936.*

> [2], 62, 11 ff.; plates.   29 cm.   Typescript.   Includes 11 ff. bibliography.   Alvarenga Prize Essay no. 32, 1936.   *[10d/131]*

279. **Edgar, John Marion,** b. 1858.   Record of the anomalies found in the dissecting rooms of the University of Pennsylvania.   *Philadelphia, 1878-79.*

> 1 v.; drawings, part col.   25 cm.   Offered in competition for a student prize awarded by Hugh Lenox Hodge, who presented this ms.   *[10a/54]*

280. **Edwards, William Aloysius,** 1860-1933.   The ovarian cell, is it pathognomonic.   *Philadelphia, 1880?*

> [35] ff.; 3 plates.   26 cm.   Brief historical overview of ovariotomies; clinical reports dated May 1880.   Published in *Amer. Jour. Med. Sci.*, n.s., v. 83: 428-33 (1882). — Author's unsigned presentation inscription to W.F. Atlee, who presented volume to Lewis Library.   *[10a/305]*

281. **Eggers, Harold Everett,** 1882-1966.   Bibliography: the etiology of cancer.   *Omaha, Neb., 1931-32.*

> 234 ff.   30.5 cm.   Bibliography used by Eggers in preparing his review "The Etiology of Cancer" pub. without bibliography in *Archives of Pathology*, v. 12-13 (1931-32).   Typewritten copy, one of eight deposited in U.S. libraries. — Presented by Harold L. Stewart, National Cancer Institute.   *[ZZ 10c/20]*

282. **Eklund, Abraham Fredrik,** 1839-1898.   Three abstracts, in French.   *Stockholm, 1888-89.*

> 3 ff.   21-22 cm.   Autograph.   On writings of C.F. Rossander (sickness of Friedrick III, German emperor), L. Wolff (trachea) and B. Howard (artificial respiration).   *[10a/412]*

283. **Elmer, Jonathan,** 1745-1817. Adversaria medica, or common-place book, containing extracts, remarks, and observations on all the several branches of physic under their proper heads, viz, anatomy, materia medica, chemistry, physiology, pathology [and] nosology. *Philadelphia and New Jersey, ca. 1768-87.*

1 v. 20.5 cm. Inscription on front fly-leaf "Ex Libris Jonathni Elmer."
[10a/392]

284. — — — — —. A compleat system of the materia medica methodi-cally arranged according to the indications they serve to answer. Vol. 1: Containing necessary preliminaries — order and division of the work — history of the first class, the *nutrientia* or the dietetic part of the materia medica. *Philadelphia, ca. 1775.*

V. 1 only (275 ff.). 25.2 cm. Inscription on front fly-leaf "Ex Libris, J. Elmer", "Ipsomet manu scripsit." *[10a/393]*

285. — — — — —. Praxis medica, extracted chiefly from the writings of the most eminent practicioners in Europe, interspersed with the practice of the principal physicians in the city of Philadelphia, particularly of Drs Redman, Bond & Morgan. *Philadelphia, ca. 1775.*

1 v. 19 cm. Contains also "Dissertation on a phthisis pulmonalis, by Doct^r John Morgan, read before the Medical Society at Edinburgh-1762"; brief anonymous lectures, "Of the air", "small pox," "of the dropsy", "of a frozen member", "of poisonous vapors & resuscitation", possibly delivered at the Pennsylvania Hospital by Thomas Bond. — Inscription on front fly-leaf "Ex Libris Jonath. Elmer ejus manu scripsit." *[10a/391]*

— — — — —. See also no. 704.

286. **Elsberg, Louis,** 1836-1885. Pneumatometry as a means of diagnosis in diseases of the respiratory organs. *New York, ca. 1876.*

27 ff. 32 cm. Typescript. Text refers to illustrations (not enclosed). Similar to an apparatus developed by Louis Waldenburg. *[10d/12]*

287. **Emerson, Gouverneur,** 1796-1874. Case histories, notes on medical topics, transcripts of letters, drafts of medical papers, newspaper clippings, etc. *Philadelphia, 1821-27.*

239 pp. 25.5 cm. Author identified by correspondence and references to Phila. Board of Health, on which Emerson served. This material seems not to have been used in any of Emerson's publications. — Gift of Mrs. David A. Cooper. *[10a/446]*

— — — — —. See also nos. 806, 1128.

288. **Emerson, Haven,** 1874-1957. Survey of hospitals and health services of Trenton and Mercer County, N.J. *N.p., 1944.*

    51, [1] ff. 28 cm. Typewritten (carbon copy). Study undertaken at the request of the Trenton Community Chest and Council.   *[ZZ 10d/17]*

289. **Emlen, Samuel,** 1789-1828. Notes on a tour through England, Wales, Ireland, Scotland, etc. Note Book no. 2 . . . . *V.p., 1813-14.*

    1 v. 15 cm. Includes typewritten transcript (9 pp.) of Extracts from the diary of the late Samuel Emlen, with a short memoir by [Charles Delucena] Meigs (London, Harvey and Darton, 1830; 23 pp.); photostat copies of postal receipt (New York, Oct. 9, 1814), and Emlen's letter of same date, to James Monroe, Secretary of State, transmitting the receipt, for six packets of despatches carried by Emlen from the American representatives at Paris and London; correspondence to W.N. Bradley from the National Archives (March, 1945) concerning these copies and the despatches. — Presented by J.T. Emlen through Wm. N. Bradley.   *[10c/52]*

—————. See also no. 804.

290. **Emmerez, Paul,** d. 1690. Copie du mémoire sur lequel Mons[ieu]r Emmerez, médicin de Paris, a donné la consultation. *Paris, 17th cent.*

    2 ff. 24 cm. Patient suffers from "incom[m]odité à la teste [for tête]." Fragile. — Shelved with 18th-cent. French consultation (Judications).   *[10a/312]*

291. **Erwin, Joseph H.,** d. ca. 1823. Notes on sixteen lectures by unnamed teacher. *Philadelphia, 1797?-98.*

    [1] f., 220 pp., [1] f. 20 cm. Signature of student, dated "February 16th Anno Domini 1798" on prel. f. According to information, supplied by the archivist of the Univ. of Pennsylvania, Erwin was not a regular student, but did take a course with Benjamin Rush in 1798. It is likely that the notes record Rush's lecture on the practice of medicine. More than one-half of the manuscript deals with fevers and contagious diseases (bilious fever, yellow fever, the plague, typhus, small pox, hepatitis); further lectures cover hemorrhages, rheumatism, gout, nervous diseases, apoplexy, etc. Rubber stamp "Presented by Dr. R. Nebinger" on first f. (recipient unknown, but not the College of Physicians of Philadelphia).   *[10a/443]*

292. **[Extra-uterine pregnancy].** The diagnosis and treatment of extra-uterine pregnancy; five papers. *V.p., 188—.*

    5 envelopes. 30-37.5 cm. Handwritten and typewritten. All except one without indication of authorship, but identified by motto or term; probably submitted in a competition. Contents: 1, ms. and typewritten copy, with motto "To the victor belong the spoils." — 2, ms. and typewritten, motto "Endlich, endlich kommt einmal." — 3, typewritten, marked "Hungary" and No. 1. — 4, ms., marked "Hungary," name and date at end: Dr. Frigyes Schwarz, Pécs . . . 1888. — 5, carbon copy, title: Extra-uterine gestation, marked "Scotland."   *[Z 10/146]*

293. **Fackenthall, Howard,** d. 1918. Record of anomalies found in the anatomical rooms of the University of Pennsylvania, 1875-76. *Philadelphia, 1876.*

> 1 v. 10 cm. Author's signed letter of transmittal to Hugh Lenox Hodge (2 copies) at end. — Pasted on flyleaf printed notice of the anatomical prizes for which this manuscript was entered.   *[10a/49]*

294. **Fahnestock, Samuel,** fl. 1798. A collection of medicinal preparations . . . together with the virtues and dosis. *Yorktown, Pa., June 22d, 1798[—1819, 1867].*

> 1 v. 21 cm. Inscription on front flyleaf, in another hand, presenting this volume as a wedding gift to Ellen Bowman and "the Bishop of Kansas," Apr. 23, 1867[?], signed Geo. Fahnestock, sen. Inscription on back flyleaf "George Fahnestock. Receipt book, commenced April 8th 1819." Includes formulas for "Dr. Rush's nervous pills," "Dr. Physick's cough mixture". — Gift of F.S.J. Stoddart.   *[10a/202]*

295. **Falconar, Magnus.** A synopsis of a course of lectures on anatomy and surgery. *London, before 1777?*

> 42, [106] pp. (interleaved throughout). 24 cm. Title taken from the printed edition, London 1777 which is textually practically identical with this manuscript, written in a formal hand, probably a copy prepared for one of Falconar's students. Contents: Section 1. On the component parts of an animal body. — 2. On osteology. — 3. On myology. — 4. On angiology.
>   *[10a/294]*

296. **Feldman, Jacob B.,** 1884-1954. Dark adaptation (retinal illumination in photons). *Philadelphia, 1936-39.*

> 3 v. 30 cm. Use of pre-printed forms by Dr. Feldman. Doctors' and hospitals' reports (handwritten and typed) attached, reporting tests, diagnoses, treatment, etc. V. 1 includes typed list of diseases, v. 2 inscription "[William J.] Ezickson's Urologic Clinic," and printed article by Feldman, entitled "An Instrument for Qualitative Study of Dark Adaptation," repr. from *Archives of Ophthalmology* v. 18: 821-26 (1937).   *[10a/496]*

297. **Fernández Cruzado, José.** Memoir; theories practical on the endemick yellow fever on the island of Cuba. *Cuba?, ca. 1840?*

> 8 ff. 26 cm. Anonymous translation of *Memoria teórico-práctica sobre la fiebre amarilla endémica en la isla de Cuba.*   *[Z 10/108]*

298. **Ferrein, Antoine,** 1693-1769. Matière medicale (interne...). *Paris, 1763.*

> 1 v. 18 cm. "Préliminaire" entitled "Extrait des leçons de Mʳ Ferein [spelling in the ms.] sur la matière medicale;" this part badly trimmed. Inscribed at end of volume "Fin du 1ᵉʳ volume ce 15 de juillet[!] 1763 Gaynor scripsit." — "Wm Darrach from P. Russell Cruise [or Cruice], July 23. 1829," at beginning of volume. Gift of J. Darrach.   *[10a/187]*

99. **Fetterolf, George,** 1869-1932. The anatomy of the pressure factor in the etiology of cardiac hydrothorax. George Fetterolf... and H.R.M. Landis . . . . *Philadelphia, 1909.*

[1], 18 ff. 28 cm. Typescript (carbon copy) with ms. corrections. Read before the Philadelphia Pathological Society, May 27, 1909. *[n.c.]*

Fidelity Mutual Aid Association, *see* **Alta Friendly Society.**

00. **Finch, Heneage,** Earl of Nottingham, 1621-1682(?). Commonplace book. *England, ca. 1647.*

589 pp., [4] ff. 28 cm. The volume begins with alphabetically arranged, largely classical, quotations (pp. 9-394), followed by irregularly arranged entries (pp. 395-413; in Latin); notes on Bible passages; classical authors, etc. (pp. 465-70; Latin and English); entry on moneys received Dec. 20, 1647 (p. 548). Of medical interest are recipes (pp. 581-87), those on pp. 582-83 signed Harvey and those on pp. 584 and 587 Mearne. A list of authors and entries to the first part concludes the volume. — A large number of pages are blank. Pages 1-8 include 6 pp. of modern genealogical notes; pp. 585-86 are missing. Page 1 contains a testimonial by W.J. Harvey (ca. 1900), claiming that the Harvey who signed the recipes (pp. 582-83) is identical with William Harvey (various letters dealing with the authenticity are on file). It has been questioned whether the early compiler and owner of the commonplace book was Heneage Finch; his arms with explanatory text (printed) are pasted in at the beginning of the volume. — Bookplate Almack and ownership entry Richard Almack inside front cover. Gift of S. Weir Mitchell. *[10c/18]*

01. **Finlay, Carlos Juan,** 1833-1915. Summary of the work . . . done since 1881 with regard to the transmission of yellow-fever through the culex mosquito. *Havana?, 1902?*

3 ff. 27.5 cm. Typewritten. Bound with several of the author's printed articles on yellow fever. *[10a/510]*

————. See also no. 679.

02. **Fisher, Henry Middleton,** 1851-1939. Notes on microscopic technology, taken in Vienna during the winter of 1879-80. *Vienna, 1879-80.*

100 pp. 22 cm. German text, in various hands. Techniques used in making histological observations. — Gift of the estate of H.M. Fisher. *[10a/229]*

————. See also nos. 1063, 1091.

03. **[Flick, Lawrence Francis,** 1856-1938]. Letters and documents received by Lawrence F. Flick, bound in 54 volumes, and one undated volume, labeled "Tuberculosis Letters." *V.p., 1888-1908.*

55 v. 28 cm. *[10a/368]*

— — — — —. See also nos. 207, 1063.

304.   **[Food Inspection].** Inspection of the food of the soldiers (52nd Pennsylvania Volunteers, 2nd Brigade). *Morris Island, South Carolina, 1864.*

>1 f. 25 cm. Inspectors: Surgeon John B. Crawford, Lieut. William V. Hollingworth.   *[10c/150]*

305.   **Formulas for medicines,** various household preparations, paints, etc. *Barnsley (Engl.), 1836-1859.*

>1 v. 19 cm. Bound in vellum pocket-book with metal clasp. F. 1 removed. Inscription on p. 1, "J. White, Barnsley, July 17th, 1836." Entry near end dated 2 Aug. 1859. Barnsley and Holbeck (towards end) are in the West Riding. Some mixtures identified by source. — Gift of Francis X. Dercum.
>   *[10a/216]*

306.   **Fothergill, Anthony,** 1732?-1813. Copy of the will of the late Dr. Anthony Fothergill. *London, 1817?*

>[1] f., 12 pp., [2] ff. 33 cm. Manuscript copy prepared for Arthur Croxton. Newspaper clipping inserted. — Presented by Sir William Osler.   *[Z 10/50]*

307.   — — — — —. Meteorological observations on the climate of Philadelphia, with remarks on the population, longevity, predominant diseases. *Philadelphia, 1806-10.*

>Envelope (addressed to Sir Joseph Banks, London), title, 5 ff. 32-40.5 cm. Partly autograph.   *[Z 10/127]*

308.   **Fothergill, John,** 1712-1780. Recipes. *London?, 1768.*

>1 p. 23 cm. Gift of E.B. Krumbhaar.   *[10a/354]*

309.   **Foulkrod, John K.** A collection of 90 anomalies . . . presented to Dr. H. Lenox Hodge, demonstrator of anatomy. *Philadelphia, 1878.*

>[61] ff.; illus. (part col.), 1 col. plate. 21.5 cm. Offered in competition for a student prize at the Univ. of Pennsylvania, Department of Medicine, offered by Hodge.   *[10a/56]*

310.   **Fox, George Howard,** 1873-1954. Lecture notes on dermatology. *New York, ca. 192—.*

>118 ff. 29 cm. Typewritten (carbon copy). Inside front cover printed obituary of Fox from *JAMA*; letter from former owner and donor, Samuel D. Allison.   *[10a/473]*

311. **Fox, Herbert,** 1880-1942. James Darrach, 1828-1923, a memoir. *Philadelphia, 1923.*

xii ff. 28 cm. Typewritten. Published in *Proceedings of the Pathological Society of Philadelphia,* v. 44: 60-67 (1924).   *[10c/113]*

312. —————. Samuel Stryker Kneass, a memoir. *Philadelphia, 1929.*

6 ff. 28 cm. Typewritten.   *[10c/114]*

313. **Fox, Lawrence Webster,** 1853-1931. Notes on ophthalmology lectures, etc. *Vienna, 1879.*

1 v.; illus. 17 cm (in envelope). Lectures, primarily by Ludwig Mauthner, but also by Ernst Fuchs, Moritz Kaposi, etc., and notes (of lecture?) on "Symmetrie und Analogie des Körpers" and "Die Asymmetrie des Gesichts bei menschlichen Embryonen," written by Fox, without name of lecturer or author. — Incl. attendance cards.   *[10a/474]*

314. [—————]. Reviews and acknowledgements of his *Diseases of the Eye* (1904) and *A Practical Treatise on Ophthalmology* (1910). *V.p., 1904-12.*

1 v. 38 cm. Clippings, typed and handwritten letters.   *[10c/145]*

—————. See also no. 1137.

315. **Frazier, Charles Harrison,** 1870-1936. Fifty years of neurosurgery (fiftieth anniversary of the Philadelphia Neurological Society), January 25, 1935. *Philadelphia, 1935.*

41 ff. 28.5 cm. Published in *Proceedings of the Philadelphia Neurological Society* and *Archives of Neurology and Psychiatry,* v. 34: 907-22 (1935). — Presented by the author.   *[10b/55]*

316. **French, Douglas George.** Observations on the hypochromic anaemia of pregnancy. *Durham (Engl.), 1949.*

1 v.; tables. 26.5 cm. Typewritten (carbon). M.D. thesis, Univ. of Durham. — Gift of Smith, Kline & French.   *[4H Durham 1949]*

317. **[Friedrich III, German emperor].** Magazine, journal and newspaper clippings on the throat condition of the then crown prince (soon to be crowned German emperor) Friedrich III. *V.p., 1887.*

4 notebooks. 28 cm. Articles in English, German and French, many signed. Among authors are Theodor Billroth, Eugen Hamilton Hahn, Sir Morell Mackenzie, Rudolf Virchow and Heinrich Gottfried Waldeyer.   *[n.c.]*

—————. See also nos. 282, 395.

318. **Fries, John William,** 1846-1927. Disease — a neglected factor in history. *N.p., 1914.*

11 ff. 28 cm. Typewritten (carbon copy).   *[10d/75]*

319. **Fritchey, John Augustus,** 1858-1916. Record of anomalies found in the anatomical rooms of the University of Pennsylvania. *Philadelphia, 1879.*

1 v.; illus. 15 cm. Offered in competition for a student prize awarded by Hugh Lenox Hodge, who presented this ms.   *[10a/50]*

320. **Fritze, Hermann Eduard,** 1811-1866. Miniatur-Abbildungen der wichtigsten akiurgischen[!] Operationen, mit erklärendem Text, nach Dr. H.E. Fritze. *Germany, 1845-46.*

3 prel. ff., 76 pp., 3 blank ff., 30 printed tables, colored by hand. 17 cm. Title-page signed Hofmann. Not identical with the author's printed editions.
[n.c.]

321. **Fry, George S.** Memorandum book. *Philadelphia, 1820-49.*

48 ff. (f. 2 badly torn). 16 cm. "Doctor James's lecture on midwifery," 1821, occupies ff. 1-16, followed by "Doctor Fry's treatment on the placenta," 1822, ff. 17, and recipes in Fry's hand (incl. a prescription by Dr. Parrish, 1832) and that of others (one on ff. 38-39 in German).   *[10a/465]*

322. **Furness, Horace Howard,** 1833-1912. Address before the College of Physicians on the presentation of a loving-cup. *Philadelphia, 14 April, 1886.*

[6] ff. 26 cm. "Presented in anticipation of . . . [College of Physicians of Philadelphia] centennial."   *[Z 10/224]*

————. See also nos. *185.2110*, 346.

323. **Galen,** 130-ca. 200 A.D. De crisibus libri tres, in the translation of Gerardus Cremonensis. *Italy, late 13th or early 14th cent.*

31 ff. (in the last quire the 8th f., presumably blank, missing); vellum; decorated initial *E* on f. 1r. 24 cm.   *[10a/233]*

324. ————. Galen's Method of physick; or, his great master peece being the very marrow and quintessence of all his writings .... (Transcript of the translation by Peter English of the De methodo medendi ad Glauconem, printed in Edinburgh in 1656). *Philadelphia, 1915.*

[2], 256 ff. 24 cm. Typewritten. Prepared for Joseph Walsh. "Much abridged," pencilled note on t.-p. With few notes by J. Walsh; his gift.   *[10d/22]*

325.   — — — — —. The third book of Galen, called in Greek [!] Methodus medendi. *Philadelphia?, ca. 1915.*

> 280 pp.   27.5 cm.   Typewritten transcript of the London 1586 edition, translated into English by Thomas Gale (?).   Some corrections and notes by Dr. Joseph P. Walsh.   *[Z 10/200]*

— — — — —. See also nos. 451, 958, 1063.

326.   **Gartrell, Ellen May Gruenberg,** b. 1951.   Medical societies of Philadelphia, 1865-1918; an introduction and bibliography. *Philadelphia, 1979.*

> 23 ff.   28 cm.   Typescript (photocopy).   Term paper, Univ. of Pennsylvania, 1979.   *[P-K 10d/157]*

— — — — —. See also no. *185.62.*

327.   **Gassaway, James Morsell,** 1848-1939.   Patient record cards. *Philadelphia, 1881.*

> 41 cards.   Printed cards, filled in by Gassaway, listing personal data about patients, disease, and dates of admission and discharge, at the U.S. Marine Hospital Service, Philadelphia.   *[n.c.]*

328.   **Gellhorn, Ernst,** b. 1893.   The influence of parathormone on the neuromuscular system; an experimental analysis. *Chicago, 1934.*

> 22, [10] ff.; 9 plates.   30 cm.   Typescript.   Letter from Dr. Gellhorn to William R. Nicholson enclosed.   Awarded the Alvarenga Prize, 1934; published in *American Journal of Physiology,* v. 111: 466-76 (1935). — Presented by the author.   *[10d/43]*

329.   **George, Silas.**   Notes on lectures at the Department of Medicine of the University of Pennsylvania. *Philadelphia, Nov. 1817-Feb. 1818.*

> 2 v.   20 cm.   Contents: Dr. Dorsey's lectures on materia medica, v. 1, pp. 21-84, v. 2, pp. 5-92. — Dr. Physick's lectures on surgery, v. 1, pp. 67-104, v. 2, pp. 47-92. — Dr. Chapman's lectures on the institutes and practice of medicine, v. 1, pp. 131-79, v. 2, pp. 101-75. — Appended to v. 2 "Mineral tonics" by unnamed lecturer or author, pp. 47-57.   Additions to Dorsey and Physick, v. 1, pp. 5-7.   Alphabetical indexes interspersed.   It is likely that one further volume with similar contents had belonged to Silas George, since his bookplate in v. 1 is numbered 13 and in v. 2 No. 15. — Presented by the heirs of Herman B. Allyn.   *[10a/232]*

330.   **Gerhard, William Wood,** 1809-1872.   Announcements of lectures and practice (n.d., and 1844), application to Board of Managers, Pennsylvania Hospital (1837), legal and financial items (1843, 1845) and letters to Gerhard. *V.p., 1834-45.*

1 envelope. 37.5 cm. Partial contents: Legal papers consist of release by E. Merrihen and Lewis Thompson, publishers of the *Medical Examiner* (2 ff.; 1843) and 6 letters settling suit Gerhard versus Dr. J.E. Wendell over money to support a bastard child (all signed R.G. Ellis; 1843). — Letters to Gerhard by A.W. Cenas (subj. charity hospitals; book on auscultation, commentary on G.'s "Cerebral Affection of Children"); James Jackson (transl. of Louis' on pulmonary consumption; peritonitis, etc.); P.C.A. Louis (2 extensive letters); Étienne Rufz de Lavison (trip to Martinique, yellow fever epidemic; Société Médicale d'Observation, Paris; cholera, etc., etc., together 10 letters); G. Robert Smith (compares French and U.S. life); Thomas Stewardson (Louis and his colleagues; 3 letters); a few others, some unidentified. — Several letters torn, fragile.   *[n.c.]*

331. ————. Journal médical. *Paris and Philadelphia, 1833-39.*

1 v. ([1] f., 172 pp., [4] and blank ff.), 1 envelope (20 items, various sizes). 38 cm. Autopsy reports, case histories, few office examinations, some in French. Volume 1 begun March 11, 1833 at the Hôpital des Enfants Malades, Paris, and continued in Philadelphia, primarily at the Pennsylvania Hospital. Further reports and miscellaneous items, incl. "Tubercules — feuille 1re," previously loosely inserted in volume, now filed in envelope.   *[Z 10/11]*

————. See also nos. 21, 203, 761, 765, 774, 1109, 1112.

332. **Germantown Dispensary and Hospital.** Correspondence. *Philadelphia, 1903-08.*

1 envelope. 26.5 cm. Mostly correspondence of Burton K. Chance, with notes and memoranda primarily concerning the medical staff of the hospital.   *[10a/390]*

333. **Getchell, Francis Horace,** 1836-1907. The renaissance of obstetrics — illustrated by the life & works of Ambroise Paré. *Philadelphia, 1872.*

[1], 34 ff. 25 cm (in envelope). Introductory lecture to the spring course of 1872 at Jefferson Medical College. — Pencilled note on cover: "Dr. F.H. Getchell?"   *[10a/404]*

334. **Ghinopoulo, Sophocles.** Pediatrics in Greece and Rome. *Philadelphia, 1936.*

[3], 120, [4] ff. 28 cm. Typescript (carbon copy). Part 13 of the *Jena Medico-Historical Contributions,* issued by Theod. Meyer-Steineg (Jena, Fisher [i.e. Fischer], 1930). — Translated by Samuel X Radbill.   *[10d/50]*

335. **Gibb, Joseph Scribner,** 1859-1914. Papers, chiefly concerning the Northern Medical Association. *Philadelphia, 1884-90.*

1 envelope. 32 cm. Contents: Constitution and by-laws, NMA, 1888 (printed); list of speakers and topics at NMA meetings; list of 72 NMA members (some not in NMA centennial membership list). — Paper on Hodgkin's

disease (delivered to NMA Dec. 14, 1888).   Presidential farewell address to the NMA, Feb. 14, 1890.   Four lectures, evidently designed for non-medical persons, on circulation and first aid.   Treatment of pseudo-membranous laryngitis (unpublished).   Gibb was Secretary, 1884-87 and President of the NMA, 1889-90. [ZZ 10c/17]

336.   **Gibson, William,** 1788-1868, comp.   List of physicians in the United States, compiled by William Gibson.   *Philadelphia, 1836.*

1 v.   27.5 cm.   Listed by state and county; thumb-indexed at the beginning (see also G.B. Wood's similar compilation of the same year). — Presented by Horatio C. Wood. [Z 10/103]

— — — — —.   See also nos. 459, 823.

337.   — — — — —.   Notes from lectures on surgery, taken by Henry Hartshorne.   *Philadelphia, ca. 1843-45.*

1 v.   20 cm. [10a/456]

338.   — — — — —.   Notes taken from Gibson's lectures on surgery . . . winter of 1841-2, by Joseph Leidy.   *Philadelphia, 1841-42.*

34 pp.   19 cm.   Volume also contains Notes on diseases of the eye and its appendages . . . taken from the lectures of Dr. Johnson (beginning June 23rd, 1842); Dr. Samuel Jackson's lectures - Oct. (1842?); Notes chiefly on poisons, especially from Dunglison's Therapeutics ([8] pp.); miscellaneous notes, chiefly from T.D. Mütter. — Gift of Joseph Leidy II. [10b/11]

— — — — —.   See also no. 384.

339.   **Gilbert, William Kent,** 1829-1880, comp.   Gilbert collection.   *V.p., 1729-1842.*

4 v. (ca. 750 items).   45 cm.   Autograph letters of John Bartram, Aaron Burr, Benjamin Chew, John Redman Coxe, Israel Pemberton, and other American and European 18th-early 19th-cent. scientific figures; personal and institutional documents, and material relating to yellow fever vaccination and other medical topics.   Described in College of Physicians of Philadelphia *Fugitive Leaves,* n.s., nos. 11-15 (1957).   With name index.   Gift of S. Weir Mitchell, 1888. [Z 10/18]

340.   **Girvin, John Harper,** 1869-1938.   Zoological notes.   *Philadelphia?, 1887-88.*

1 envelope (88 ff.).   23 cm.   Fragile.   Contents: Vertebrate animals; notes on the frog (n.d.) — Lecture on biology by Dr. Leidy; vermi[n]s (1888). — Anatomy (in German; 1887). — Notes on the crayfish (n.d.) — Notes on the crab (1887). — Gift of Helen Girvin. [10a/228]

341.   **Gleason, Edward Baldwin,** 1854-1934.   Reports of the otological clinics, held by Prof. Gleason.   *Philadelphia, etc., 1901-12.*

8 v.; illus. 25-29 cm. Typewritten. Titles and contents vary (otology clinical notes; clinics and lectures on otology and laryngology; etc.). — Reports written, illustrated and submitted by J.L. Loutfian (1901), P.A. Zoelle (1901-02), J.H. Hinchcliffe (1902-03), C.M. Strotz (1904), H.W. Levengood (1904-05), G.K. Levan (1906-07), P.A. Deckard (1908), M.S. Bheden and J.E. Kalodner (1908-09), M. Segal (1911-12). — From the library of A.C. Morgan.   *[10d/137]*

342.   **Goddard, Paul Beck,** 1809-1866. Receipt book. *Philadelphia, after 1857.*

137 ff. 22 cm. Cover title: Private recipes. Contains prescriptions and recipes, some for household compounds, etc. — Gift of S. Weir Mitchell.

[10a/43]

343.   **Goodell, William,** 1829-1894. Notes, abstracts and memoranda. *Philadelphia, 1856-89.*

1 v. 25.5 cm. Inscribed in a copy of John Todd's *Index rerum: or Index of Subjects* . . . (13th ed., Northampton, Mass., 1849), a book of blank pages, indexed alphabetically, with a preface suggesting methods for keeping a commonplace book. Goodell's entries, on obstetrical and gynecological topics, summarize articles in journals of the period.   *[10a/206]*

— — — — —. See also nos. 1014, 1079-80.

344.   **Goodman, Nathan Gerson,** b. 1899. Biography of Benjamin Rush. *Philadelphia?, ca. 1932-33.*

1 box. 31.5 cm. Pencilled draft of biography which appeared in bookform in 1934; corrections throughout.   *[Z 10/158]*

Gordon, Bernard, *see* **Bernardus de Gordonio.**

345.   **Gould, George Milbry,** 1848-1922. Letters, newspaper clippings, obituary notices, etc., collected for his wife (Laura Stedman Gould). *V.p., 1906-27.*

1 v.; illus., portraits. 24 cm. Manuscript and printed items. Scrapbook of material about Dr. Gould, ophthalmologist and editor, in preparation for a biography. Incl. letters by and to Gould, some of his poems, and advertisements for his *Medical Dictionary.*   *[10c/57]*

346.   — — — — —. Scrapbooks consisting primarily of printed items (clippings, reprints, pamphlets, etc.), but including correspondence in selected volumes (see below). *V.p., ca. 1886-1932.*

v. 54-61, 63-76, 79, 84-90; illus. 25-28 cm. Covers a great variety of subjects; of special interest are ophthalmology, evolution, history of medicine, and health examinations. The correspondence is largely in vols. 68-9, 71-6, 79, 87-9, with letters from G.E. de Schweinitz, H.H. Ellis, H.H. Furness, L.S. Gould, W.S. Halsted, F.W.E. Hare, T.P.C. Kirkpatrick, P. Loti, J.K. Mitchell, W.J. Morton, T.B. Mosher, W. Osler, W. Pepper, S. Solis-Cohen, S. Stephenson, A.

Stillé, S.H. Thayer, J. Trumbull, H. Van Dyke, W.H. Welch, A.D. White, and H.V. Würdemann. Furthermore included: Gould's critical memo to the Board of Trustees of the Jefferson Medical College, Jan. 1, 1893 (corrected to 1892. — 30 ff.; typewritten draft?, with ms. corrections); letters of Gould commenting on criticism of his book, *The Meaning & Method of Life*; Norman Roberts, A correct solution of the eyestrain problem (8 ff., 1909, carbon); Thomas F. Staley, Eye strain (4 ff., 1912, carbon); T. Percy C. Kirkpatrick, Eye strain (7 ff., n.d., typewritten); Herbert C. Mooney, On eye strain (3 ff., 1907?, typewritten); carbon of Gould's letter to Sydney Stephenson on article in *Lancet*, 1910, On mathematics & eyestrain (6 ff., Ithaca, 1911); material concerning Laura Stedman Gould (letters from and to, poetry).   *[10c/56]*

347.   **Gould, Laura Stedman,** comp.   Letters, poems, obituaries, etc., in memory of, or concerning George M. Gould. *V.p., 1921-23.*

1 v.; illus. 24 cm. Manuscript and printed items. Includes clippings, articles, photographs and other memorabilia.   *[10c/58]*

348.   **Gowers, William Richard,** 1845-1915.   Post-graduate lecture on neuralgia delivered at the National Hospital for the Paralytic and Epileptic. *London, 1894.*

30 ff. 34 cm. Typescript. Heavily edited text, probably the copy used by the printers; published in *International Medical Magazine*, v. 4: 113-23 (1895). — Presented by *International Medical Magazine*.   *[Z 10/12]*

349.   **Grahame, Thomas J.,** b. 1830?   An inaugural essay on influenza, presented to the faculty of the Philadelphia College of Medicine, for the degree of doctor in medicine. *Philadelphia, 1857.*

Title, 17, 3 blank ff. 25 cm.   *[n.c.]*

350.   **Grant, James Robertson.**   Valedictory address to the graduating class of the Medical Department of the Pennsylvania College, March 7, 1848. *Philadelphia, 1848.*

[32] ff. 25.5 cm (in envelope). Corrected copy. Published (Phila., 1848). Includes schedule of examinations, with names of students and draft of letter to a correspondent in Halifax, Nova Scotia. — Presented by Charles E. Rosenberg.   *[10c/138]*

351.   **Greater Philadelphia Committee for Medical-Pharmaceutical Sciences.** Papers. *Philadelphia, 1963-70.*

3 v. (loose-leaf). 28 cm. Collection of typewritten correspondence, minutes, reports, reprints and scientific papers; presented 1973-74 by Thomas M. Durant, chairman (1963-68). The Committee, described as "under the aegis of the College of Physicians . . .," concerned itself broadly with "medical-pharmaceutical research in all its phases," other health-related matters, especially including national legislation on drugs.   *[ZZ 10d/21]*

————. See also no. *185.18.*

352. **Green, Aaron Samuel,** 1879-1941. Case reports from the Greens' (i.e. Aaron Samuel and Louis David Green's) Eye Hospital. *San Francisco, 1916-19.*

41 ff.; 4 illus. (perimeters) attached. 28 cm.   *[n.c.]*

353. **Gregory, James,** 1763-1821. Notes . . . on practice of physic, 1817-18. *Edinburgh, 1816-18.*

1 v. 22 cm. Lectures 1-113 (29 Oct. 1817-20 Ap. 1818), with gaps. Writer notes (20 Ap.) that Gregory was injured and "thus prevented from finishing a course of lectures . . ." Notes resume (in a different hand?) with lecture 7 (15 Nov. 1816) and continue to lecture 98 (20 Mar. 1817); some lectures missing. Folio 104 followed by ff. 195-417, but text appears continuous. — Prov.: J. Solis Cohen.   *[10a/279]*

354. **Gregory, John,** 1724-1773. Lectures on clinical medicine. *Edinburgh, 1771-72.*

323 ff. 24 cm. Notes on 22 lectures, dated from Feb. 10th, 1771 (i.e., lecture no. 4; earlier ones undated) to February 18, 1773 (i.e., 1772). Consists of histories and observations on ward patients. On f. [322] Gregory says, "I have now resigned the care of the patients . . . to . . . Dr. Cullen." — Prov.: Jos. S. Neff, Philadelphia, 1875.   *[10a/44]*

—————. See also no. 111, 232.

355. **Griffith, John Price Crozer,** 1856-1941. Case books. *Philadelphia, 1886-91.*

v. 3-4 only. 24 cm. With graphic clinical charts, designed by Griffith, and used at the Hospital of the University of Pennsylvania; cf. *Trans. & Stud.*, ser. 3, v. 11: 244-50 (1889). Cases arranged alphabetically by patient. — Presented by the author.   *[10a/318]*

356. —————. Correspondence. *Philadelphia, 1914-32.*

17 v. 31 cm. Copies of typewritten letters. Apparently complete record of correspondence, incl. business and private affairs, etc.; large number of letters to colleagues, e.g. C.W. Burr, H.D. Carpenter, M.S. Councill, H.A. Hare, A.G. Mitchell, H.K. Pancoast, William Pepper, David Riesman,Alfred Stengel, as well as to some hospitals and medical associations and to the publishing firm W.B. Saunders, Philadelphia.   *[10d/138]*

357. —————. An essay on the histology of the testis (its coverings and appendages), for the degree of doctor of medicine in the University of Pennsylvania, . . . preceptor, W.W. Keen, . . . Presented Jan. 24th, 1881. *Philadelphia, 1881.*

150 ff.; 42 plates. 24.5 cm.   *[10a/234]*

358. —————. Notebooks. *Philadelphia, 1885-1900?*

> 2 v.; illus. 18-19 cm. V. 1 deals primarily with microscopic observations, v. 2 with "Important notes of diagnosis, treatment, microscope, etc." Includes notes on post-mortem examinations (pp. 69-89).   *[10a/235]*

—————. See also no. 1014.

359. **Griffitts, Samuel Powel,** 1759-1826. Diary, 1798, July 20-Nov. 30. *Philadelphia, 1798.*

> 26 (i.e., i, 29) ff. 19.5 cm. Concerned with the epidemic of yellow fever. Label on cover: "Ship Fever 1798." Discussed, with quotations, by Wm. S. Middleton in *Ann. Med. Hist.,* n.s., v. 10: 474-90 (1938).   *[10a/196]*

—————. See also no. 1127.

360. **Gringoire, Pierre.** La coqueluche. Poem on an epidemic in Paris, ca. 1510. *France, 18th cent.?*

> 7 ff. (vellum). 14.5 cm. Facsimile of the copy of printed volume in the Rothschild Coll., Bibliothèque nationale (Paris, Pierre le Dru, Aug. 14, 1510), imitating the style of the original.   *[10a/265]*

361. **Gross, Samuel David,** 1805-1884. Correspondence. *Louisville and Philadelphia, 1854-83.*

> 1 envelope. 30 cm. Includes acknowledgement of election to the American Philosophical Society (letter to René La Roche, 1854), several to G.W. Norris (incl. 1 on biographical sketch of Dr. P.S. Physick [1856] for an *American Medical Biography,* unpublished?; printed prospectus included) and to John Ashhurst (reference to a chapter on the history of surgery for the *International Encyclopaedia of Surgery;* letter 1881).   *[n.c.]*

362. —————. Wounds of the intestines. *Philadelphia, 1884.*

> 26 pp. 20 cm. "Last paper written by Prof. S.D. Gross . . ." Read before the American Surgical Association by Dr. T.G. Richardson, April 30, 1884 (ASA, Minutes). Published with some revisions in *Trans. ASA,* v. 2: 1-15 (1884). — Presented by I. Minis Hays.   *[10b/5]*

—————. See also nos. *185.613,* 589, 796, 980.

363. **Gross, Wilhelm.** On the anatomy and physiology of lymph follicles, Peyer's plaques, and appendices (animal experiments). *Hamburg, 1929.*

> 15 ff. 33 cm. Typewritten. Submitted for the Alvarenga Prize; letters of transmittal included. German version published under title, "Über die Anatomie und Physiologie der Lymphfollikel," in *Arch. f. klin. Chir.,* v. 157: 812-21 (1929).   *[Z 10/150, box 3]*

364. **Guillou, Charles Fleury Bienaimé,** 1813-1899. Collection of manuscripts and drawings, etc., by Guillou; letters, family memorabilia, etc. *V.p., ca. 1830-56?*

2 v. (text), 3 v. (illus.), 7 envelopes. 27-39 cm. Partial contents: Reminiscences, 1818-30 (89 ff.); experience in Terra do Fogo, 1839, with additions dated 1842 (35 ff.). — Autobiographical notes, one in response to a letter from Emma Brewster Guillou (20 ff.; 16, 4, 2 pp., etc., placed in folder). — Transcript of Guillou's reminiscences of W.C.P. Barton (4 ff.). — Illustrations: Sketches taken during exploratory voyages in the Western Hemisphere, 1838-41 (86, few in color). — Sketches taken during the cruise of the U.S. Flagship *Columbus* to China, Japan and around the world, 1845-47 (65 drawings). —Various sketches and paintings (a few numbered) from the Mediterranean area and Honolulu, etc. (loose, broken binding, in folder). — Handcolored lithographed view (Naples and Vesuvius?; 132 cm. wide, in 4 pieces, in folder). — Gift of Mrs. C.T. Blackmore.   *[10d/152]*

365. **Guitéras, John,** 1852-1925. Notes on general pathology and morbid anatomy from the lectures to the medical class of '93 at the University of Pennsylvania. *Philadelphia, 1890-93.*

5 v.; illus. 21-23 cm. Notes taken by John M. Swan; his autograph in v. 2-5. Few ff. inserted.   *[10a/331]*

—————. See also no. 1013.

366. **Guthrie, Douglas James,** b. 1885. The philosophical basis of medicine; an address delivered on 15th April 1949 . . . at the College of Physicians of Philadelphia before the Section on Medical History. *Philadelphia, 1949.*

[2], 2-20 ff. 27 cm. Manuscript introduction, typewritten text with ms. emendations. — Presented by the author.   *[10a/357]*

367. **Haase, Wilhelm Andreas,** 1784-1837. Materia medica; lectures at the University of Leipzig by W.A. Haase, C.F. Ludwig and S.C.F. Hahnemann, recorded by J.I.(?) Müller. *Leipzig, 1815-16?*

Title page, 481 (irregularly numbered) pp., [7, 6 blank, 73, 7 blank] ff. 21.5 cm. The dates 1815-16 were consistently (but mistakenly) changed to 1803. Haase's lectures (481 pp.), divided into 11, Ludwig's (ff. 1-57, f. 2 removed) into 3 notebooks. Hahnemann's lecture (ff. 59-71) is followed by prescriptions dealing with problems of gynaecology (ff. 71-73), also written by Müller, but with a different pen. Index of Haase's lectures on 7 ff. after p. 481.   *[10a/293]*

368. **Haggard, Howard Wilcox,** 1891-1959. What a frail sunday-school teacher (Dorothea L. Dix) did for medicine and humanity. *Philadelphia, 1933.*

Title, 28 ff. 29 cm. Typescript, with pencilled additions. Deals with efforts to establish mental hospitals. Read before the Section on Medical History of the College of Physicians and the Philadelphia Psychiatric Society, November 13, 1933.   [10d/37]

369. **Hahnemann Medical College and Hospital of Philadelphia. Nurses' Training School Committee.** Minutes, May 20, 1915-Sept. 21, 1921. *Philadelphia, 1915-21.*

[1] f., 301 (i.e. 295) pp., largely blank, 23 ff. 26 cm. Typewritten documents and letters inserted.   [n.c.]

370. **Hall, William Kearney,** b. 1918. History of dermatology in St. Louis, Missouri. *St. Louis, 1973.*

206, [2] ff. 30 cm. Typewritten, with photocopies included. Prepared for delivery before the St. Louis Dermatological Society in 1973; copies of journal and newspaper obituaries, etc., inserted. Presented by the author to the American Academy of Dermatology Collection of the College of Physicians; correspondence attached.   [10d/150]

371. **Hamilton, James,** 1825-1892. Recipes. *Chambersburg, Pa., ca. 1850-80.*

113 pp., [8] ff. 28 cm. Recipes cited from various journals and professors; some clippings pasted in. Presentation inscription to Richard H. Shryock from Mrs. Julia Allerman, Jan., 1951, inside front cover. Also inscribed to Dr. J.L. Suesserott, Sept. 4, 1864.   [ZZ 10c/14]

372. **Handley, William Sampson,** 1872-1962? Origin of bone deposits in breast cancer. *London, 1927.*

12 ff. 26 cm. Corrected copy of lecture delivered at Philadelphia General Hospital and published in *Surgical Clinics of North America,* v. 7(1): 4-6 (1927). With presentation letter from John B. Carnett.   [10a/288]

373. **Harris, Henry Albert,** 1886-1968. Cod liver oil and the vitamins in relation to bone growth and rickets. *London, 1930.*

60 ff.; 2 envelopes of photogr. 23-37 cm. Typescript (carbon copy). Alvarenga Prize Essay, 1930. Published in *Amer. Jour. Med. Sci.* v. 181: 453-78 (1931).   [10d/27]

374. **Harris, Henry Fauntleroy,** 1867-1926. On the alterations produced in the large intestines of dogs by the amoeba coli, by heat, and by various chemic substances, with notes on the anatomy and histology of this viscus. *Atlanta, 1901.*

[8], 224 ff., incl. plates. 28 cm. Typescript. Research carried on under the auspices of the Nathan L. Hatfield Prize Committee of the College of Physicians of Philadelphia, 1901. Published in *Trans. & Stud.,* ser. 3, v. 23 (1901).   [10a/151]

375.   **[Harte, Richard Hickman,** 1885-1925]. Bibliography, 1889-1907, by unidentified compiler. *N.p.d.*

3 ff. 27 cm.   *[10c/77]*

————. See also nos. *185.13*, 859.

376.   **Hartman, Frank Wilbur,** b. 1890. Studies on the pathology and prevention of anoxia; the methods for, and clinical application of, continuous recording of blood oxygen. *N.p., 1947.*

15 ff. 28 cm. Typescript. Mary Scott Newbold Lecture, College of Physicians of Philadelphia, 1 October 1947.   *[Z 10a/3]*

377.   **Hartmann, Philippe.** Cahier d'histoire naturelle appartenant à Philippe Hartmann. *Bruxelles, le 4 octobre, 18——[?].*

102 pp.; illus. 20.5 cm. Title-page waterstained, date unreadable. A student's outline, with handsome pen-and-ink drawings of some of the phyla, classes, and orders of the animal kingdom.   *[10a/147]*

378.   **Hartshorne, Henry,** 1823-1897. Account books, including daily notes on patients, receipts and expenditures. *Philadelphia, 1848-51.*

3 v. 16.5-17.5 cm. All vols. begin with reports on patients' progress, and payment records at one end, expenditures at other end. Comments on patients and personal affairs accompany some entries.   *[10a/455]*

379.   ————. Case book, Pennsylvania Hospital. *Philadelphia, 1846-47.*

229, 27 pp. 19 cm. Signature of Henry Hartshorne on flyleaf. Written from either end of book. Contains medical and surgical cases from 4/46 to 11/47, with table of contents.   *[10c/129]*

380.   ————. Chemical catechism for the use of students of medicine. *Philadelphia, 1850?*

1 v. 20 cm. Inscription inside front cover "unfinished rough draft — written about 1850; perhaps sooner, H.H." In form of questions and answers. Table of contents mentions parts I-VII; part VII not included. Section of metals (part of Section VI) loose, laid in.   *[10c/128]*

381.   ————. Memoir of Edward Hartshorne. *Philadelphia, 1886.*

[1], 30, [1 blank] ff. 21 cm (in envelope). Published in *Trans. & Stud.*, ser. 3, v. 9: xxv-xxxiv (1887).   *[10c/146]*

382.   ————. Random notes. *Philadelphia, 1844-45.*

[26] pp. 15 cm. Medical commonplace book, citing prescriptions, etc., from Joseph Hartshorne, N. Chapman, G.B. Wood, S. Jackson, and others. Notes cover wide range of medical topics.   *[10a/454]*

————. See also nos. *185.51*, 337, 383, 1112.

383. **Hartshorne, Joseph,** 1779-1830. Prescription record book. *Philadelphia, 1838.*

1 v. 16 cm. Bears signature of JH's son, Henry Hartshorne.   *[10c/131]*

384. **Hatfield, Nathan Lewis,** 1806-1887. Medical notebooks; miscellaneous personal papers. *Philadelphia?, ca. 1823-26 and later.*

1 box. 36.5 cm. Contains, among others, notes from lectures by John Eberle, George McClellan, Benjamin Rush Rhees, Francis S. Beattie, Jacob Green, William Gibson, John Redman Coxe, and Nathaniel Chapman; also ms. notebook (20 cm.) with title on cover, librarian's book, apparently the circulation record of a private society library, with mathematical or medical notes on verso of some pages; passport of Nathan Hatfield, bearing his signature and that of Hamilton Fish. Contents more fully described in 3-page list, filed with the collection.   *[Z 10/229]*

————. See also no. *185.234.*

385. **Haw, Walter Herbert.** An essay upon bilharzia haematobia or endemic African hamaturia. *Barberton, South Africa, 1898.*

77 ff.; xv and [2] plates. 33 cm. Submitted for Alvarenga Prize in 1898, under the motto "Eendragt maakt magt."   *[10a/504]*

386. **Heat** possesses the properties of matter; unsigned document. *N.p., 1807-08.*

8 pp. 24 cm (in envelope). Agrees with Lavoisier's position (cf. p. 2).   *[n.c.]*

387. **Heller, Edward Peter,** 1892-1948. A treatise on echinococcus disease; incorporating the report of the second case of the disease to be revealed in the ape, cynocephalus porcarius. *Kansas City, Mo., 1923.*

59 ff.; 16 plates. 27 cm. Typewritten. Published (with some illustrations omitted) in *International Clinics*, ser. 33, v. 4: 253-98 (1923). — Alvarenga Prize Essay no. 21, 1923.   *[10d/7]*

388. **Henderson, William Gates,** 1821-1852. Note-book while attending Jefferson Medical Coledge[!] .... *Philadelphia, 1840-41.*

94 ff. 20 cm. Consists chiefly of notes on lectures, operations, and cases by members of Jefferson's faculty (Dunglison, Pancoast, Revere, Pattison, Huston, and Green). Folios 81v. to 94 list patients' accounts, June-Aug. (year unspecified). — Gift of Helen E. Keep (her letter with biogr. info. on Henderson pasted in).   *[10a/211]*

389.   **Henry, Frederick Porteous,** 1844-1919.   Notes, largely quizzes. Autobiographical sketch. *Philadelphia, ca. 1916.*

[28, 2, 5] ff.   13-26 cm.   Topics range from jaundice to cancer of the stomach; fragmentary? — According to pencilled note in Dr. Henry's hand the autobiographical sketch was "written by request for publication in a pamphlet" (i.e. biographical sketches of members of the class of 1866, Princeton Univ.).   Three versions of the first leaf.   *[10a/505]*

390.   — — — — —. Notes on clinics and clinical lectures. *New York, 1865-66.*

[38, 90] pp.   21 cm.   Notes from clinics and lectures of Austin Flint, Thomas Masters Markoe, Joseph C. Hutchison, Willard Parker, Dr. Clarke (Alonzo Clark?), Robert Watts, and Dr. Thomas at Long Island College Hospital and the College of Physicians and Surgeons, N.Y.   Topics include cholera, lung diseases (Flint's lectures).   *[10a/173]*

391.   — — — — —   — — — — —. Notes on clinics and clinical lectures. *New York, 1865-66.*

1 v.   23 cm.   Notes taken at Long Island College Hospital from lectures of William Gilfillan on therapeutics, De Wit C. Enos on anatomy, Austin Flint on practical medicine, Darwin G. Eaton on chemistry and Joseph C. Hutchison on surgical anatomy.   *[10a/500]*

392.   — — — — —. Observations with the haemacytometer upon the globular composition of the blood and milk. *Philadelphia, 1881.*

92 ff.; illus.   25.5 cm.   Cartwright Prize Essay of the College of Physicians and Surgeons of New York, published Philadelphia, F.A. Davis, 1881.   *[10a/45]*

— — — — —. See also nos. 389, 505, 963, 1021.

393.   **Herbarius** continens simplicia ad medicinam utilia.   Alphabetically arranged dictionary of medicinal plants, largely with extensive explanatory notes and with indication of sources, especially Matthiolus (Mattioli), Dorsten and Wecker. *Germany?, early 17th cent.*

92 ff. (87v-92r, an appendix, numbered pp. 1-10), followed by 21 blank ff.   28.5 cm.   *[10a/282]*

394.   **Herbst, John A.,** 1735-1812.   Autograph letter transmitting his "Prayer on the day of dedication of Franklin [and Marshall] College" (not included). *Lancaster, June 18, 1787.*

[1] p. (16 lines text).   23.5 cm.   Addressed "Dear Sir," probably Benjamin Rush, since the name "John Herst" [!] seems to be in Rush's hand.   One-fourth of a second blank leaf (probably containing name and address) removed.   Added: Extract from Arthur Young's Travels, 1787-1790, pp. 221-23, description of Venice (2 ff., unidentified scribe).   *[10a/250, no. 14]*

395. **Heredity** and its general influence. *N.p., 1888.*

9 (vero 10) ff. and 3 smaller ff., 2 with diagrs. 27 cm. Lecture for "professional [i.e. medical] or lay men;" name of author and place of delivery of the lecture not established. Authorities cited: Theolule A. Ribot, Frank M. Deems, Sir Francis Galton, Prosper Lucas, Herbert Spencer and Henry Drummond. Lord Byron and German crown prince Friedrich serve as named examples of the author's theory. Since the name Deems appears separately and distinctly twice (ff. 3 and 5) it is suggested that he may be the author.   *[10a/502]*

396. **Herpel, John Kling,** b. 1946. Landmarks of ophthalmic publishing, 1474-1941. *Philadelphia, 1976.*

20 ff. 28 cm. Reproduced from typescript. — Resident talk, Scheie Eye Institute, Philadelphia.   *[10d/153]*

397. **Hewson, Addinell,** 1828-1889. Photographs of patients operated on by Addinell Hewson. *Philadelphia, 1861-65.*

1 envelope. 29 cm. Seven photographs, with brief notes, of six patients of Hewson, of whom one was also (Joseph?) Pancoast's patient, and one T.G. Morton's. Procedures include rhinoplasty, removal of fragments of stone without trephining in fracture of parietal bone, amputation of thigh, and treatment of cancer of the breast and of the leg. Two pictures show a patient with a growth on the right shoulder; dimensions of the tumor are given.
                                                                        [10b/46]

— — — — —. See also nos. 112, *185.632,* 940.

398. **Hewson, Thomas Tickell,** 1773-1848. Observations on the treatment of varicose veins of the lower extremities. *Philadelphia, 1833.*

[6] ff. 25 cm. Read before the College of Physicians of Philadelphia, Oct. 29, 1833.   *[n.c.]*

— — — — —. See also nos. 171, *185.13,* 481, 787-8.

399. **Hewson, William,** 1739-1774. The state of the dispute. *London, 1767-68.*

[32] pp. 38.5 cm. Hewson's rough draft of the major portion of his Appendix, relating to the discovery of the lymphatic system in birds, fish, and the animals called amphibious. Being a vindication of the author's right to these discoveries, in opposition to the claim of Dr. Alexander Monro . . . . — This manuscript begins with the 3d paragraph of the version printed as "Appendix" [etc.] (pp. 159-218) of his *Experimental Inquiries, Part the Second . . . .* (London, 1774). Text altered in the printed version. Both manuscript and text begin with a discussion of priority (Hewson vs. Monro) in proposing a procedure for paracentesis of the thorax. — Photostat copy of pp. 1-3 enclosed.   *[Z 10/166]*

400.   —————. Syllabus of a course of anatomical and chirurgical lectures. *London, third quarter 18th cent.*

[4] ff. 19 cm. Incomplete, nos. 33-74 (of 78) missing. According to the "Advertisement" (f. 1v) the present Syllabus is part one, covering anatomy. With corrections and deletions.   *[10a/506]*

—————. See also nos. 114, 479.

401.   **Higbee, William S.,** 1852-1939. Two addresses: 1. Health and welfare in business organizations. *Philadelphia, n.d.* — 2. An outline of obstetrical experience, remarks delivered at the meeting of the Obstetrical Society of Philadelphia. *Philadelphia, May 5, 1938.*

[4, 4] ff. 22 cm. Typewritten; the second address in photocopy. On cover of the first address: [To] The President and Officers of the Market Street Title and Trust Company."   *[10d/76]*

402.   **Hill, Archibald Vivian,** b. 1886. The present tendencies and methods of physiological teaching and research. *London?, ca. 1924.*

16 ff. 33 cm (in envelope). Autograph (ink and pencil, with many corrections, some deletions, and generally much edited). Gross lecture (Nov. 13, 1924), published in *Proc. of the Pathological Soc. of Phila.*, n.s., v. 27: 60-79 (1925), and a revision of *The Present Tendencies and the Future Compass of Physiological Sciences* (London, 1923); edited copy of *The Present Tendencies*, pp. 11-32 enclosed. — Gift of E.B. Krumbhaar.   *[Z 10/145]*

—————. See also nos. 507, 514.

403.   **Hinsdale, Guy,** 1858-1948. Anomalies found in the anatomical rooms of the University of Pennsylvania. *Philadelphia, 1879-81.*

1 v.; illus. 20 cm. Offered in competition for a student prize awarded by Hugh Lenox Hodge, who presented this ms.   *[10a/51]*

404.   —————. Howard A. Kelly, M.D. *Lewisburg, W. Va., ca. 1943.*

3 ff. 28 cm. Typewritten.   *[10d/57]*

405.   —————. Syringomyelia. *Philadelphia, 1895.*

1 v.; illus., diagrs. 27.5 cm. Typewritten and manuscript. Awarded the Alvarenga Prize of the College of Physicians of Philadelphia in 1895. Published in the Nov. and Dec., 1896, and Jan., 1897, issues of the *International Medical Magazine* and reissued separately.   *[10a/46]*

—————. See also nos. *185.63*, 1075-6.

406. **Hippocrates,** 460-375 B.C. A translation of the Aphorisms of Hippocrates, by George Sharswood, for Geo. W. Norris. *Philadelphia, 1830.*

[35] pp. 19.5 cm. Pasted on flyleaf Sharswood's holograph letter [Phila.] 1830 Apr. 26, to Norris. *[10a/207]*

— — — — —. See also nos. 695, 958.

407. **Hirsh, Abraham Bernheim,** 1888-1928. Philadelphia medical societies directory. *Philadelphia, 1911, 1913-14.*

2 parts in 1 v. 21.5 cm. Pasted-in printed notes with list of officers; handwritten headings, entries and additions. *[1h/56]*

408. **Hirst, Barton Cooke,** 1861-1935. Note-book; lectures on labor and dystocia. *Philadelphia, between 1889-1927.*

2 v. 27-28 cm. Printed charts and sheets of instructions to nurses, etc., bound in. *[10a/184]*

— — — — —. See also nos. 1014, 1085.

409. **Hirst, John Cooke,** 1875-1925. Gynecology quiz, University of Pennsylvania. *Philadelphia, 1908.*

24 ff.; illus. 23 cm. With notes by E.B. Krumbhaar. *[10a/425]*

— — — — —. See also no. 136.

410. **Histadruth ha-Refu'ith be-'Yisrael. American Physicians' Fellowship Commitee. Philadelphia Chapter.** Forms, letters, membership lists, etc. *Philadelphia, etc., 1953-62.*

1 box. 32 cm. Deposited, 1953. *[ZZ 10a/2]*

411. **Hitchens, Arthur Parker,** 1877-1949. Seventh Congress of the Far Eastern Association of Tropical Medicine, held in Calcutta, December 5 to 10 inclusive, 1927. *N.p., ca. 1928.*

12 ff. 19 cm. Informal account of the history of the association and the proceedings of this congress. *[10a/430]*

412. **Hodge, Hugh Lenox,** 1796-1873. Notes from Hodge's lectures on the principles of surgery. *Philadelphia, 1830.*

132 ff., pp. 133-244, [7] ff. 25 cm. Notes taken by Thomas Forrest Betton (M.D., 1832, Univ. of Pennsylvania). Table of contents after p. 244. — Presented by the City of Philadelphia. *[10a/472]*

413.   —————. Notes on Hodge's lectures on tokology. *N.p., 1842-43.*

> 2 v. 19 cm. Inside front cover of v. 1 a printed confederates' souvenir label, dated 1902, containing portrait of Stout aet. 80. — On verso of front cover of v. 2 inscribed "Samuel H. Stout Nashville, Tenn.," author of the Notes.
>
> *[10a/376]*

414.   —————. Notes on medical lectures. *Philadelphia, 1861.*

> [60] ff. 16 cm. Written on rectos and versos, the latter beginning at end of volume. Includes besides notes on Hodge's lecture on obstetrics, those on Wm. Pepper's on skin diseases, F.G. Smith's on ophthalmology and respiration, and Samuel Jackson's on the respiratory system. May also include notes on Leidy (see f. 60v: "Leidy 9 Saturday"). Leaf [3] contains list of students (at University of Pennsylvania) "Thirtenth[!] Class."   *[10a/418]*

415.   —————. Original photographs taken for book on obstetrics. *Philadelphia, 1856?*

> 1 v. (chiefly illus.). 45 cm. Scrapbook; photographs followed by lithographic prints, as they appeared in Hodge's *The Principles and Practice of Obstetrics* (Philadelphia, Blanchard and Lea, 1864).   *[Z 10/235]*

416.   —————. Papers. *Philadelphia, etc., 1818-70.*

> 2 boxes. 39.5 cm. Largely autograph. Contents: Box 1. Cash accounts, 1820-1821 (12 ff., partly blank; 18 cm.). — Cholera papers, incl. "Observations on the review of cholera maligna" (Phila., 1833), published in *Trans[ylvani]a Journal of Med[icin]e*, v. 6: 559-78 (1833, printed copy enclosed); the ms. consists of 5 conjugate ff.; review anonymous, but by Charles Caldwell. — Cholera epidemics in India, with case histories (of 1819; 10 ff., 34 cm.); other notes and clippings. — Correspondence: Two letters to René La Roche, 1828 (one announcing his marriage); others to Joseph Carson (1852?-71) appear in his son's hand (HLH, Jr., acting as amanuensis because of his father's failing eyesight). — "Notes and references:" On the peculiar duties of a physician to his Creator and to the public. On the conduct of physicians to their patients. On the patient or his friend suggesting a remedy to his physician. On professional conduct relative to hospitals or other medical charities (n.d., 15 pp., followed by many blank ff.; bound, 35 cm.).
>
> Box 2. Catalogue of medical library of H.L. Hodge (1870?; not in his hand; 20, blank ff.; 1 f. towards end "Tracheotomy on account of croup;" bound, 34 cm.); 1,118 books, and about as many pamphlets; also anatomical and obstetrical plates. — Case-book no. 5. Philadelphia and Calcutta, 1817-1819 (368 pp., bound, 21.5 cm.); cases numbered 85-153, they include a few patients seen at sea and in Calcutta late in 1818 and 1819. — Notebook of prescriptions, Philadelphia, 1818-31 (48 pp., 15 cm.) and various miscellaneous notes and memoranda (in envelope). — Gift of Dr. Edward B. Hodge.   *[Z 10/144]*

—————. See also nos. 70, 74-5, 1032.

417.   **Hodge, Hugh Lenox,** 1836-1881. Note book for cases of ovarian tumors and other abdominal enlargements. *Philadelphia, 1875-80.*

5 v.; diagrs. 22 cm. Collection of note-books (35 pp. each), filled in by hand and dated 1876-80. Bound in are details of cases, patients' and physicians' letters, prescriptions, etc.   [10b/57]

––––––. See also nos. 110, 188, 193, 221, 293, 309, 431, 589, 717, 758, 765, 847, 979.

418. **Hoffman, Frederick Ludwig,** 1865-1946. Cancer and diet; with facts and observations on related subjects. *Philadelphia, 1935-36.*

5 parts in 5 vols. 27 cm. Author's typewritten copy. Parts 2-3 entitled "Cancer in relation to diet and nutrition." Published with some changes (Baltimore, 1937).   [ZZ 10a/16]

––––––. See also nos. 235, 952.

419. **Holcomb, Richmond Cranston,** 1874-1945. Copies of source materials, photostats, photographs, other illustrative materials, text, notes, etc., almost exclusively concerned with the history of syphilis. *Pennsylvania, etc.?, ca. 1920-37?*

237 v.; illus. 25-29 cm. and 3 oblong (12 × 22 cm.). Contents: V. 1-43, 46-190, I-XIV, 4 unmarked v. and 3 oblong v. are primarily textual. – V. 1-2, 4-13, 15-19, 21-28, one unnumb. v. and 2 v. shelved with the notebooks (a total of 28 v.) are facsimiles of source materials and illustrations of bone deterioration; most illus. are accompanied by legends and many by commentaries. – The unnumbered volumes may correspond to the missing nos. 3, 14 and 20. – Gift of the author.   [ZZ 10a/7]

420. ––––––. An evolutionary perspective of the treponemiases (syphilis and syphiloids). *Philadelphia, 1944.*

[1], 31 ff. 28 cm. Typescript (carbon). "Corrected copy." Precis of an address planned by the Institute for the Control of Syphilis of the Graduate School of Medicine, Univ. of Pennsylvania and the Philadelphia Board of Education.   [ZZ 10a/8(1)]

421. ––––––. Bone growth. Bone growth – illustrations. *Phila-delphia, 1944.*

[4], 79, [5]; [8, 73] ff. 28 cm. Typescript (carbon copies). Contents: Text (corrected copy). – Description of illus. (see his Miscellany and the collection of photostats, photographs, etc.). Letter of transmittal to Capt. G.U. Pillmore contains direction to deposit "reprints" with Wistar Institute as his "associate member thesis." Unpublished? The 73 ff. are descriptions of illustrations (not present, but see photostats, photographs, etc. in this collection and/or in the volumes entirely devoted to illustrations).   [ZZ 10a/8(2)]

422.   — — — — —. Syphilis the venereal leprosy of the Middle Ages. *Philadelphia?, 194—.*

[2], 74, [3] ff.; illus., with unnumb. descriptions. 28 cm. Typescript. Contents: The evidence of bones. — The evidence of medical texts.
[ZZ 10a/8(3)]

423.   — — — — —. Correspondence (primarily with Dr. E.W. Rodenheiser), documents, etc. concerning the Emergency Medical Services, Zone 3. *Upper Darby, Pa., 1942.*

Several items in large envelope. 30.5-37 cm. Includes in separate folder photostats from Salicetus, *Summa conservationis et curationis; chirurgia,* Venice, 1490.
[ZZ 10a/8(4)]

424.   **Holscher, Georg Philipp,** 1792-1852. Venerische Krankheiten, Syphilis. Vorgetragen im Wintersemester 1829/1830 . . ., nachgeschrieben von J.N. Hinrichs. *Hanover, 1829-30.*

[1] f., 91 pp., [1] blank f., 55 pp. 20 cm. Part 2 (55 pp.) entitled Systema nervorum, Nervensystem. Neurologie, Nervenlehre, in the same hand as part 1, and probably by the same author.
[n.c.]

425.   **Holt, Jacob Farnum,** 1831?-1908. Anatomy and physiology, volume 1. Notes taken by Gustave A. Baumann, Central High School, Philadelphia. *Philadelphia, 1872?*

1 v. 21 cm. Tipped in Monthly reports of Gustave A. Baumann, term ending July 3, 1872.
[10a/373]

426.   **Home, Everard,** bart., 1756-1832. Lectures on the principal operations of surgery. *London, 1811[-12?].*

[12], 164 ff. 20 cm. Notes taken by W.H. Neville (cf. signature, dated 1812 on fly-leaf). Table of contents on prel. leaf, signed J. Solis-Cohen. Lectures probably delivered at St. George's Hospital, London. — Gift of J. Solis-Cohen, with his bookplate.
[10b/31]

427.   **Home, James,** 1758-1842. Clinical cases and dissections with remarks by Jas. Home. *Edinburgh, 1815-16.*

[viii], xlii, 853 pp.; [ii], 70 pp. 20 cm. Half-title: Clinical cases. Vol. I. 1815-16, and in another hand: Reported by Robley Dunglison (aged 17 years). Added: Clinical cases by Dr. Rutherford and Dr. Hamilton Senr. of the Royal Infirmary, Edinburgh, 1816. — Note in v. II. 1816 in another hand: Reported by Robley Dunglison (aged 18 years). Described and discussed by M.J.A. Jones and C.L. Gemmill in "The notebook of Robley Dunglison, student of clinical medicine in Edinburgh, 1815-1816," *J. Hist. Med. and Allied Sci.,* v. 22: 261-73 (1967).
[10a/143]

— — — — —. See also no. 111.

428. **Homoeopathic Medical and Surgical Hospital** and Dispensary Association, Reading, Pa. Minute book. *Reading, Pa., 1893-1911.*

> 300 pp. 27 cm. Constitution and by-laws, pp. 269-99. *[ZZ 10a/26]*

429. —————. Miscellany covering the years 1893-1914. *Reading, Pa., 1906-14.*

> 32 ff. and 2 clippings. Various sizes in envelope (37 cm.). Hand- and typewritten. Folder contains correspondence, 1906-08; draft of resolution; lists of staff, 1893-1906; financial statements, 1906-08. List of attending physicians at the Home for Friendless Children, 1914; clippings.
> *[ZZ 10a/26 (env.)]*

430. **Hosack, David,** 1769-1835. Lectures on the theory and practice of physic. *New York?, 1815 or later.*

> 2 v. 19 cm. Student not identified. Notes parallel the first six of the eight classes of Hosack's nosology, with introductory notes in v. 1. *[10a/60]*

> —————. See also nos. 42, 112, 1127.

431. **Hospital and Dispensary for the Relief of Diseases of the Rectum and Genito-Urinary Organs,** Philadelphia. Papers. *Philadelphia, 1875-87.*

> 1 box. 39 cm. Surgeons: E.C. Hine and L.S. Clark; consulting surgeon: H. Lenox Hodge. — Contains Charter, Dec. 6, 1875; Indentures, bills, checks, etc.; Papers relative to the dissolution of the Hospital, Dec. 1887; Prospectus; Minutes of the Board of Governors, July 10, 1875-86; Drafts of annual reports to the contributors; Account book, 1875-87; Bank book. — Gift of Mrs. Howard L. Lewis. *[10c/26]*

432. **Hough, John Stockton,** 1845-1900. Catalogue of his library as purchased after his death by the Library of the College of Physicians. *Philadelphia, 1901?*

> 362 pp. 33.5 cm. Typewritten. 2402 nos., 15th-19th cent. — Items outside the interest of the College (incl. duplicates) were disposed of, largely or entirely to the University of Pennsylvania, cf. *Trans. & Stud.*, ser. 3, v. 28: 298 (1906). *[Z 10c/19, box 1]*

433. ————— —————.

> 362 pp. 33.5 cm. Carbon copy of the same. Coded to show disposition of books (blue, items retained; brown, items disposed). Cover-title missing, f. 1 incomplete; fragile. *[Z 10c/19, box 2]*

434. —————. Catalogue of the medical library of John Stockton Hough. *Trenton, N.J., 1875-1900?*

> 1 v. 17 cm. *[10a/157]*

435. — — — —. Vital statistics of Philadelphia, 1860-71, with comparative data for 1820-31. *Philadelphia, ca. 1872.*

> 1 envelope (86 pieces). 39 cm. Manuscript and corrected and edited galley proof. Published in *Penn Monthly*, Philadelphia, Sept. 1873. Presented by the Historical Society of Pennsylvania (letter of transmittal enclosed).
>
> *[10a/160]*

— — — —. See also nos. *185.614*, 277, 618, 1094.

436. **Howe, Herbert Marshall,** 1844-1916. Medical notes. *Philadelphia, 186—?*

> 1 v. 18 cm. Incomplete; begins in mid-sentence.   *[10a/386]*

437. — — — —. Notes on hospital cases. *Philadelphia, 1865-6.*

> 1 v. 18 cm.   *[10a/387]*

438. — — — —. The organizable elements of the blood. *Philadelphia, 1865?*

> [25] pp. 31.5 cm. At head of title: "On fibrin as a plastic element." Presumably a draft of his thesis submitted to the Medical Department of the University of Pennsylvania, 1865.   *[10a/381]*

439. — — — —. Notes taken from clinical lectures delivered at Pennsylvania Hospital in the Spring of [18]63. *Philadelphia, 1863.*

> [1], 52 ff. (ff. 45-51 blank, f. 28 removed; col'd illus.). 10 × 17 cm (oblong). Cases presented by Drs. E.G. Smith, E. Hartshorne, J.J. Levick and J. Pancoast. H.M. Howe refers to himself on the title-page as "acting U.S.A. cadet." Partial index on f. 52 (a last f. missing?).   *[10a/378]*

— — — —. See also nos. 125, 777-8, 782, 961, 966, 968.

440. **Howship, John,** 1781-1841. Drawings of morbid anatomy. *London, 1804.*

> 274 colored drawings on ff. 2-85, with explanatory legends. 47.5 cm. Inscribed on verso of f. 1: "These drawings . . . were all taken from diseases in my [i.e. John Heaviside's] collection in 1804 — by Mr. J. Howship, then a house pupil of mine — London 1805." Ff. 2, 3-8 with signature "I. Howship Del?." A few specimens are dated (1794, 1797, 1799), sex and age of patients is indicated in many cases, and one is identified as "Mr. Thomsons patient." — Gift of Henry K. Pancoast.   *[Z 10/92]*

441. **Hughes, William Ellery,** 1857-1944. A record of anomalies found in the dissecting rooms of the University of Pennsylvania,

offered in competition for the prize to be awarded by H. Lenox Hodge. *Philadelphia, 1880.*

2 v.; illus. 21.5 cm.   *[10a/57]*

––––––. See also no. 88.

442.   **Human longevity.** *N.p., 1784?*

219 pp. 23 cm. Phillipps Ms. 9402. Examples of longevity, A.D. 66-1784. The manuscript described by James Easton as "by a gentleman deceased," which formed the basis of Easton's *Human Longevity* (Salisbury, 1799). Many entries correspond word-for-word with Easton's.   *[10a/281]*

443.   **Hunter, John,** 1728-1793. Notes from physiological lectures delivered by John Hunter, recorded by Benjamin Waterhouse. *London, 1777-78.*

319 pp. 22.5 cm. Signed or initialled notes by Waterhouse on pp. 210-12 and 224. – Signature of William Ashmead on flyleaf.   *[10a/165]*

444.   ––––––. Prescription, beginning "Venitian soap, a dram . . . ." *London?, ca. 1780.*

1 p. (mounted and bound). 19.4 × 14.7 cm. Inscribed on leaf following prescription: "This prescription of John Hunter was obtained by Simon Gratz Esq. of Phila. from the collection of autographs belonging to the late Rev. Wm. B. Sprague. It had been sent to him some fifty years ago by Dr. Yellowly of London. Given to the College of Physicians of Phila. by J.M. DaCosta, Jan. 4, 1882." Patient and disease not identified.   *[10a/134]*

445.   ––––––. Surgery and venereal diseases, notes compiled from the lectures of Dr. Hunter by Caspar Wistar. *London, 1783-84.*

302, [9 blank] ff. 23.5 cm. Signed C. Wistar on f. 1. "Having premised Mr. Hunters intention [in the introduction] it is necessary to observe that it was impossible to take a verbatim copy, therefore I have neither followed his language . . . nor his order, but have altered both as best suited my own plan . . . ." (advertisement, f. 4). "Index to Hunter Surgery" inserted between ff. 220-21. "From Dr. Caspar Wistar's medical library. Presented to the College of Physicians in the name of Dr. Mifflin Wistar. 1887."   *[10b/6]*

––––––. See also nos. 269, 447, 449, 587, 644.

446.   **Hunter, William,** 1718-1783. An abstract from Dr. Hunter's lectures on the gravid uterus. *Salem, Mass., 1786.*

58, [8] pp. 20.5 cm. Inscribed on p. 58 "Salem. Decr 23^d - 1786 - AP scripsit." A.P. may be Abiel Pearson, 1756-1827 who studied under Dr. Edw. A. Holyoke of Salem, beginning practice in Andover in 1787. At end: 8 pp. of notes, on Benjamin Rush's "Observations on the Cause & Cure of the Tetanus" (American Philosophical Society, *Transactions*, v. II, p. 225), and on Wm. Wright's "The Antiseptic Vertues of Vegetable Acid & Marine Salt Combined in Various Disorders Accompanied with Putridity" (*ibid.*, v. II, p. 284). — Inscribed on the front flyleaf: "This book belonged to the late Gov. Winthrop Sargent. W.V.(?) Sept. 18, 1856." — Pasted on front flyleaf: Ed.(?) Penington, Jr., letter to Samuel Lewis, Philadelphia, March 21, [18]71, stating that "Mrs. Duncan gave some of Sargent's books & papers to Mr. Townsend Ward and myself."   *[10a/62]*

447.   ————. From Dr. Hunter's course of lectures. *London, Jan. 19, 1763.*

> 1 f. 37 cm. Edges frayed, with loss of text. Contains summaries of the following lectures: The rise and progress of anatomy; The blood; The arteries & anastamosis of arteries; The teeth (by John Hunter). — Presented by the heirs of Dr. Carson.   *[n.c.]*

448.   ————. Notes taken from Dr. Hunter's lectures on anatomy. *London, ca. 1783.*

> [1 blank] f., 520 pp., [1] f. table of contents. 25 cm. "From Dr. Caspar Wistar's medical library, presented . . . in the name of Dr. Mifflin Wistar" (inside front cover). C. Wistar's signature on p. 1, and written by him during his stay in London, before he went to Edinburgh.   *[10a/63]*

449.   ———— **(or John Hunter).** Lectures. *London, 178—.*

> 1 v. 20.5 cm. Frequently mentions "Dr. Hunter," without indicating whether he is to be identified with William or John. Content corresponds roughly to parts of the outline of anatomy appearing on pp. 84-85 of Two introductory lectures, delivered by Dr. William Hunter, to his last course of anatomical lectures (London, 1784).   *[10a/61]*

450.   **Hyde Collection** of medical letters, incl. some prescriptions, receipts, documents, etc. and collection of portraits. *V.p., 1763-1925.*

> 2 boxes. 39 cm. Various lists describing the contents in box 1. Among items in the extensive collection are letters by H.I. Bowditch (1846-70), F.H. Garrison (1911, 1916), E. Jenner (1821), B. Rush (1808); approximately 50 letters to Lyman Spalding; investigation and trial of Samuel Thompson for the murder of Ezra Lovett (16 ff., 1809), etc. Box 2 contains the portraits. For a brief summary description see *Trans. & Stud.*, ser. 4, v. 43: 62-63 (1975-6). — Gift of Mr. and Mrs. A.P. Hyde.   *[ZZ 10a/24]*

451.   **Ilberg, Johannes,** 1860-1930. Essays on Galen and his writings . . . Translated into English for personal convenience between 1910 and 1937 by Joseph Walsh. *Philadelphia, 1937-39.*

> 1 v. 27 cm. Typewritten. Contents: (1). Ilberg's "Über die Schriftstellerei des Klaudios Galenos . . ." abstracted and sometimes slightly modified (131 ff.); together with (2). reprints of the original (*Rheinisches Museum für Philologie,* N.F., v. 44, 47, 51-52). — (3). J. Walsh, "Date of Galen's Birth" (repr.: *Annals of Medical History,* n.s., v. 1: 378-82 [1929]), with (4) Engl. transl. of Ilberg's "Wann ist Galenos geboren?" (ff. 132-38, originally printed in *Archiv für Gesch.*

d. Medizin, v. 23, Heft 3 [1930]; answer to the foregoing). — (5). Joseph Walsh, "Refutation" (of no. 4, repr.: *Annals of Med. Hist.*, n.s., v. 4: 126-46 [1932]). — (6). Ilberg, "Aus Galens Praxis" (repr.: *Neue Jahrb. für das Klass. Altertum, Gesch. u. d. Lit.*, v. 15: 276-312 [1905]), with (7). abridged translation by Walsh (ff. 139-63). — (8). J. Walsh, "Galen's Writings and Influences Inspiring Them" (repr.: *Annals of Med. Hist.*, n.s., v. 6: 1-30, 143-49 [1934]). — (9). J. Walsh, "Essays on Galen furthering Ilberg's Studies" (bibliography; ff. 164-5).

[Z 10/176]

452. **Imperatori, Charles Johnstone,** 1878-1949. Commentary on Leonardo Da Vinci's contribution to laryngology, rhinology and phonetics. *New York, 1941.*

1 v. ([16] ff.); illus. (photogr.). 18 cm. Illustrations in miniature and descriptions; compiled for E.B. Krumbhaar. Full text and illustrations published in *Annals of Otology, Rhinology, and Laryngology*, v. 50: 979-94 (1941).

[10a/388]

453. **International Medical Congress,** Philadelphia, 1876. Minutes, accounts, registration records, scrapbooks. *Philadelphia, 1874-78.*

7 v. 14.5-36 cm. Ms. and printed items. Minute book and financial accounts, 1876-78, of the IMC's Committee on Publication. Registration book, 1876, of delegates to the Congress, arranged alphabetically, and including signature, address, and affiliation; visitors' register, 1876, from the Congress. Scrapbook, with printed announcements, forms, etc., and also containing correspondence, 1874-76, with committee members, delegates, and others, concerning plans and activities of the Congress. *[10c/10-11]*

————. See also nos. 36, 586.

454. ————, 9th, Washington, D.C., 1887. Extracts from minutes of Executive Committee, circulars, etc. *Washington, D.C., 1884-85.*

25 hectographed ff., 1 f. (list of chairmen; handwritten), 2 ff. (2nd blank; handwritten letter, signed by John S. Billings and addressed to S. Weir Mitchell). 25-32 cm. Material issued by Billings as secretary general of the committee organizing the congress, and, in the case of the present set, sent to S. Weir Mitchell as member of the Executive Committee and chairman of the Section of Nervous Diseases and Psychiatry. *[Z 10c/4]*

455. **International Society of Internal Medicine,** 5th Congress, Philadelphia, 1958. Official record. *Philadelphia, etc., 1958 and later.*

1 v. 29 cm. Typescript and printed material. Partial contents: unsigned typed introd. statement, list of donors; letters from President Eisenhower, Vice-President Nixon; news releases; programs; reprints of papers read at the Congress (parfial only), etc. Autograph of T. Grier Miller on front flyleaf. — Gift of T. Grier Miller. *[n.c.]*

456. **Ireland, Merritte Weber,** 1867-1952. The achievement of the Army Medical Department in the World War in the light of general medical progress. *Philadelphia, 19[20-]21.*

[1], 25 ff. 28 cm. Typescript (carbon). Fourth Mary Scott Newbold Lecture of the College of Physicians of Philadelphia, delivered February 4, 1921. Published in *Trans. & Stud.*, ser. 3, v. 43: 394-414 (1921). — Presented by William J. Taylor. *[10d/136]*

— — — — —. See also no. 253.

457. **Isaacs, Raphael,** 1891-1965. On the nature of the action of Roentgen rays on living tissues. *Boston, 1925.*

32, [3] ff.; tables, plates. 28 cm. Typewritten; two tables missing. — Alvarenga Prize Essay no. 23, 1925. Published under title: "Effect of Roentgen Ray Irradiation on Red Blood Cell Production in Cancer and Leukemia," *Am. J. Med. Sci.,* v. 171: 20-37 (1926). — Gift of the author. *[10d/16]*

458. **Ivervex (Juerves?),** supposed Swedish physician. Recepte du fameux docteur Juerves(?) . . . trouvée dans les papiers après sa mort l'age de 104 ans. . . (Elexir suedois de longue vie). *N.p., 18th cent.*

2 ff. in French dealer's cover. 22.5 cm. Described in *Trans. & Stud.*, ser. 4, v. 5: 28-9 (1937). Gift of E.B. Krumbhaar. *[n.c.]*

459. **Jackson, Alexander,** ca. 1803-1879. Lecture notes taken at the Medical School of the University of Pennsylvania. *Philadelphia, 1824.*

[2], 338 (vero 341) pp.; illus. 20 cm. Notes on lectures by J.R. Coxe, W. Gibson, N. Chapman, R. Hare, P.S. Physick, T.C. James and W.P. Dewees. "List of 26 professional books taken . . . 1824" and "[literary] Books . . . that belong to STM" on prel. leaf. — Gift of William P. Ridley. *[10c/154]*

460. **Jackson, Chevalier,** 1865-1958. Curriculum vitae. *Philadelphia, 1954?*

11, [1] ff. 28 cm. Typewritten. *[ZZ 10d/15]*

461. **Jackson, Samuel,** 1787-1872. Notes of a course of lectures on the materia medica . . . . To which are added three lectures on the stethescope[!] by the same, AD 1827, vol. 2nd. *Philadelphia, 1826-28.*

391, [3] pp. 24.5 cm. "This case I saw; R.R. Dorsey" (p. 350); Dorsey also inscribed repeatedly on flyleaves, and also "Richard Maris — 1835." Contains "Lectures 33-54." *[10a/366]*

462.   —————.   Notes on Dr. Jackson's lectures, delivered during session 1839-40. Taken by Henry Selden. *Philadelphia, 1839-40.*

1 v.; illus. 20 cm. Pencilled notes on facing pages; subject matter often not directly related to topics of Jackson's lectures.   *[10a/429]*

463.   —————.   Notes taken on Dr. Jackson's lectures on the institutes of medicine, during the session of 1850-51, by F.W. Sargent. *Philadelphia, 1850-51.*

145, [3] pp. 19 cm.   Binder's title: Letters.   *[10a/64]*

464.   —————.   Reports of cases and inquiries sent to Dr. Jackson; two letters by him, a few prescriptions and one bill. *V.p., 1834-64.*

1 envelope. 37.5 cm. Several clinical cases concern epilepsy. Letter by Jackson, dated May 18, 1864, congratulates Brigadier General W.A. Hammond on having successfully silenced his detractors. — Added: Printed cover of Samuel Jackson (1788-1869), *Memoir of Isaac Parrish* (Phila., 1853) with handwritten dedication to Dr. Rush Van Dyke.   *[n.c.]*

465.   [—————].   Collection of 20 holograph letters addressed to Samuel Jackson from various correspondents, chiefly physicians, asking advice relating to the epidemic of cholera. *East coast of the U.S., 1832.*

1 box (20 folders). 39 cm. 11 letters from Virginia, 4 from Pennsylvania, 2 from Washington and 1 each from New Jersey, Maryland and South Carolina.   *[Z 10/143]*

—————.   See also nos. 82, 112, 114, 338, 382, 414, 795, 804, 979, 1032.

466.   **Jacobi, Abraham,** 1830-1919. Correspondence. *New York, etc., 1879-1906.*

1 envelope. 37.5 cm. Letters by Dr. Jacobi include acknowledgement of election to College of Physicians of Philadelphia (1891), letters to Dr. W.W. Keen (1906) and S.W. Mitchell (n.d.); those to him involve in many cases the Mount Sinai Hospital in New York. Also included a few items only indirectly connected with Jacobi, and a letter of transmittal (1968) from Joseph Hirsh of Temple University.   *[n.c.]*

467.   **Jacobs, Merkel Henry,** b. 1884. Lectures on physical chemistry and physiology, University of Pennsylvania, School of Medicine; notes taken by E.B. Krumbhaar. *Philadelphia, 1923.*

1 v.; diagrs. 19 cm. Physical chemistry on rectos. Text on physiology, mainly the transfer of energy, on versos, beginning at end of volume.

[10c/87]

————. See also no. 547.

468.   **Jaeger, Eduard,** Ritter von Jaxtthal, 1818-1884. Augenspiegel Bilder. *Vienna, ca. 1851-55.*

3 v., 2 boxes; plates, port. 29-32 cm. One hundred forty-two hand-colored drawings published in Jaeger's *Ophthalmoskopischer Hand-Atlas* (Vienna, 1869). Case notebook, incl. correspondence and documents concerning the transfer of the material to William Fisher Norris. Jaeger's illustrations were removed from the 2 volumes and are kept in boxes. — Presented by George W. Norris.   *[Z 10/36]*

469.   **James, Thomas Chalkley,** 1766-1835. Medical commonplace book. *Philadelphia, 1800.*

316 pp. (incl. many blank pages). 23 cm. Bookplate of Hugh Lenox Hodge. Consists of notes from various published works, with footnotes and acknowledgements.   *[10a/82]*

470.   ————. Notes from the lecture ... on midwifery. *Philadelphia, ca. 1800.*

1 v. 16-24 cm. Six lectures, the last ending in mid-sentence; next 8 pp. (16 cm) fragmentary; followed by 22 pp. (20.5 cm) entitled "Of pains" in a different hand. — Name at head of title "Dr. I. Hays." — "Vol. 1st" (front flyleaf).   *[10a/66]*

471.   ————. Notes on the lectures on midwifery in the University of P[ennsylvani]a, delivered by Drs. James & **[William Potts] Dewees,** etc. *Philadelphia, 1826-36?*

[79] ff. (ff. 21-69 blank, 1 f. at beginning removed). 33 cm. 39 lectures, notes varying in length, some with references to "Dewees' Syst. Mid." Further lectures omitted, since they were "nearly verbatim" taken from Dewees' book (f. 20). At the opposite side of book are notes on physics (mercurial thermometer; molecular forms; light; heat; lengthy section on electricity, etc., f. 70 to end), interspersed by 2 pp. (f. numb. 96) entitled "Remarks, chiefly surgical made by Dr. Physick in his lectures on anatomy ... 1826." The notes on physics contain many corrections, alterations and additions, possibly in preparation of Daniel B. Smith's *Principles of Chemistry* (Philadelphia, 1837). Laid in 4 folded, colored drawings of geological formations. According to letter from Haverford College, pasted in front, the notes were taken by Daniel B. Smith; but it is uncertain whether both parts are in the same hand. Inscribed on front cover "For William Richardson." — Gift of Haverford College.

[Z 10/55]

472. ————, comp. Philosophical and medical miscellanies, no. 1. *Philadelphia, 1787-92*.

146, [4] pp. 16 cm. Bears bookplate of Hugh Lenox Hodge, by whom it was presented. — Contains notes and observations from the works of various authors.
[10a/65]

————. See also nos. 74-5, *185.13*, 221, 459, 751, 901.

473. **Janowitz, Henry David,** b. 1915. Studies in the regulation of hunger and appetite. *Chicago, 1949*.

[3], 87, 6, [12] ff.; tables. 28 cm. Typewritten (carbon). Thesis — M.Sc.(Med.) — University of Illinois. Printed title page. Bookplate of A.C. Ivy. Gift of Smith, Kline & French.
[4X Illinois 1949]

474. **Jefferson Medical College.** Alumni Association and W.S. Forbes Anatomical League records. *Philadelphia, 1886-1918, 1943*.

V. 1 ([69] pp., 26 cm.); 23 ff. in envelope (27 cm.); v. 2 (501 pp.,incl. many blank; 36 cm.). Alumni Association, Executive Committee minutes, 1886-99, with some related notes and correspondence. List of Jefferson's faculty and teaching corps who were officers in the service of the U.S. during the war of 1918; list, 1943, of Jefferson men in the service. — W.S. Forbes Anatomical League. Constitution and by-laws, 1895; amendment of Oct. 26, 1900; minutes, 1896-1907 (pp. 79-271); list of League presidents, 1893-1908 (p. 51); membership roll, 1895-1910 (pp. 19-32); membership attendance, 1896-1907 (pp. 470-94); members awarded anatomical prizes, 1895-1905 (p. 55); members receiving honorable mention, 1895-1905 (p. 57).
[10a/217; 10c/51; Z 10c/3]

————. See also nos. 12, 26, 56, 91, 212, 228-9, 234, 271-3, 275, 333, 346, 388, 714, 785, 830, 844, 935, 943, 1047, 1062, 1128.

475. **Jelenffy, Z.** What is veritable paralysis of the posticus (posterior cricoarytenoid)? *Budapest, ca. 1888*.

1 envelope (6 pp., 11, [2] ff.; diagrs.). 26-34 cm. Manuscript and typescript (carbon copy). "Read by Dr. J. Solis Cohen in the Laryngological Section, Am. Med. Assn., June, 1889," printed in *N.Y. Medical Jour.*, v. 50: 225-27 (1889). Two slightly different versions.
[10a/490]

476. **Jenks, William Furness,** 1842-1881. Manuscript notes on interleaved printed copy of Joseph Carson's *Synopsis of the Course of Lectures on Materia Medica and Pharmacy*... (3d ed., Philadelphia, 1863). *Philadelphia, 1863[-64?]*.

244 pp. (many written and blank ff. interspersed). 22.5 cm. Notes begin on 2 ff. between pp. 18-19 and end on f. following p. 206. Pencilled annotations on printed pages.
[10a/484]

————. See also nos. 128, *185.233*.

477. **Jenner, Edward,** 1749-1823. Holograph letters to Charles Murray. *London, 1806-17.*

> 1 v. 24 cm. Seventeen letters dealing with activities of the National Vaccine Establishment, of which Murray was secretary; also concerning other persons involved with vaccinations; some brief discussion of experiments, papers, annual reports. Recorded in W.R. LeFanu's *Bio-Bibliography of Edward Jenner* (London, 1951); 10 were published by S. Weir Mitchell in *Trans. & Stud.*, ser. 3, v. 22: 101-11 (1900). — Presented by S. Weir Mitchell and J.M. da Costa.
> *[10a/142]*

————. See also nos. 112, 450, 805t.

478. **Johns Hopkins University,** Baltimore. William H. Welch Medical Library. Proposed course for medical librarians. *Baltimore, 1946.*

> Folder (5 ff.). 28 cm. Typescript (carbon copy). Revised, June 15, 1946.
> *[Z 10/181]*

————. See also no. 79.

479. **Jones, John,** 1729-1791. Lectures on surgery by the late John Jones M.D. presented to me [James Mease] by Mrs. Clark (ff. 1-109). With Jones' notes on lectures of William Hewson (ff. 111-46). *New York and London, 1769-74?*

> [148] ff. (ff. 2, 18, 46, 91, 110, 114, 147-48 blank [modern numbering]; with partial, irregular contemporary pagination). 25 cm. Autograph manuscript, with corrections. The Lectures on surgery were delivered at King's College, New York. The Notes on Hewson's lectures were taken during Jones' stay in England, 1772-74. For text of the introduction (serving also as lecture 1), detailed contents and explanations of dates see W.B. McDaniel's article in *Trans. & Stud.*, ser. 4, v. 8: 180-90 (1940). Hewson refers to a variety of authorities, frequently to Percival Pott (see among others Pott on ophthalmology, especially cataract, ff. 125-26). Gift of George William Norris who received the manuscript from a Mrs. Randolph. *[10b/23]*

————. See also no. 166.

480. **Judications,** qui se présentent sur l'incommodité dont Mad[a]me Cl. . . . se trouve affectée. *France, 18th cent.*

> 1 f. 24 cm. Consultation in a case of "fibres nerveuses et musculeuses, qui se trouvent crispées et racornies." Shelved with 17th-century consultation (Emmerez). *[10a/312]*

Juerves, *see* **Ivervex.**

481. **Kane, John Kintzing,** 1833-1886. Notebook. *N.p., ca. 1865?*
[58] ff. 15 cm. Notes on patients, and medical texts. *[10a/460]*

⸺⸺⸺. See also nos. 270, 765.

482. **Kappa Lambda Society of Hippocrates.** Constitution and by-laws, minutes, committee records, correspondence, memorials, and accounts. *Philadelphia, 1821-35.*

9 v., 2 boxes. 31.5-39 cm. Constitution and by-laws of the Kappa Lambda Society of Hippocrates of Philadelphia, and also of the Pennsylvania Society, both signed by members. Minute book, 1822-32, 1835, describing society business; journal, 1823, recording presentations of case histories at meetings, and minute book, 1828-31, containing abstracts of written and verbal society communications. Minutes, 1824-30, 1835, of the Editorial Committee of the *North American Medical and Surgical Journal,* published by the society, with some related extracts from the society's minutes. Correspondence, 1822-32, including a group of letters from the Kappa Lambda Societies of New York and Washington, and some correspondence about the *North American Medical and Surgical Journal.* List, 1825, of Kappa Lambda members throughout the world, incl. dates of admission, society membership, and residence; eulogies, 1827-32, of society members J.H. Ewing, S. Wilson, and J.G. Whilldin; records, 1829, of the case of Drs. Caleb B. Matthews and J.M. Paul. Account books, 1822-33, 1835, of society; account book, 1825-35, of the *North American Medical and Surgical Journal.* Misc. pamphlets and broadsides. — Presented by the society. *[Z 10/141]*

⸺⸺⸺. See also no. *185.222.*

483. **Kates, Herbert S.,** 1894-1947. Drawings (clinical) and sketches of buildings, exteriors and interiors. *Camp Upton, N.Y., 1917-18.*

1 box, 3 envelopes. 39-52 cm. Drawings in pastel, watercolor, and crayon. Of the clinical drawings, 58 illustrate dermatological disorders, 27 disorders of the head and neck, especially hyperthyroidism (14). A series in watercolor illustrates the progression of a laboratory test injection from 6 minutes to 5 weeks later. The drawings were made of cases under the care of H. Harlow Brooks, Chief, Medical Service, Camp Upton Base Hospital; none appeared in papers publ. by Brooks on his cases at the hospital. Detailed outline with the collection. — Gift of Jerome S. Kates (correspondence included). *[Z 10c/22]*

⸺⸺⸺. See also no. 94.

484. **Keats, John,** 1795-1821. Anatomical and physiological note book. *London, 1815-16 (reproduced in 1923).*

1 folder (irregular, original numbering: 50, 18 pp.). 27 cm. Photographic reproduction. Based on lectures by Astley Cooper at Guy's Hospital, cf. William Hale-White, *Keats as Doctor and Patient* (New York, etc., 1938), pp. 24-6. Letter of transmission, W. Hale-White to W.W. Keen, enclosed. *[n.c.]*

485.   **Keeler, Harold Raudenbush,** 1894-1953.   Notes on pathology.
       Philadelphia, ca. 1918.

> 10 ff., pp. 11-50, [1] f., pp. 51-171, [31] ff.; illus.   20 cm.   Name Keeler taken
> from signature on binder (no longer extant).   Lecturer not mentioned; Keeler
> received a M.D. from the University of Pennsylvania in 1921.   *[10a/481]*

486.   **Keen, William Williams,** 1837-1932.   Correspondence, notes,
       etc.   *V.p., 1885-1926.*

> 22 folders in box.   31 cm.   Much of the material deals with the controversy
> over vivisection.   Incl. also W.W. Keen's efforts on behalf of the College of
> Physicians of Philadelphia, incl. purchases and exchange arrangements
> during his European journey (1908); some printed items and clippings. –
> Among the correspondents are H.P. Bowditch, W.B. Cannon, Alexis Carrel,
> E.G. Conklin, Simon Flexner, W.C. Gorgas, S.W. Lambert, S.J. Meltzer, W.H.
> Welch, and among members of Congress especially Eugene Davis and J.H.
> Gallinger.   *[10c/105]*

487.   —————.   Correspondence, reports, etc., largely items address-
       ed or submitted to him.   *V.p., 1891-1925.*

> 2 boxes.   39 cm.   Material concerned with Keen's *American Textbook of Surgery*;
> opposition to anti-vivisection campaign and the Gallinger bill (incl. letters
> from W.J. Mayo, L.C.A. Calmette, W.H. Welch, etc.); information on supposed
> mortality from rabies inoculation (incl. reprints and letters from V. Ushakoff,
> reports from various Pasteur institutes, statistics from Palermo); letters from
> Marie Curie (folder 11), A. Carrel, Simon Flexner, etc. (folder 14) and file of
> letters from the editor of *JAMA*, 1899-1900 (envelope no. 15).   Some of the
> items relate to Keen's activities as president of the AMA, the American
> Philosophical Society or his various official capacities at the College of
> Physicians of Philadelphia. – Gift of Florence Keen.   *[n.c.]*

488.   —————.   Correspondence and documents relating to efforts
       of anti-vivisectionists to prevent typhoid inoculation of Ameri-
       can soldiers and to prevent an appropriation of $100,000 for
       medical research by the American Red Cross during 1918.   *Phila-*
       delphia, etc., 1918-19.

> 1 box.   31.5 cm.   Arranged by date.   Contents of this collection indexed by
> addressee, with two other collections of Keen papers.   Includes 1 envelope of
> misc. items.   *[10a/320]*

489.   —————.   Draft for a "book on artistic anatomy, or better
       anatomy for artists."   *Philadelphia, ca. 1900.*

> [14], 66 ff.   34 cm.   Four chapters and unnumbered, unfinished chapter "On
> the proportions of the human body." – Presented by W.W. Keen.   *[Z 10/99]*

490.   —————.   Notebook . . . on Dupuytren's contracture.   *Philadel-*
       phia, after 1878?

[1] f., 92 (vero 93) pp., [1] f. 17 cm (in boards, 26.5 cm). Notes taken from journals, theses, etc., published between 1831 and 1878. – Gift of the author.   *[10b/48]*

491.   – – – –, compiler. Reports, correspondence and clippings relating to the operation of President Cleveland on board the yacht Oneida in 1893. *Philadelphia, 1893-1927.*

1 box; illus. 27 cm. Manuscript and printed material. Contemporary, as well as later items connected with Dr. Keen's article on the operation in the *Saturday Evening Post* (Sept. 22, 1917) and his publications in book form (1917 and 1928) constitute a major part of the collection, incl. furthermore letters to and from some of the attending physicians (J.D. Bryant, R.M. O'Reilly, J.F. Erdmann, F. Hasbrouck, Francis F. Cleveland Preston, etc.). Photographs of the cheek retractor used included. Gift of W.W. Keen.   *[10b/37]*

– – – – –. See also nos. 138, *185.13,* 253, 466, 507, 603, 609, 669, 675, 684, 765, 1024.

492.   **Kimbrough, Robert Alexander, Jr.,** 1899-1967. Presidential address consisting of observations on the Obstetrical Society of Philadelphia. *Philadelphia, 1939.*

4 ff. 28 cm. Mimeographed. "Read . . . May 4th, 1939 . . . and endorsed by the Council of the Society . . . July 11, 1939." With second copy.   *[n.c.]*

493.   **King, Edgar Samuel John,** 1900-1966. The nature of the stroma of the ovary. *Melbourne, 1931.*

54 ff.; illus. 33 cm. Typewritten, photographs pasted in. – Alvarenga Prize Essay, no. 29, 1931. Unpublished.   *[ZZ 10d/3]*

494.   **[King, Rufus,** 1755-1827]. Collection of letters from English and European physicians on yellow fever. *London, 1798-1802.*

1 v. 24 cm. Addressed to King during his tenure as American Minister to the Court of St. James, following the Revolutionary War. Writers, with dates of their letters: Coenraad Gerard Ontyd, Sept. 3 and Dec. 16, 1798; April 25, 1799. – Benjamin Farmer, Nov. 4, 1798. – John Gooch, Dec. 21, 1798. – Sir Gilbert Blane, Dec. 30, 1798. – John Coakley Lettsom, Aug. 5, 1802. – William Martin Trinder [clergyman], Oct. 26, 1802. – Gift of King's grandson, Charles R. King, through W.F. Norris.   *[10a/146]*

495.   **Knight, Richard Payne,** 1750-1824. A discourse on the worship of Priapus and its connection with the mystic theology of the ancients . . . . To which is added an essay on the worship of the generative powers during the Middle Ages of western Europe. *Philadelphia, 1883-84.*

xvii, 256 pp.; xl plates. 30 cm. Handwritten by Abraham C.W. Beecher. Copy of the privately printed volume (London, 1865). – Presented by the heirs of Mrs. Louisa Webb.   *[Z 10/45]*

496.   **Knipe, Norman Leslie,** 1879?-1961.   Gynecology notes and quizzes (in connection with lectures of John G. Clark at the University of Pennsylvania).   *Philadelphia, 1903.*

1 v.; illus. 22 cm. Two ff. at end (presumably questions 1-6 of final examination) removed.   *[10a/462]*

497.   **Knopf, Siegmund Adolph,** b. 1857.   Modern prophylaxis of pulmonary tuberculosis and its treatment in special institutions and at home.   *New York, 1897?-98.*

[1], 133, [1] ff.; 8 folded tables, illus., plates. 36 cm. Typescript. Alvarenga Prize Essay, no. 7, 1898. Published, revised and enlarged (Philadelphia, 1899).   *[Z 10/30]*

498.   **Koch, Robert,** 1843-1910.   L'Etiologie de la tuberculose.   *Berlin, Juillet 1883.*

601 pp. 22 cm. Apparently unpublished translation of his *Die Aetiologie der Tuberkulose*, finished by Koch in July 1883, but not published until one year later in *Mitteilungen aus dem Kaiserlichen Gesundheitsamt*, vol. II. Assuming that the place and the date on the title and on p. 583 are correct, the manuscript antedates the first printing (this text is not to be confused with the much shorter version which appeared in 1882, cf. B. Möllers, *Robert Koch*, Hanover, 1950, pp. 551-52, 733-34). The French translation was written by a Frenchman (cf. the typically French number 5 and the style) for an unidentified recipient. The 53 illus. described on pp. 584-601 are not included.   *[10a/433]*

499.   **Kolbé, D.W. & Son.**   Illustrations of orthopaedic apparatus with explanatory texts.   *Philadelphia, late 19th cent.?*

Fragment of 15 ff. 24 cm. Not identical with the printed pamphlet of the same title, 2nd ed., 1871. Dr. G.G. Davis mentioned as designer of one (or more?) apparatus. — Very fragile.   *[10d/155]*

500.   **Koller, Hermann.**   Vorträge in Ophthalmologie.   *Berne?, ca. 1860.*

242 pp. 25 cm.   *[10a/67]*

501.   **Kolmer, John Albert,** 1886-1962.   Biographical notices, to 1941.   *Philadelphia, 1941.*

1 envelope. 28 cm. Typewritten. Besides brief biographical accounts, contains bibliography of papers published 1938-41, and of his books; two addresses given at commencement exercises; paper entitled "Dr. John A. Kolmer and Calvin Coolidge, Jr." (a first-person account of Kolmer's attendance on young Coolidge during his final illness).   *[10a/448]*

502.   —————. Collection of lectures on public health, preventive medicine, and syphilis, letters (chiefly to Fred B. Rogers) and schedules. *Philadelphia, 1952-57.*

1 box. 28 cm. Mainly typescript, some autograph.   *[10a/435]*

503.   —————. Outline of lectures, demonstration questions, exercises in bacteriology and parasitology at Temple University Medical School. *Philadelphia, 1938-39.*

[41] ff. 28 cm. Typescript and 5 ff. manuscript. Includes schedules and a letter of inquiry.   *[10a/471]*

504.   —————. Syphilis and marriage in relation to specific therapy. *Philadelphia, 1926.*

1 envelope ([1], 10 ff.). 37.5 cm. Typescript (carbon copy). Published in *Trans. & Stud.*, ser. 3, v. 48: 178-85 (1926).   *[10d/156]*

—————. See also nos. 244, 962.

505.   **Konkle, Burton Alva,** 1861-1944. A history of the medical profession of Philadelphia, from 1638 to 1897. *Philadelphia?, 1897.*

520 pp. 32 cm. Unrevised manuscript of five main chapters written for the history of the medical profession of Philadelphia, edited by Dr. Frederick P. Henry in 1897. Presented to the College of Physicians by the author. The published version corresponds closely in its first 433 pages; it includes also several chapters by other writers. Konkle, however, is not named, described only as "an experienced historian in the employ of the publishers." — Fragile: paper brittle.   *[10a/158]*

506.   **Krecker, William Henry,** b. 1860. A list of anomalies found… in the dissecting room of the University of Pennsylvania. *Philadelphia, 1880-83.*

40, [4 blank] ff.; xii col. plates pasted on ff. 29-40. 25 cm. Presented by J. Montgomery Deaver.   *[10a/251]*

507.   **Krumbhaar, Edward Bell,** 1882-1966, comp. Autograph collection. *V.p., 1799-1947.*

2 boxes (ca. 1200 pieces). 32 cm. Includes autographs of J.L.M. Alibert, Claude Bernard, Robley Dunglison, T.D. Mütter and letters to EBK from: F.G. Banting, W.B. Cannon, Alexis Carrel, H.W. Cushing, J.F. Fulton, F.H. Garrison, A.V. Hill, Cordell Hull, W.W. Keen, W.T. Longcope (50 letters), W.G. MacCallum (10), R.T. McKenzie, Wm. Osler, D'Arcy Power, David Riesman, G.C. Robinson (29), F.D. Roosevelt (4, 1933-1936), F.P. Rous (12), George Sarton, C.J. Singer, Wm. H. Taft, N.P. Tendeloo (9), and Wm. H. Welch (12). The main strength is in the period 1910-40. An alphabetical name index is filed with the collection. — Gift of E.B. Krumbhaar.   *[Z 10/124]*

508.   —————. Autopsies, inquests, and post mortems in colonial New England. *Philadelphia, ca. 1946-47.*

> 31, [3] ff. 28 cm. Typewritten (carbon copy, with some handwritten corrections and annotations). 3 ff. notes in E.B. Krumbhaar's hand, undated letter on autopsies from Eva L. Butler (2 ff.), typewritten extracts (4 ff.); reprint of his "History of the Autopsy and Its Relation to the Development of Modern Medicine" (*Hospitals*, April 1938; 4 ff.) enclosed.   *[ZZ 8c/20]*

509.   —————. Bills, correspondence, packing lists, reports, concerning Base Hospital Unit no. 10. *Philadelphia, etc., 1917.*

> 1 box. 39 cm. Typewritten (incl. carbons). Primarily orders from Arthur H. Thomas Company, Philadelphia for laboratory equipment, charged to the American Red Cross, Southeastern Division of Pennsylvania.   *[ZZ 10d/11]*

510.   —————. Collected reprints, book reviews, abstracts, historical and other miscellaneous medical papers. *Philadelphia, etc., 1913-61.*

> 7 v. (v. I-IV bound [29 cm], V-VII in boxes [32 cm]). Printed, typewritten and handwritten. Contents: v. I-II, printed items. — v. III, book reviews, 1913-31 (280 pp.); abstracts, 1923-25 (pp. 281-301); misc. papers incl. "Experimental and Clinical Studies in Hemolytic Jaundice . . . with Special Reference to the Effects of Splenectomy," address before the N.Y. Academy of Medicine, 1916? (30 pp., pp. 302 to end). — v. IV, reprints; book reviews, 1932-39; abstracts, 1933-37. — v. V, reprints, 1937-49. — v. VI, reprints; historical texts (Philadelphia Heart Assoc., General Hospital [Blockley], University of Pennsylvania Pathology Department), eulogies, etc. — v. VII, reprints; book reviews, 1951-61; paper on the role of the spleen. V. I-IV with E.B. Krumbhaar's detailed index.   *[Z 10/232]*

511.   —————. Comparative histology of spleen and other hemopoietic organs. *Mt. Desert, Me., etc., 1928-31.*

> 11 ff. 32 cm. Handwritten notes and drawings. With a letter from Harry M. Kaufman, 1931 July 22, Washington, D.C. (1 p., 28 cm., typescript signed).   *[ZZ 10c/8]*

512.   —————. Comparative psychology (examination paper). *Cambridge, Harvard University, ca. 1904.*

> 8 ff., 2 ff. laid in. 23 cm.   *[10c/88]*

513.   —————. A comparison of the method of thought of the alchemists and of the chemists of the 18th century. *Philadelphia or Cambridge, Mass., 1902.*

> 13 pp. 26.5 cm. Paper written for course in history of chemistry at Harvard University.   *[ZZ 10c/10]*

514.   — — — —. Correspondence. *V.p., 1944-48.*

1 envelope (17 folders). 39 cm. Among correspondents in this group are James B. Conant, George W. Corner, John F. Fulton, Archibald V. Hill, Chauncey D. Leake, Roger I. Lee, Warfield T. Longcope, Joe V. Meigs, George R. Minot, and Isidor S. Ravdin.   *[n.c.]*

515.   — — — —. Correspondence and reports, etc. *V.p., 1900-64.*

1 box. 31 cm. The collection contains visiting cards of S.W. Mitchell and Sir Lander Branton (3) introducing Dr. Krumbhaar; many letters by him and colleagues, incl. those of Paul Diepgen (1939, 2 ff.), John F. Fulton (1931-57, 4 ff.), F.H. Garrison (1927-34, 29 ff.), F.L. Gates (1924-25, 3 ff.), W.E. Gye (1925, 2 ff.), R.H. Halsey (with K.'s carbons, 1920, 9 ff.), E.R. Long (1949-56, 5 ff.), W.T. Longcope (1915-50, 13 ff. and reprint), G.R. Minot (1927-46, 4 ff.), G.C. Robinson (1919-50, 12 ff.), Theobald Smith (1933, 4 ff. and facs.), and Hans Zinsser (1929-37, 3 ff.); letters and documents relating to Dr. K.'s service with the Medical Corps of the Pennsylvania National Guard (1912-14); reproductions of 5 letters from Franklin D. Roosevelt (1933-36); few miscellaneous items.   *[10d/146]*

516.   — — — —. Correspondence as editor of the *American Journal of Medical Sciences*. *V.p., 1929, 1936.*

4 boxes (xviii folders). 39 cm. Besides letters to a wide variety of actual and potential contributors, the correspondence includes letters from sponsors or advisers, and many from and to the publisher, Lea and Febiger. — In approximate alphabetical order.   *[n.c.]*

517.   — — — —. Correspondence between the editor of *Clio medica* and contributors (potential and actual), advisors, etc. *V.p., 1927-43.*

6 boxes; illus. 31 cm. Typewritten (incl. carbons) and handwritten; few printed items. Box 6 is confined to correspondence, etc., with the publisher Paul B. Hoeber.   *[ZZ 10d/7]*

518.   — — — —. Correspondence file, Miscellany I. *V.p., 1926-39.*

1 box (5 folders). 37 cm. Includes mimeographed and printed items. Contents: Folder 1. *Physiological Reviews*, incl. Dr. Krumbhaar's classified list of articles printed, and of suggested articles (1926). — 2. 13th International Physiological Congress, Boston (1929), largely concerned with local financial support for the Congress. — 3. Medical museums, with emphasis on pathological specimens (1930-31). — 4. Medical Library Association (1933-39). — 5. Sigma XΛ (1930-32).   *[n.c.]*

519.   — — — —   — — — —, Miscellany II. *V.p., 1919-38.*

1 box (6 folders). 37 cm. Includes a few mimeographed items. Contents: Folder 1. Medical history lectures, University of Pennsylvania Medical School, etc. (1931-32), incl. correspondence with John F. Fulton, Francis R. Packard, David Riesman, Joseph P. Walsh, Eugene F. Du Bois, Charles W.

Burr, George W. Corner, Warfield T. Longcope, etc. — 2-3. Open medical positions (1930-38). — 4. Resolutions upon the death of Thomas B. Holloway (1936). — 5. F.H. Garrison correspondence (1919-29). — 6. William Pepper correspondence (1927-32). *[n.c.]*

520.   ————— —————, Miscellany III, incl. some extraneous items. *V.p., 1924-44.*

3 folders in box. 31 cm. Contents: Folder 1. Correspondence relating to the meeting of the American Society for Experimental Pathology (1924); correspondence relating to the Federation of American Societies for Experimental Pathology (1929-32). — 2. Miscellaneous correspondence (1927-44, but mainly 1933), incl. G.R. Minot, Victor Gomoiu, W.T. Longcope, Louise Pierce, J.F. Fulton, etc. — 3. Correspondence re position of superintendant at Chestnut Hill Hospital (1931-32); bacteriologist at Dept. of Medicine, University of Pennsylvania (1931-32), and pathologist (*ibid.*, 1931-33); items (incl. correspondence) re University of Pennsylvania Bicentennial (1940); certification by American Board of Pathology (1936-38); W.H. Lewis' election to honorary membership in the Philadelphia Pathological Society; correspondence to and by Dr. Krumbhaar as editor of the *American Journal of the Medical Sciences* (1929); letter by Dr. Krumbhaar to Dr. Fishbein on hemolytic jaundice (1936). *[ZZ 10d/10]*

521.   ————— ————— relating to cancer research and radium poisoning. *V.p., 1923-31.*

1 box (5 folders). 39 cm. Incl. mimeographed, photostated and printed items. The two folders on cancer research and the "Glover Serum" include letters from Francis C. Wood; three on radium poisoning, many from James Ewing; folder marked III contains photostat of hearings in the Chancery of New Jersey, Grace Fryer, Albina Larice, *et al.* against the U.S. Radium Corp. (1927; 103, 26 ff.). *[n.c.]*

522.   ————— ————— relating to medical institutions in Philadelphia. *Philadelphia, etc., 1928-39.*

1 box (4 folders). 39 cm. Incl. mimeographed and printed items. Contents: Thomas W. Evans Museum and Dental Institute, School of Dentistry of the University of Pennsylvania (2 folders, 1937-39). — Chestnut Hill Hospital (1937-39). — Henry Phipps Institute, Philadelphia (1928-32). *[n.c.]*

523.   ————— ————— relating to medical societies. *V.p., 1921-32.*

1 box (5 folders). 39 cm. Incl. mimeographed and printed materials. Societies represented: American Heart Association, Philadelphia Heart Association, Pathological Society of Philadelphia, Medical Society of the State of Pennsylvania, Society for Protection of Scientific Research (incl. printed vol., *Hearing on Senate Bill S. 4497*), Federation of American Societies for Experimental Biology. *[n.c.]*

524.   ————— ————— relating to the College of Physicians. *Philadelphia, etc., 1937-38.*

1 box (2 envelopes). 27 x 40 cm. Incl. considerable correspondence between Dr. Krumbhaar and W.B. McDaniel; most of the items relate to the library and the garden of the College of Physicians of Philadelphia. Contains some mimeographed and printed materials, incl. copy of the Charter of 1935 with pencilled annotations.   *[ZZ 10d/8]*

525.   ————— ————— relating to the Philadelphia General Hospital. *V.p., 1920s-1930s.*

1 box (6 folders). 39 cm. Incl. many reports, printed and mimeographed items, clippings, etc. Contents: General correspondence (2 folders). — Clinical-pathological conferences (2 folders). — Radiology Department (2 folders).   *[n.c.]*

526.   —————. ————— relating to the University Hospital and the Medical School of the University of Pennsylvania. *V.p., 1920s-1930s.*

2 boxes (13 folders). 39 cm. Incl. reports, statistics, printed items, etc. Contents: I. University Hospital; Hospital Medical Board; Graduate School of Medicine; School of Medicine, Pathology Dept. — II. School of Medicine, Pathology Dept. (cont.); G.W. Wagoner, "Experimental Pathology"; autopsy reports; staff and staff positions; Journal Club; research and misc.   *[n.c.]*

527.   ————— ————— relating to the University of Pennsylvania (excl. Medical School and Hospitals). *Philadelphia, etc., 1925-39.*

2 boxes (10 envelopes). 27 × 40 cm. Incl. mimeographed and printed items.   *[n.c.]*

528.   ————— —————, United States Army Officers' Reserve Corps (1923-27) — New York World's Fair, Committee on Blood Diseases and Medicine and Public Health (1937-39). *V.p., 1923-39.*

1 box (2 envelopes). 27 cm. Incl. mimeographed and printed items.   *[10c/153]*

529.   ————— ————— with colleagues, publishers, booksellers, institutes, foundations, etc. *V.p., 1931, 1935-39.*

9 boxes (150 folders). 27 × 32 cm. Contents: Boxes 1-2, 1931. — Boxes 3-4, 1935 and 1936 (A-K). — 5, 1936 (L-Z). — 6-7, 1937 and 1938 (A-L). — 8, 1938 (M-Z). — 9, 1939. Incl. correspondence with Charles W. Burr, Charles S. Burwell, Elliott C. Cutler, Warfield T. Longcope, Eugene P. Pendergrass, Henry E. Sigerist and George W. Wagoner, the American Association for the Advancement of Science, the American College of Physicians, and the International Congress of the History of Medicine, 1935. — More detailed list is on file.   *[ZZ 10d/9]*

530.   —————. Diaries, and notes during Krumbhaar's journey to France and service at Base Hospital no. 10, Le Tréport, Normandy, May 19, 1917 to 1919. *Le Tréport, 1917-19.*

3 v. 12-15 cm. Includes notes of cases, arrivals of wounded, activities of Mrs.
Krumbhaar, who accompanied him, off-duty trips, etc.   *[10c/111]*

531.   — — — — —. Documents relating to his career. *Philadelphia, etc.,
1912-17, 1951, 1961.*

11 ff. 28-32 cm.   *[10c/69]*

532.   — — — — —. Early personal correspondence, photographs, memorabilia, etc. *V.p., 1899-1916.*

1 envelope. 31 cm. Incl. visiting card of S. Weir Mitchell, introducing E.B.
Krumbhaar, letters from German relatives, etc.   *[ZZ 8c/32]*

533.   — — — — —. Editorial (on the Pennsylvania Hospital). *Philadelphia, 1951.*

1 envelope. 31 cm. Manuscript and typescript (2 carbons, with notes). Published in *Annals of Internal Medicine*, v. 34: 1280-83 (1951). Included are letters
to the author from Garfield G. Duncan and others, concerning the editorial.
                                                              [ZZ 8c/38]

534.   — — — — —. Fish blood studies. *Salisbury Cove, Me., etc., 1929-33.*

1 envelope; illus. 32 cm. Notes, drawings, etc., and correspondence with
Warren H. Lewis, Margaret Reed Lewis, M.M. Wintrobe and Joseph D.
Aronson (1929-33).   *[ZZ 8c/30]*

535.   — — — — — — — — —. Notes and sketches on blood cells of
fishes, with 1 frog toad. *Ibid., 1937.*

1 folder; illus. 34 cm.   *[ZZ 8c/31]*

536.   — — — — —. Gassed autopsies at 16 Gen. Hospital, B.E.F., France,
May 1917 to February 1919. *V.p., ca. 1918-42.*

1 v., 1 portfolio ([13, 2] ff., 7 ff. proofs, 1 folded graph). 28.5 cm. Typewritten.
The author's collection of case histories and autopsy reports. Some published
in his paper, "The Blood and Bone Marrow in Yellow Cross Gas (Mustard Gas)
Poisoning... [with Helen D. Krumbhaar]," *J. Med. Res.* 40: 497-507 (1919), and
plates XXI and XXII; reprint pasted in. Page proof of Leukocythosis Induced
by Methyl-Acetamide with P-Chloro-Xylenol, by B. Zondek and Y.M.
Bromberg included. Accompanied by portfolio of mss. and notes related to
Krumbhaar's article.   *[ZZ 8c/35]*

537.   — — — — —. Histology, general pathology and histopathology
drawings. *Philadelphia, 1904-06.*

3 v. (envelopes); illus. 21 cm (box, 32 cm). Pencil drawings made by Dr.
Krumbhaar while a medical student, University of Pennsylvania. Contents:
V. 1. Histology and embryology, 168 drawings. — V. 2. Pathology, 103
drawings. — V. 3. Histopathology, 50 drawings.   *[ZZ 10a/11]*

538. –––––. A historical sketch of the School of Medicine of the University of Pennsylvania. *Philadelphia, etc., 1952-53.*

1 envelope. 31 cm. Typescript (carbons) with manuscript corrections, notes, and correspondence with W.D. Stroud, etc., concerning the article, published in the July 1953 issue of *Postgraduate Medicine,* v. 14 (1): 1-5 (1953).

[ZZ 8c/25]

39a. –––––. History of the pathology of the heart. *Philadelphia, etc., 1950-53.*

1 envelope; illus. 38 cm. Manuscript, typescript (carbons), films and photostats, and correspondence with S.E. Gould. Published as chapter in the original edition of Gould's *Pathology of the Heart* (Springfield, Ill., 1953).

[ZZ 8c/21]

39b. –––– –––––. *Philadelphia, etc., ca. 1956.*

1 envelope; illus. 34 cm. Incl. correspondence with S.E. Gould concerning publication of the second edition (1960). *[ZZ 8c/26]*

40. –––––. Lecture notes, 2nd half first year at the Department of Medicine, University of Pennsylvania. *Philadelphia, 1904-05.*

201 pp. (pp. 95-6, 121-2, 143-4, 151-2 removed; 2 loose ff. inserted between pp. 19-20 and 66-7); illus. 27 cm. Contents: Anatomy (G.A. Piersol). – Physiological chemistry (John Marshall [cf. inside front cover, Taylor named on p. 91 not included]). – Etiology (A.J. Smith). *[ZZ 10a/13]*

41. –––––. Material for a third edition of Castiglioni-Krumbhaar's *History of Medicine* (never published), consisting of correspondence, notes, pamphlets and clippings. *V.p., ca. 1948-53.*

1 box; illus. 30 cm. Among letters are few by A. Castiglioni, J.F. Fulton, and E.B. Krumbhaar. Notes and commentary on printed items by E.B. Krumbhaar. Added a folder with text and another with photographs, on myasthenia gravis. *[10c/76]*

42. –––––. Medical progress in the past 50 years. *Philadelphia, 1954.*

6 ff. (2 copies, ff. 10-17), [3] ff. 28 cm. Typescript (carbon) with manuscript corrections, of talk given at reunion of Class of 1904, Harvard University; notes and correspondence included. *[ZZ 8c/29]*

43. –––––. Memoir of Balduin Lucké (1889-1954). *Philadelphia, 1954.*

1 folder. 33 cm. Manuscript, typescripts, galley proof, representing several versions, notes, and correspondence. Published in *Trans. & Stud.,* ser. 4, v. 22: 146-48 (1955) and elsewhere. With these is: "Osmotic Properties and Permeability of Cancer Cells. I.", by Balduin Lucké and Arthur K. Parpart (reprinted for private circulation from *Cancer Research,* v. 14: 75-80 [1954]).

[ZZ 8c/17]

544. —————. North American medical superstitions. *Philadelphia?,*
      1950.

      1 envelope. 38 cm. Summary, notes, and correspondence, prepared for the
      Sixth International Congress of the History of Science, Amsterdam, 1950.
      [ZZ 8c/18]

545. —————. Notebook. *Holland and Philadelphia, 1917-27.*

      17 ff., xxi-lxxi (verso; incl. blank) pp.; illus. 21 cm. Notes on classification of
      kidney disorders, by Ludwig Aschoff and N.P. Tendeloo, on the latter's
      Allgemeine Pathologie, 1919; M.H. Jacob's graduate class in physical chemistry,
      University of Pennsylvania (1927).   *[10c/90]*

546. —————. Notes and correspondence for an unfinished histori-
      cal article on "The Care of the Wounded," and correspondence
      with Arthur M. Walker, etc. *Philadelphia?, 1952-54?*

      11 ff. and pamphlet. 26.5 cm. With this is "Military Preventive Medicine"
      by James Stevens Simmons (extract from *Armed Forces Medical Journal*, v.
      2: 785-97 [1951]) and catalogue of the series *Technical Bulletins of the Department
      of Medicine and Surgery of the Veterans Administration.*   *[ZZ 10c/7]*

547. —————. Notes on lectures by members of the medical faculty,
      University of Vienna, in the summer courses, 1906. *Vienna,*
      1906.

      59 ff. (numbered I-LX in reverse, XXVI and LVI omitted); diagrs. 20 cm. In
      German. Notes on rectos and versos. Includes Alfred Fuchs, Pathologie und
      Therapie der Nervenkrankheiten; Walther Pick, Hautkrankheiten; Anton
      Ghon, Grosse Pathologie; Otto Marburg, Histologie des menschlichen Zentral-
      nervensystems; Leo von Zumbusch, Dermatologie; Karl von Stejskal, Innere
      Medizin.   *[10a/420]*

548. —————. Notes on the halometer, eriometer, and other meth-
      ods of cell measurement. *Philadelphia, 1933-35?*

      1 envelope; graphs, illus. 37 cm. Manuscript notes, diagrams, and typed
      copies of book reviews by various authors.   *[ZZ 8c/39]*

549. —————. Notes taken during a journey to England, Holland &
      Germany, in 1927. *V.p., 1927.*

      105 pp., [7] ff. incl. blanks, 18 pp., [3] ff.; illus. 13.5 cm. Notes visits to
      laboratories and lectures. Ff. 1-18 at end, numbered in reverse, list Leyden
      theses of the 16th and 17th centuries, and include notes on the Elzevier
      publishing firm.   *[10c/110]*

550. —————. On collecting Elzeviers; with notes on the Elzevier
      Collection in the University of Pennsylvania Library. *Philadel-*
      phia, 1956.

1 envelope; illus. 32 cm. Includes correspondence, portrait of Dr. Krumbhaar, and reproduction of an Elzevier printer's block. Published in *The Library Chronicle*, v. 23: 1-15 (1957).   *[ZZ 10c/28]*

551.   —————. On the history of extirpation of the spleen. *Philadelphia, 1914.*

1 envelope. 30 cm. Manuscript and 2 versions of typescript (carbon). Read before the Historical Section of the College of Physicians of Philadelphia, November 12, 1914, and published in *New York Medical Journal*, v. 101: 232-34 (1915).   *[ZZ 8c/19]*

552.   —————. Osler in Philadelphia. *Philadelphia, 1948?-49.*

1 envelope. 33 cm. Typescript (22, [1] ff.) and two carbons (12 ff. each), notes, and correspondence with N.C. Gilbert concerning the article. Published in *Archives of Internal Medicine*, v. 84: 26-33 (1949) under title "Additional Notes on Osler in Philadelphia."   *[ZZ 8c/27]*

553.   —————. The Pennsylvania Hospital. *Philadelphia, 1951-52.*

1 folder; illus. 38 cm. Contains primarily the ms. of "The Pennsylvania Hospital" (incl. correspondence with L.P. Eisenhart) written for *Transactions of the American Philosophical Society*, v. 43, pt. 1: 237-46 (1953). Added: *Pennsylvania Hospital . . . Founded 1751* (printed pamphlet); "Babel in Medicine," by O.H. Perry Pepper (repr.: *Proceedings, Amer. Phil. Soc.*, v. 94, no. 4: 364-68 [1950]) and EBK's "Days at the Pennsylvania Hospital During Its First Century" (repr.: *Amer. Jour. of Med.*, v. 11: 540-45 [1951]).   *[ZZ 8c/12]*

554.   —————. Physiology experiments, University of Pennsylvania, School of Medicine. *Philadelphia, 1906.*

1 envelope; diagrs., graphs. 30 cm.   *[10c/86]*

555.   —————. Polygraph records. *Philadelphia, 1914.*

1 v. ([1], 39 ff., rest blank); illus. 22 cm. One hundred and thirteen patient polygraphs with annotations pertaining to cardiovascular conditions. With index and table of contents; 16 further records laid in.   *[10a/419]*

556.   —————. Radium in pituitary. *Philadelphia, 1924.*

1 envelope (50 small and 8 lettersize ff.); illus., 3 photographs. 30 cm. Notes of experiments on dogs made in cooperation with J.E. Sweet. Unpublished.   *[ZZ 10a/10]*

557.   —————. Relic list and bibliography of the Siamese twins, at the College of Physicians of Philadelphia. *Philadelphia, 1923.*

[8] pp. 22 cm. Typewritten.   *[10a/447]*

558. —————. Repeated agglutination tests by the Dreyer method in the diagnosis of enteric (fever) in inoculated individuals, by E.B. Krumbhaar with the assistance of W.B. Smith. *Philadelphia?, 1918.*

> 37 ff. 33 cm. Incl. notes, and correspondence with F.F. Russell, Eugene R. Whitmore, and J.F. Siler.   *[ZZ 10a/15]*

559. —————. Review of *Letters of Benjamin Rush*, ed. by L.H. Butterfield. *Philadelphia, etc., 1951.*

> 1 folder. 32 cm. Incl. correspondence with Owsei Temkin. Published in *Bulletin of the History of Medicine*, v. 26: 393-7 (1952).   *[ZZ 8c/13]*

560. —————. Some notes on the early days of the American Association of the History of Medicine. *Philadelphia, etc., 1945.*

> 1 envelope. 37 cm. Typescripts (2 versions) with manuscript corrections, galley-proofs, and correspondence with Benjamin Spector and Owsei Temkin. Read at the 1949 annual meeting of the Association and published in *Bulletin of the History of Medicine*, v. 23: 577-82 (1949).   *[ZZ 8c/14]*

561. —————. Special B[one] M[arrow] studies. *Philadelphia, etc., 1942.*

> 1 envelope. 38 cm. Incl. reports of collaborators. — Largely animal experiments. — Fragile.   *[n.c.]*

562. —————. The spleen. *Philadelphia, 1949-50.*

> 1 envelope. 32 cm. With notes, and correspondence with Michael G. Wohl and Frederick A. Coller, etc. Published, in collaboration with R. Philip Custer, as chapter "The Reticulo-Endothelial System and Spleen" in John H. Musser, ed., *Internal Medicine* (5th ed., 1951). Added: "Pan-Marrow Hematopoeiesis (L. Casei Factor) and Splenic Hematopenia: Experimental and Clinical Studies", by Charles A. Doan, reprinted from *Proceedings of the Institute of Medicine of Chicago*, v. 16, no. 6 (June 15, 1946).   *[ZZ 8c/15]*

563. —————. The state of pathology in the British colonies of North America. *Philadelphia, etc., 1946-47.*

> 1 envelope. 33 cm. Incl. notes, photostats and negatives, and correspondence with John R. Paul and E. Ashworth Underwood concerning the article. Several versions. Read as Carmalt Lecture to the Beaumont Medical Club, New Haven and published in *Yale Journal of Biology and Medicine*, v. 19: 801-15 (1947) and reprinted, with alterations, in *Science, Medicine and History; Essays... in Honor of Charles Singer* (Oxford, 1953), v. 2: 129-40.   *[ZZ 8c/22]*

564. —————. Thoughts on bibliographies and Harvey's writings. *Philadelphia, etc., 1956-57.*

> 1 envelope. 31 cm. Incl. correspondence with John F. Fulton, etc., concerning the article and carbon copy of W.B. McDaniel's "Harvey and the College of

Physicians of Philadelphia." Published in Harvey issue of *Journal of the History of Medicine and Allied Sciences*, v. 12: 235-40 (1957).   *[ZZ 8c/28]*

565.   —————. Tissue cultures. *Philadelphia, 1928.*

[2], 17 ff.; illus. 28 cm. Handwritten notes and drawings.   *[ZZ 10c/9]*

—————. See also nos. 45, 86, 101, 178, 183, *185.13,* 189, 409, 452, 467, 581, 754, 792, 1018, 1040, 1051, 1053, 1067, 1085.

566.   **Kuhn, Adam,** 1741-1817. Introductory lectures. *Philadelphia, last quarter 18th cent.?*

1 v. 22 cm. Inscribed on leaf following the title-page: "Dr. Adam Kuhn's lectures when professor in University of Pennsylvania W Kuhn."   *[10a/73]*

567.   —————. Lectures on the institutes of medecine[!]. *Philadelphia, 1789-97.*

2 v. in 1. 21.5 cm. Inscribed on title-page of v. 2: "W Kuhn." – Presented by John H. Packard.   *[10a/68]*

568.   —————. Lectures on the materia medica. *Philadelphia, last quarter 18th cent.*

2 v. 27.5 cm.   *[10a/70]*

569.   ———— —————. *Ibid., same period.*

1 v. 22.5 cm. This ms. and the preceding gifts of John H. Packard.   *[10a/71]*

570.   ———— —————, written by Marcus Kuhl. *Ibid., ca. 1790.*

3 v. 20.5 cm.   *[10a/74]*

571.   —————. Lectures on the practice of medecine[!]. Vol. I. *Philadelphia, 1789-97.*

1 v. 21.5 cm. Presented by John H. Packard.   *[10a/69]*

572.   —————. Lectures on the practice of physic . . . . *Philadelphia, 1794.*

90, [1] pp. 20.5 cm.   *[10a/75]*

573.   —————. Lectures on yellow fever. *Philadelphia, 1794.*

1 v. (17 pp., pp. [17-97]; 11, [10] ff.). 34.5 cm. Autograph. The date 1794 is derived from the statement on p. [71] "last summer 1793." The manuscript deals with origin, prophylaxis, treatment and spread of yellow fever, with references to published literature and opinions of medical authorities, among these extracts from "Essay on Fevers" by Dr. Robert Robertson (p. 7), statements of Robert Jackson, Noah Webster, Colin Chisholm, William

Hillary, Benjamin Moseley, William Cullen, James Lind, Jean Devèze, William Currie, etc. The lectures refer to outbreaks in many areas, but especially in the West Indies and Philadelphia (cf. mention of the sloop *Amelia*, the warship *Sans Culotte* and the ship *Flora*). Pages [79-89, 95] deal with the case of Dr. James Hutchinson, involving Samuel Coates (misspelled Coats) and Kuhn's controversy with Benjamin Rush. Various references to the hospital at Bush Hill. [Z 10/6]

574. —————. Notes from a course of lectures on the materia medica. *Philadelphia, last quarter 18th cent.*

269, [7] pp. 24 cm. Signature of Thos. C. James on front flyleaf. Bookplate of Hugh Lenox Hodge inside front cover. [10a/72]

575. —————. Notes from Dr. Kuhn's lectures on materia medica. *Philadelphia, 1778-79?*

v. 2 (only). 20 cm. Inscribed in pencil on title-page: "by Dr. Morris," who may be John Morris, 1759-93. — The dates are uncertain; Kuhn is said to have left Philadelphia for the West Indies after the withdrawal of the British in June, 1778, not returning until 1780. [10a/76]

576. —————. Notes from the lectures on the practice of physic . . . taken by Mr. Stratton. *Philadelphia, last quarter 18th cent.*

136 pp. 21.5 cm. Interleaved; some blank leaves with additions. — On front flyleaf: Thomas C. James. [10a/77]

—————. See also nos. *185.13, 224, 1049.*

577. **Laënnec, Réné Théophile Hyacinthe,** 1781-1826. Cours de medecine . . . 1ère année. *Paris, 1825.*

[1], 157 ff. 26 cm. Title (f. [1]r) signed Dufour, presumably identifying the student. Main headings: Anatomie pathologique (f. 1); Des maladies générales (f. 42); Des maladies locales (f. 116v). Lectures delivered at the Collège de France. "Cours de l'année 1825 . . . (f. 156v)." [Z 10/96]

—————. See also nos. *57, 605.*

578. **La Roche, Réné,** 1795-1872. Material on music. *Philadelphia, 1830s-1840s?*

1 box (3 folders, 9 small envelopes). 39 cm. Autograph with corrections, additions (attached in a variety of ways) and footnotes in envelopes. In 3 sections: Observations of the ancient music of the Chinese; Use of music in the practice of religious worship; Music around the world (characteristic differences; icplt.). Summary description, unsigned but by Karen Adelmann, filed with collection. [n.c.]

579.   ─────. Treatise on fevers. *Philadelphia, ca. 1855-58.*

   3 boxes. 31.5 cm. Incomplete draft of an unpublished work on fevers,
   including chapters on acclimatization, temperament, treatment, malaria,
   periodicity, and idiopathic fever. Lengthy sections on yellow fever (Box 1 and
   2) are in part taken from his *Treatise on Yellow Fever* (1855); some are altered and
   expanded. Mentioned in F.P. Henry, *Standard History*, p. 209, also in
   correspondence of Ayres P. Merrill, Nashville, Tenn.; photocopies attached
   (originals in La Roche Papers, American Philosophical Society). ─ Box 3
   contains material on paludal, periodic, malarial, intermittent and remittent
   fevers, treated in the same fashion as yellow fever; also fugitives, miscellany,
   footnotes, and 3 drafts of a bibliography for the projected treatise.
   [ZZ 10a/19]

580.   [─────]. Collection mainly of letters to R. La Roche. *V.p.,
   1818-69.*

   2 boxes. 39.5 cm. The main part is alphabetically arranged and accompanied
   by typewritten list (168 nos.). A few extraneous items (e.g. a letter of "Ventose
   an 6" [Feb. 1799] by L.D.A. Boceffey to a botanist colleague) are included. Added to box 2: folder with 31 letters and envelope with few originals and with
   photocopies. ─ The letters cover a wide range of subjects, among them
   publications, appointments, medical problems, etc.   *[n.c.]*

   ─────. See also nos. 154, 361, 416.

581.   **Larrabee, Ralph Clinton,** 1870-1935. Chronic congestive splenomegaly. *Boston, 1934.*

   1 envelope. 38 cm. Correspondence (involving F. Parker, Jr., the author, and
   E.B. Krumbhaar), history, case records, galley proofs, etc. Concerns cases and
   observations at the Mallory Institute of Pathology of the Boston City
   Hospital. The galley proofs are from the *American Journal of the Medical Sciences*
   (publ. in v. 188: 754-60 [1934]). ─ Fragile.   *[ZZ 10a/14]*

582.   **Lataste, J.** The condition of fractured limbs after union. *Philadelphia, 1885.*

   [1], 47, 33 ff. 33 cm. Handwritten and typed (corrected) translation by Émile
   Perrot of Lataste's thesis, originally published under the title *De l'etat des
   membres fracturés après la consolidation* (Paris, 1880). Presented to the Lewis
   Library by W.F. Actee.   *[Z 10/105]*

583.   **Latimer, Matthias Randolph,** b. 1833. An inaugural essay on
   scarlet fever, presented to the faculty of the Philadelphia College
   of Medicine, for the degree of doctor in medicine, by M.
   Randolph Latimer, . . . Maryland. *Philadelphia, May 1855.*

   Title, 1 blank, 32 ff. (last blank), 25 cm.   *[n.c.]*

584.   **Latta, William Sutton,** d. 1872. Entries in Physicians' Registry
   of Births and Deaths. *Chester County, Pa., 1852-55.*

   1 v. 20 cm. Incl. copy of Registration Act (1852).   *[10c/137]*

585. **Lawrence, John,** 1747?-1830. Oratio sive sermo academicus, de honoribus quos gentes sapientissimae et maximè celebres, in veros medicinae cultores contulerunt. *Philadelphia, 1768.*

[1], 11 ff.; port. 19 cm. Thesis — MB (University of Pennsylvania). "A Johanne Lawrence habita — primis publicis Academiae commitiis, ad gradus medicos conferendos, qui pro gradu baccalaureatus in medicina prostitit." Signature of Lawrence (spelled here Laurence) on f. 11 verso. The original text and an English translation were published in *Fugitive Leaves* of College of Physicians of Philadelphia, n.s., nos. 2-4 (1956) and in *Trans. e² Stud.*, ser. 4, v. 25: 41-52 (1957-58). Pasted in as frontispiece portrait of Lawrence after a painting by Sully. *[10a/79]*

586. **Lazarevich, Ivan Pavlovich,** 1829-1902. Atlas of gynaecological and obstetrical instrument . . . for the International Medical Congress, Philadelphia 1876. — On the three most important obstetrical instruments. *Kharkov, 1876.*

2 v.; plates. 32 and 27 cm. Vol. 2 was published in the *Trans. Int. Med. Congress* (Phila., 1876). Deposited by the Obstetrical Society of Philadelphia.
[Z 10/21]

587. **Leidy, Joseph,** 1823-1891. Note book. *Philadelphia, 1841-42.*

1 v. 19 cm. Contents: Notes taken from (John) Hunter on the blood; commenced July 6 (-Oct. 8) 1841 (15 pp., unfinished). — (Beginning in back of volume:) Notes from the Principles and practice of surgery by Sir Astley Cooper, 5.19.42 (106 pp.) — Notes taken from the lectures of Dr. (George Bacon) Wood on the proximate principles of plants, etc., Univ. of Penna., October 1842 (19 pp.). — Gift of Joseph Leidy, Jr.   *[10b/12]*

588. **————.** Notes to his course on anatomy at the University of Pennsylvania Department of Medicine. *Philadelphia, n.d.*

1 box (183 pieces in 14 envelopes). 31.5 cm. Contents: Envelope 1. Circulatory system (13 pieces). — 2. Digestive system (14). — 3. Ears and nose (5). — 4. Eye (15). — 5. Glandular system (7). — 6. Introductory lectures and embryology (6). — 7. Muscular system (10). — 8. Nervous system and brain (55). — 9. Respiratory system (2). — 10. Skeletal system (23). — 11. Skin (7). — 12. Urogenital system (16). — 13. Various tissues (10). — 14. Miscellany, incl. proofs of chapter of Leidy's *Human Anatomy*, 2d ed., and receipts signed by Leidy to William Horner. Notes are written on backs of invitations, letters, handbills, etc., among which are autographs of William Hunt, Thomas H. Andrews, Anna Lea Merritt, Isaac Jones Wistar, George Washington Tryon, and others. — Gift of Oscar V. Batson.   *[10c/130]*

589. **[————].** Correspondence. *V.p., 1850-90.*

6 boxes (ca. 2,900 items). 31.5 cm. Assembled by Joseph Leidy, Jr., and presented to the College in 1944, by his son, Philip Ludwell Leidy, who gave one half of Leidy's correspondence, without regard to date or source, to the Academy of Natural Sciences (largely letters by Leidy). Photocopies of the College of Physicians of Philadelphia's collection (mostly letters to Leidy) are

at the Academy, which described both collections in its *Guide to the Manuscript Collections* (1936). The letters concern Leidy's wide scientific and professional interests in all phases of biology and related fields. Typewritten list of the correspondents, prepared by David L. Wenrich in Box 1, include Alexander E. Agassiz, D. Hayes Agnew, S.F. Baird, Elliott Coues, Thos. S. Foulke, Albert Frické, Traill Green, S.D. Gross, F.V. Hayden, H. Lenox Hodge, Jr., Isaac Lea, Edw. H. Magill, S. Weir Mitchell, J.C. Nott, John H. Packard, Robt. E. Rogers, H.D. Schmidt, Alfred Stillé, James Tyson, and Geo. B. Wood. — Box 6 contains some papers by Leidy's nephew, Joseph Leidy, 1867-1932, including a short biography of his uncle (18 pp.), a 202-page biography of him, and a large group of clippings about the elder Leidy. *[Z 10/236, boxes 1-6]*

590. **[————]. —————. Supplement. *V.p., 1882-87.***

2 boxes (6 folders); illus. 39.5 cm. Alphabetically arranged collection of letters (and some miscellaneous items) addressed to, or concerning, Joseph Leidy, supplementary to the larger collection. Some of the letters with drawings, usually on the verso. Concerns specimens, supplies, publications, royalties, personal affairs, etc. Handwritten lists of writers, and letter by J. Percy Moore on the Leidy correspondence, filed with the collection. — A second box (no. 8) contains clippings and other printed items relating to the Leidy family, and a letter from Provost Edgar Fahs Smith to Joseph Leidy Jr. (1915). *[Z 10/236, boxes 7-8]*

—————. See also nos. 110, 114, 253, 338, 340, 414, 592-4, 834, 846, 945, 1032, 1074, 1080, 1112.

591. **Leidy, Joseph,** 1867-1932. Manuscript notes for a biography of Joseph Leidy sen., genealogical, biographical and scientific. *N.p.d. (Philadelphia?, 1920s?).*

1 box (12 folders). 39 cm. Includes copies of letters to S.F. Baird, material on evolution (Lamarckian theories, T.H. Huxley), paper on "American science in the 4th decade of the 19th century with particular reference to the beginning of modern biology," few printed items, etc. Detailed index of contents filed with the notes. *[Z 10/214, box 3]*

592. —————. Memoir of Joseph Leidy senior, to 1867. *N.p.d. (Philadelphia, 1920s?).*

385 pp. (incl. blank pp.), 134 ff. 33-38 cm. Autograph in ink and pencil; in fragile condition. 17 original letters by Leidy sen. (to A.A. Gould, J. Wyman), by G.A. Piersol, F.E. Forsey, J.D. Dana, Jeffries Wyman, F.P. Henry, F.V. Hayden, S.F. Baird and F.B. Meek (all concerned with Leidy's scientific work) filed in separate folder at end of Memoir. *[Z 10/214, box 2]*

593. —————. Papers, correspondence, clippings, other printed materials. *V.p., 1869?, 1879-1932.*

16 folders in box; illus. 32 cm. Contents: Leidy's activity in the U.S. Army Medical Corps (3 folders, 1917-18, 1922-30). — Printed and manuscript items relating to the Joseph Leidy Memorial Fund, incl. list of contributors (1896-

1913, 1923). — Correspondence, largely relating to Joseph Leidy sen. (9 folders, 1879-1932), incl. letters from Harvey W. Cushing, E.S. Dana, Albert Ehrenfried, F.H. Garrison, Archibald Geikie, J.C. Hemmeter, S.W. Mitchell, H.F. Osborne (incl. letters by Leidy to Osborne), William Osler, Mary E. Powel, E.A. Spitzka. — Miscellany, largely printed items, incl. clippings (3 folders in 1). — Alphabetical list of correspondents filed at the beginning.

[Z 10/214, box 1]

— — — — —. See also nos. 589-90, 1074.

594.   **Leidy, Philip,** 1838-1891.   Miscellaneous collection relating to Philip Leidy, partly by him. *Philadelphia, etc., 1880-86.*

43 ff.   Various sizes in envelope (46 × 35.5 cm).   Contents not analyzed.   Includes a paper read on cases of abnormal behavior (nervous diseases) before . . . Medical Society (5 ff., n.d.), letter by P.L. as port physician on the public bath house (1 f., 1881), letter from a former soldier (musician) in the 119th platoon of the 5th Penna. Reserve, with reaction by P.L. (2 ff., 1885), post mortem (1 f., 1886), letter by Leidy on the Philadelphia Insane Asylum (4 ff., 1886), and pencilled biographical notes on Joseph Leidy in diary form, with references to pages of a biography (printed?, unidentified; 20 ff., n.d.).   Fragile.   *[n.c.]*

595.   — — — — —.   Papers. *Philadelphia, ca. 1878-86.*

[21] ff.   32.5 cm (envelope, 37.5 cm).   Contents: 1.   Paper on foreign bodies in the air passages, illustrated with cases (1878?, 4 ff.). — 2.   Original communication on diagnosis of syphilis, with case histories (1885; 6 ff.). — 3.   Letter to Philip C. Garrett, chairman of the Lunacy Commission, on Philadelphia Insane Asylum where Leidy served as "physician in chief" (1886; autogr. copy, signed, 5 ff.). — 4.   Paper read before unnamed group (Board of Guardians of the Insane Asylum?) on the teaching of psychiatry in Philadelphia (n.d., 4 ff.). — 5.   Paper on general paralysis of the insane (n.d., 2 ff.).   *[10a/483]*

596.   **Lemer, Lerue.**   Commonplace book. *New Haven, Conn. and Harrisburg, Pa., 1828-32.*

1 v.   25 cm.   Notes on diseases of children by Prof. Ives, 1828, pp. 7-[34].   Professor Tully's lectures on materia medica in Yale College, pp. [35-43].   *[10a/442]*

— — — — —. See also no. 153.

597.   **Le Moyne, John Julius (Jean Jules),** 1760-1849.   Book of prescriptions, remedies, recipes. *Paris? and Washington, Pa., late 18th cent.-ca. 1840.*

1 v. ([1] f., 263 pp.), 1 envelope.   17.5-31.5 cm.   The volume is written in at least two different hands; the text is in French and English.   The contents incl. extraneous directions, e.g. for "foiling glass mirrors" and "plating" (pp. 193-94).   It is likely that entries were made by John Julius Le Moyne (born near Paris, left France in 1790) and his son Francis Julius (about the latter see the

Dictionary of American Biography, vol. 11, pp. 163-64). On the verso of the prel. f. is the inscription "John Le Moyne Junior" (in the same hand as many headings) and in a much later hand "Given to him before 1847." According to a letter from V. Le Moyne Ellicott (1977; enclosed) there is no John Le Moyne Jr. in the family. He may however be identical with John Valcoulon Le Moyne, son of Francis J. — Index on pp. 243-63, continued on pp. 239-42. Pasted in at end of volume account of money due (1812-19) to J.J. Le Moyne by Coraline Alberti. Bound in armorial 18th-cent. morocco binding (damaged), the arms with letters (G +?) W + G + W + G. Added in envelope 1-leaf account due to J.J.L. by Patrick Moore (1822-30). — Gift of Dr. V.L. Ellicott. *[10a/461]*

598. **Lendon, Alfred Austin.** . . . Nodal fever (febris nodosa). *Adelaide, Australia, 1905.*

62 ff.; charts. 27 cm. Typescript. "Aquila non capit muscas" at head of title. Submitted for Alvarenga Prize, but not accepted. Published by Baillière, Tindall and Cox, London, 1905. *[10d/44]*

599. **Leverson, Montague Richard,** b. 1830. Draft of a proposed book attacking vaccination. *New York, ca. 1907.*

1 v. (loose ff.). 35 cm. Typescript, with manuscript alterations and additions, and miscellaneous documentary data. — Attribution to Leverson and approximate date based on letters. *[Z 10d/5]*

600. **Lewey, Frederic Henry,** 1885-1950. Sickness insurance in Germany; has it been satisfactory? By F.H. Lewy [sic]. *Philadelphia, 1939.*

11 ff. 28 cm. Typewritten, with manuscript alterations. Read before the Section on Public Health, Preventive and Industrial Medicine of the College of Physicians of Philadelphia, Feb. 6, 1939. *[ZZ 10d/6]*

601. **Lewis, Fraser.** Medicine in the continental army of the Revolutionary War, 1775-1783. *Princeton, 1956.*

iv, 121 ff. 28 cm. Typewritten (carbon copy). Senior thesis, Princeton University. — Gift of the author. *[ZZ 10a/5]*

602. **Lexer, Erich,** 1867-1937. Reconstructive surgery (translation of Lexer's *Die gesamte Wiederherstellungs-Chirurgie*, Leipzig, 1911-31). *N.p.d., 193—.*

[4], 247 ff. 29 cm. Typewritten (original and carbon). "Translated by [H.J.] Schireson" on spine. *[n.c.]*

603. **Lister, Joseph Lister,** baron, 1827-1912. On vivisection. *London, 4 April 1898.*

4 pp. 34 cm. Autograph letter, addressed to W.W. Keen. Typed commentary
(1 p.) by Keen and clipping (fragile original and reproduction) from Phila.
Public Ledger, 1 Jan. 1917, laid in.   *[Z 10/67]*

— — — — —. See also nos. 32, *185.54.*

604. **Liston, Robert,** 1794-1847. Memoir on the formation and
      connexions of the crural arch. *N.p., 1847.*

      [18, 3] ff. 21 cm. Copy of the text of Liston's published *Memoir* (Edinburgh,
      1819) copied by Samuel Lewis (14 ff.). Lewis presented the volume to John
      Ashhurst, Jr., who gave it to the College of Physicians of Philadelphia.
      [10a/152]

605. **Louis, Pierre Charles Alexandre,** 1787-1872. Remarques sur
      la clinique de Mr. Louis. *Paris, ca. 1860.*

      75 ff. 21 cm. Two hundred and two remarks on clinical cases, many with
      information on number of cases treated, index of mortality, etc. Deals with a
      great variety of illnesses, e.g. typhoid, pneumonia, bronchitis, cancer, tubercu-
      losis. References in the text to Laënnec, Bayle, Cayol, A.P. Cooper, Favill and
      Pinel. — Gift of the Board of Managers of the Episcopal Hospital, Philadelphia.
      [10a/169]

      — — — — —. See also nos. 172, 330.

606. **Lowber, Edward.** Notes on diseases. *Philadelphia, 1805.*

      187 pp. 16 cm. Each disease occupies one or more pages with indication of
      source on the margins.   *[10a/80]*

607. **Lowder, William,** d. 1801. Notes taken [by Adam Seybert]
      from Doct^r. Lowder's lectures on midwifery, delivered in London
      during the summer 1793. *London, 1793.*

      264 pp. 20 cm.   *[10a/81]*

      — — — — —. See also no. 750.

608. **Lucké, Balduin Hermann Edward Wilhelm,** 1889-1954. Tu-
      mors of the kidney, renal pelvis, and ureter; Section VIII,
      Fascicle 30 (of *Atlas of Tumor Pathology of the Armed Forces Institute
      of Pathology*), by Balduin Lucké and Hans G. Schlumberger. *Phil-
      adelphia?, 195—?*

      109 ff.; 5 plates, 191 figures. 27.5 cm. Typewritten draft of published
      version.   *[ZZ 10a/18]*

      — — — — —. See also no. 543.

609. **Ludlow, John Livingston,** 1819-1888. Unilocular ovarian cyst, opening spontaneously at the umbilicus and later into the peritoneal cavity. Case report by J.L. Ludlow and W.W. Keen. *Philadelphia, 1870-71.*

> 8 ff. 30 cm. Read before the Obstetrical Society of Philadelphia, which declined publication in its Proceedings. Ff. 1-4 by Ludlow, ff. 5-8 bear Keen's signature.   *[Z 10/203]*

610. **Lurie, Max Bernard,** 1893-1966. Resistance to tuberculosis; experimental studies in native and acquired defensive mechanisms. *Philadelphia, 1964?*

> 4 loose-leaf notebooks. 29 cm. Corrected typewritten copy for the printer, with separate sheets of corrections for the galley proofs.   *[ZZ 10a/17]*

611. **Lusk, William Thompson,** 1838-1897. Diagnosis and treatment of extra uterine pregnancy. *New York, 1888.*

> 170 ff. 39.5 cm. Unpublished. A different study by Lusk appeared under the same title in *New York Jour. Obst. and Gyn.*, v. 1 (1891).   *[10d/14]*

612. **McCamant, John,** 1787-1862. Recipes, incl. General directions in curing or preventing disease (ff. 20-23). *Churchtown, Pa., ca. 1840-50.*

> 35 ff. (first and ff. 25-35 blank). 32 cm. Poor condition (reproduction enclosed).   *[ZZ 10a/9]*

613. **McCarthy, Daniel Joseph,** 1874-1958. Papers. *Philadelphia, 1924-32.*

> 2 boxes. 32 cm. Typewritten and manuscript. Papers, speeches, notes, correspondence, etc., largely on topics of psychiatry and medical jurisprudence, e.g. depression psychosis, psycho-neurotic reactions to war experiences, dementia praecox, functional neurosis, morphine habit, responsibility in the law, etc.   *[10a/486]*

614. —————. Record of his service in World War I. *France, etc., 1918-19.*

> 1 box. 27 cm. Manuscript and printed items. Consists of case record, clinical charts, circulars and correspondence of Dr. McCarthy, senior consultant in neuro-psychiatry.   *[10c/140]*

—————. See also no. 757.

615. **McClendon, Jesse Francis,** 1880-1976. Collection of papers on the physiology of digestion, fat and other substances on the diet, iodine and goiter, some of the excurses with historical information. *Minneapolis and Philadelphia, ca. 1931-45.*

13 folders. 35 cm. Typewritten (largely carbon copies), with corrections. Contains 2 items on echinochrome (6 ff.), health and disease at the time of the American Revolution, with references to Hahnemann and Franklin (3 ff.), 2 items on the physiology of digestion (5, 19 [vero 20] ff.), fat in the diet (7 ff.), fluorine in animals and plants (2 ff.), dietary fluorine (3 ff.), 4 papers dealing with iodine and goiter (24 ff.), separate ff. superseded by revisions (19 ff.) and book reviews (8 ff.).   *[n.c.]*

616.   —————. Correspondence, reports, bibliographies, etc., relating to toxic and non-toxic goiter, its biochemical and microbiologi-cal aspects. *V.p., 1925-45.*

2 boxes. 39 cm. Includes letters from physicians, chemists, health officers, pharmaceutical companies, most of these addressed to J.F. McClendon, collecting data on an international basis. Letters and reports in box 1 cover the United States, Canada; Latin America; New Zealand, Oceania and Polynesia; box 2, Africa; Asia; Europe. Much of the material was collected in preparation of the author's study, *Iodine and the Incidence of Goiter* (Minneapolis, © 1939).   *[n.c.]*

617.   **McDaniel, Walton Brooks,** 1897-1975. Recognition of the specialties in the "Organic Law" of the College of Physicians of Philadelphia. *Philadelphia, 1943.*

1 envelope. 36 cm. Typewritten (original discarded 1972, due to paper deterioration; photocopy substituted). Read before the Section of Ophthalmol-ogy, Apr. 3, 1943.   *[Z 10a/4]*

—————. See also nos. 104, 138, 184, *185.611, .62,* 524, 564, 938, 1011.

618.   **Macer Floridus.** De virtutibus herbarum et aromatum (ff. 1r-30v). — **Idem.** De virtutibus et potentiis specierum sive aroma-tum (ff. 31r-34r). — **Theodorus Priscianus.** De monitione medicorum, *inc.*: Nos frustra mortalium (Thorndike & Kibre, cols. 436, 427; ff. 34v-39r). *Italy, 1493.*

40, [1] ff. 21.5 cm. Minor corrections in a contemporary (i.e. the scribe's?) hand. Based on wording of title, and contents, it seems certain that this manuscript was not copied from a printed edition (see Hain, *Repertorium,* nos. 10417-21; Klebs 636.1-6). Written by a "Christophorus B" (entered at conclusion of texts). 8-line test on woman's ability to conceive on f. 34r; among prescriptions or tests in the third tract "Ut mulier concipiat," followed by 3 related brief statements. Christophorus B. states that the first item was written between June 17 and 27, the second in a few hours (hora 13-20). The last f. contains table of contents to f. 33; the continuation (on a second leaf) is missing. Owner's stamp Donato Silva on verso of prel. f. — From the J. Stockton Hough Library.   *[10a/159]*

619. **Macfarlan, Douglas,** 1886-1966. Collection of notes, letters, clippings, catalogues, etc., chiefly relating to herbs and their use in medicine. *Philadelphia, ca. 1951-63.*

> 1 box. 30 cm. Material for his "The History of the Use of Herbs in Medicine" (copy of paper included), read before the Section on Medical History, College of Physicians of Philadelphia, Feb. 17, 1959. Incl. translation of Christopher Sower Jr.'s "All Sorts of Useful Remedies," published in his *Almanac* for 1774 (27 pp., typewritten).   *[10c/106]*

620. — — — — —. Dr. George de Benneville, Sr., and medicine in colonial times. *Philadelphia, 1954.*

> 10, [1] ff. 29 cm. Paper read to the Section on Medical History, College of Physicians of Philadelphia, Feb. 25, 1954. Includes "Medicina Pensylvania [!], or, the Pensylvania physician," ms. by George de Benneville, Sr., reviewed by Douglas Macfarlan.   *[10c/115]*

— — — — —. See also nos. 22, 242.

621. **McFarland, Joseph,** 1868-1945. Dysontogenetic and mixed tumors of the urogenital region, with a report of a new case of sarcoma botryoides vaginal in a child, and comments upon the probable cause of sarcoma. *Philadelphia, 1935.*

> 3 folders (81 ff.); plates (photographs). 28 cm. Typescript. Submitted in competition for the Alvarenga Prize, 1935. Printed text enclosed (*Surg. Gynecol. Obstet.*, v. 61: 42-57 [1935], but without tables and bibliography).
>   *[10d/49]*

622. — — — — —. An outline of regular and special pathology as taught at the Medico-Chirurgical College. *Philadelphia, 1901-05.*

> 195 pp. 26 cm. Inscribed inside front cover: M.F. Percival, jr. "Med 05". Contains pasted-in printed outline, underlined and with extensive ms. notes by M.F. Percival on sections morbid anatomy (pp. 64-122), followed by continuous ms. notes (without outline) on diseases of lymphatics, nervous system, on tuberculosis, respiratory tract, etc. (pp. 124 to end), possibly, like pp. 10-14, by Wm. W. Babcock (cf. name Babcock on p. 10). Index at beginning of volume. Laid in instructions for fixing and staining tissues (3 ff.) and 2 hectographed folded sheets. — Gift of Mrs. M.F. Percival.   *[10a/457]*

623. — — — — —. Papers. *Philadelphia, 1900-43.*

> 3 boxes (incl. loose-leaf notebook). Contents: *Box 1.* Correspondence (list with the collection) and data on tetanus and vaccination; tumors of the parotid. — *2.* General correspondence (list with the collection); miscellaneous case notes and illustrations; W.L. Rodman's collections on cases of abnormal involution and carcinoma of the breast; miscellaneous lists concerning the course in general pathology at the Evans Dental Institute; loose-leaf notebook containing biographical memoirs of Joseph Weatherhead Warren, John

Forsyth Meigs, Arthur Vincent Meigs, David Hendricks Bergey (publ. in *Trans. & Stud.*, ser. 4, v. 6: 249-53 [1938]), Alfred Stillé, James William White, George Bacon Wood, Horatio C Wood, Theodore George Wormley, and John Richardson Young; "A Resurrection of 'Pile'," etc. (ibid., ser. 4, v. 7: 278-96 [1939]); "The Epidemic of Yellow Fever in Philadelphia in 1793 and Its Influence upon Dr. Benjamin Rush" (publ. in *Medical Life*, v. 36: 449-96 [1929], under title "Dr. Benjamin Rush and the Yellow Fever Epidemics in Philadelphia"). — 3 (oversize). Further cases of tetanus resulting from vaccination; inventories of equipment, etc., in various laboratories of the Medico-Chirurgical College, one dated December, 1915; medico-legal matters: briefs, notes, and letters relating to various cases in which McFarland gave an opinion; brief outline of the professional career of J. McFarland, with bibliography.   *[Z 10/204]*

————. See also nos. *185.63*, 631-2, 1013, 1038.

624. **Mackrill, Joseph,** 1762-1820. Bill to "The estate of the late Mr. John Pannel" for medical care. *Baltimore County?, 1798-1800.*

[4] pp. 32 cm. With notes in support of Mackrill's claim, signed by Edward Pannel, Owen Dorsey, and William Buchanan Pew(?); receipt for payment, signed by Joseph Mackrill.   *[10c/67]*

625. **McNeil, Donald,** fl. 1788. Of Natural philosophy. *Scotland or Ireland, 1788.*

544 pp.; ff. 545-67, 19 ff.; illus., plates, tables. 25 cm. Text of not clearly established origin and date, written in 1788 by Donald McNeil in his final year at a Scottish university or possibly at Trinity College, Dublin (cf. verso of last f. "Magistrand class 1788"; also f. 562v referring to 1789 as "10 years hence"). Partial contents: Of the phenomena of thunder, electricity . . ., pp. 59-82. — Of the laws of motion, commonly called Sir Isaac Newton's laws of nature, pp. 83-93. — Of elasticity & the congress of bodies, pp. 168-73. — Of the centre of gravity . . ., pp. 187-209. — Of hydrostatics . . ., pp. 343-406, unnumbered plate and 2 ff. — Of damps and pestilence, pp. 420-24. — Of optics, pp. 435-544, ff. 545-48. — Electricity (in a cursive hand), ff. 549-54. — Of astronomy, ff. 557-67, final ff. 1-19. Among the many authorities quoted are Isaac Newton (throughout) and Benjamin Franklin (pp. 52, 57). With ms. corrections and additions, partly in a different hand.   *[Z 10/73]*

626. **Magrath, George Burgess,** 1870-1938. Medical science in the service of the state; some professional experiences. Lantern demonstration. *Philadelphia, 4 March 1931.*

[2], 58 ff. 28 cm. Typescript. Prefaced by unnumbered minutes of stated meeting of College of Physicians of Philadelphia, with an introduction by Francis R. Packard. — Mary Scott Newbold Lecture.   *[10d/132]*

627. **Malaria;** a Clinical and Therapeutic Study. *Philadelphia, 1933.*

[1], 25, [1] ff. 28 cm. Typescript. Essay, with motto MEPH of unidentified author, submitted for Alvarenga Prize.   *[Z 10d/1]*

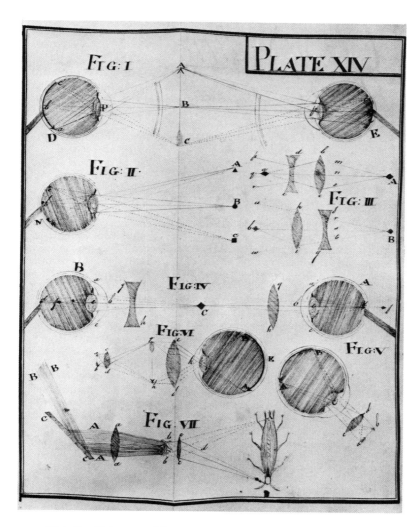

Plate 5. 624. Donald McNeil. *Of Natural Philosophy, 1788.*

628. **[Manget, Jean Jacques,** 1652-1742]. Bibliotheca chemica curiosa. . . . Notes, on this work, in Latin. *France, after 1830.*

[25] sheets. 20 cm. Written on the verso of blank forms, dated 183—, acknowledging requests for payment of expenses, etc., from "Le Directeur de l'Enregistrement et des Domaines." *[10c/107]*

629. **Mansfeld, David,** 1797-1863. Arzneimittel Lehre privatim vorgetragen nach [Justus A.] Arnemann . . . Michaelis 1825 bis Ostern 1826 in Braunschweig. I. Theil. *Brunswick?, 1826 or soon thereafter.*

[1] f., 189 pp., [1] f.   25 cm. Copied or written by A. Keitel (cf. title and recto of last leaf). — Gift of John Marshall; from the library of Jacob Marshall.
[10a/278]

630. **Marshall, Jacob,** b. 1741? Artzt und Kunst Buch. *Reading, Pa., 1807.*

[2] ff., 273 pp. (pp. 245-71 blank). 21 cm. Partial contents: Prescriptions, pp. 2-10. — Der natürlichen Dingen Eigenschaft (pp. 21-30) and Augmentatio (pp. 31ff.). — Tabella . . . Von vielerley Kranckheiten samt den nöthigen Medicamendum (pp. 133-220); interspersed Aus Zin Silber zu machen (p. 197). — Kunst Buch, pp. 221-25, 230-41. — Gift of John Marshall (1922).
[10a/277]

631. **Marshall, Jacob,** 1788-1871(?). Medical miscellany. *Philadelphia and Reading, 1817-20.*

80 ff. 20 cm. Contains instructions for dyeing cloth, ff. 1-2; notes on Nathaniel Chapman's lectures on the practice of physic, ff. 2-37, 47-53 with prescriptions from various Philadelphia physicians interspersed. In reverse, prescriptions in German ff. 77-79; lists of drugs with prices, incl. patent medicines, ff. 58-76. Written in two different hands, possibly by Jacob Marshall and Henry Witman, whose names are found on outside label, fly leaves and inside. "Bunker & Height, No. 36 Plum Street. Philadelphia, Jan 15th 1819" on back fly leaf. — Presented in 1922 by John Marshall who noted that it had belonged to his grandfather, Jacob Marshall. *[10a/276]*

————. See also no. 629.

632. **Massa, Baptista, de Argenta.** De fructibus vescendis, ff. 1r-70v, dedicated to Duke Hercules d'Este, dated 10 June 1471. — Tractatus de modo confitiendi ordaceam, ff. 70v-76r, dedicated to Petrus de Trano, dated 15 June 1471 "in felici gimnasio ferrariensi," and accompanied by a 4-line poem on the author by Francesco Ariosto. An epigram dedicated to Massa by Ariosto on f. 79r, followed by a table of contents on ff. 79v-80r. *Ferrara, June 1471, or soon thereafter.*

80 ff. 16 cm. Illuminated initial P and coat of arms on f. 1r. The two texts were printed at about the same time in Venice (Goff M344). Differences in spelling have been noticed. No attempt has been made to establish the relationship between this manuscript, others, or the printed edition. Authorities quoted entered on margins, occasional corrections, and one sizable addition on f. 34r. — Gift of G.E. de Schweinitz.   *[10a/189]*

633. **Massei, Ferdinando,** 1847-1917. Abstract of articles by G. and O. Masini and Massei. *Naples, 1888(-9?).*

4 ff. in envelope (37.5 cm). Sent by Massei as corresponding editor of an unidentified journal. Incl. abstract of C.A. Blume's Phlebectasia by a correspondent in Copenhagen.   *[n.c.]*

634. **Massey, Samuel,** ca. 1735-1793. Two letters to his daughter Ann Massey on conditions during the yellow fever epidemic. *Philadelphia, Sept. 12 and 15, 1793.*

4, 6 pp. 34 × 20.5 cm., in portfolio (35 cm). Fragile; paper torn at creases, poorly mended many years ago. Included are a near contemporary note, identifying writer and recipient, with information on Samuel Massey's death, Sept. 23; typescript copy (cf. *Fugitive Leaves* of the College of Physicians of Philadelphia, n.s., nos. 88-89, Jan.-Feb.-Mar., 1967, with text of the letters and introduction). — Gift of Francis Clark Wood, January 10, 1967.   *[Z 10c/13]*

635. **[Materia Medica].** Lectures. *N.p., 1927-31?*

47 pp., 1 blank f. 33 cm. Lecturer and student unidentified. Dates mentioned in the text extend from 1912 to 1931.   *[n.c.]*

636. **Materia Medica** and Pharmacy. *N.p., first quarter 19th cent.?*

8 ff. 20 cm (envelope, 26.5 cm). Lect. 9 on upper left corner of f. 1. Signatures A and B only, ending on f. 8 in midsentence. Earlier assigned to Nathaniel Chapman, but differs essentially from his lecture on the history of materia medica.   *[10a/416]*

637. **Mathes, William Thomas,** 1887-1966. The East Tennessee Medical Association. *Greeneville, Tenn., 1941.*

8 ff. 28 cm. Typewritten (carbon copy). Published in *Journal, Tennessee State Medical Association*, v. 34: 138-41 (1941). — Gift of S. X Radbill.   *[10d/71]*

638. **Medical and Household Recipes.** *England, 17th-18th cent.*

[24] ff. (first 2, and last blank), 167 pp., [61] blank ff. 36 cm. Pages 31-2, 39-40, 61-2, 69-70, 87-8, missing. Drawing of human skull on verso of p. 167. Extensive index on preliminary ff. In two distinct hands (pp. 1-120; pp. 121-67). One recipe, addressed to Miss Noesley, laid in between pp. 120 and 121, and bill of Mr. Lotterell to Susanna Mathews, dated June 18, 1745 pasted on verso of f. 3. Among medical recipes are prescriptions against canker, consumption, apoplexy, rickets, etc., collected from many sources, among them "ladies", and some doctors (e.g., Butler, W. Water, Wright, Smith). — Bookplate of Strickland Freeman, Fawley Court, Bucks, 1810.   *[Z 10/71]*

639. **Medical,** Chemical and Agricultural **Extracts.** *Philadelphia,* *1796-1815?*

> 3 v. 18 cm. Notebooks containing prescriptions, case histories and notes on therapeutics, in an unidentified hand. Newspaper clippings tipped and laid in. — Presented by Jacob Solis Cohen.   *[10a/270]*

640. **Medical Commonplace Book.** *Pennsylvania?, ca. 1841.*

> Pp. [9]-68 (pp. 33-4 removed; pp. 28-36, 38-9 blank). 20 cm. Incomplete at beginning; first and last leaf torn; unbound. Contents: Recipes, unguents, solutions, etc., pp. 9-22, 24-7. — Dream over a cure, p. 23. — Remedy against cancer, p. 37. — Extracts from John Brown's *Elements of Medicine,* pp. 40-8. — "On the gout taken from [not further identified] Gar[di]ner[?]," pp. 48-51. — Verses on the beneficial effects of inoculation by . . . William Lipscomb, pp. 53-68.   *[10a/350]*

641. **Medical Library Association.** Correspondence in matters of the Association, largely addressed to Charles P. Fisher, librarian of the College of Physicians of Philadelphia and member of the Executive Committee. *V.p., 1899-1926.*

> 1 box. 32 cm. Includes some carbon copies and drafts of letters by C.P. Fisher, few official documents, membership lists, programs, few printed items, etc.   *[Z 10/128]*

642. — — — — —. Regional meeting, Philadelphia, College of Physicians, 1943. Correspondence, list of participants, menus, photographs. *Philadelphia, etc., 1943.*

> 4 envelopes, 1 vol. 24-31 cm. "Report on the Regional Meeting. . .," *Trans. & Stud.,* ser. 4, v. 11: 94-6 (1943-44).   *[10c/45]*

— — — — —. See also nos. *185.62,* 518.

643. **Medical Miscellany I.** 1. **Bernardus de Guidonia** (i.e. Gordonio), d. ca. 1320. Tractatus de regimine sanitatis (part 4 of his De conservatione vitae humanae), *inc.* (text): Nullus debet sumere cibum. . . *England, 1307. 10 ff., vellum, incomplete.* — 2. **De regimine sanitatis,** *inc.*: In tractatu isto qui intitulatur de regimine sanitatis (Thorndike & Kibre, col. 339, without indication of author). *England?, ca. 1400.* 11 ff., paper. — 3. **Peers** (Pearse, Pearce, etc., or possibly Petrus, see *infra*). Wyse boke. *England, 14th cent.* 18 ff., paper, and part of 1 f. vellum.

> Three items bound in 1 vol. (contemp. vellum document), ca. 21.5 cm. Ad 1: See L.E. Demaitre, *Doctor Bernard de Gordon. . .* (Toronto, 1980). — Ad 2: Title in explicit reads Dietarius optimus. Followed by poem, beginning (title): Luna. venus. stilbons. sol saturnus jovis et mars/(text): Est aries taurus gemini. . . — Ad 3: The first paragraph reads: Here begynnyth the wyse boke of mayster Peers of Salerne as he transposyd it owte of lateyn in to englysche at ye requeste

and desyre of Margerye Fygyll [?] the qwene of spayne, and as it was affernyd
by ye opynyons of alle the maystres that tyme in Sallerne dwellyng. Followed
by recipes (ad faciendum incaustum. . ., and contra sudorem et pestem, etc.,
others in code) on verso of last and 1 following f. Attempts to identify Peers
with Petrus Hispanus have been unsuccessful. *The Medical Practitioners in
Medieval England* by C.H. Talbot and E.A. Hammond (London, 1965) lists a
physician Peter de Barulo alias Salernia, ca. 1387. Nothing more is known of
him.   [10a/215]

44. **Medical Miscellany, II.** Of the teeth. — The female parts of
generation. — Hints from Dr. [John?] Hunter on injections. *London?, 1763.*

[1] f. 37 cm (folded, in envelope, 31 cm). Fragment. Fragile.   [n.c.]

45. **Medical Miscellany, III,** with emphasis on child birth and
related matters. Probably part of a larger compilation; begins
with De hominis generatione liber 2 (*inc.*: Humani corporis
partes), followed by De humoribus lib. 4, Institutionum medicarum pars altera . . . lib. 3, De crisibus lib. 2, etc., with later chapters
on uroscopy, pulse, diet, etc. *Italy?, late 17th century.*

41 ff. 20 cm. With references to a large number of medical authorities, from
classical times to the 17th century, among them Galen, Hippocrates, Pliny,
Cardano, van Helmont, William Harvey, Bartholin and Boyle.   [10a/156]

46. **[Medical-Pharmaceutical Miscellany].** Collection of tracts
in Latin and Italian, probably put together by a practitioner. *Italy, first half 16th cent.*

45, 70-117 ff.; colored, decorated initials, illus. 20.5 cm. Contemporary
numbering. Ff. 46-69 not present; they may have been removed when the
tracts were rebound in modern times. Title on spine: Prohemium puntis
huius operis; with initials C.M.P. — Contents: Prohemium, ff. 1r-2v (1r within
decorated border). — De modus(!) medicinarum vero curacionis, ff. 3r-6v (incl.
"Cerotus . . . de magistro Ambroxio de Binascho"; icplt.?). — Joannes de Tracco
(= Joannes de Tracia), Practica chirurgiae, *inc.*: Illorum recte quod craneom
non est lesum. . ., ff. 7r-10v (cf. Thorndike & Kibre, Index, and cols. 89, 324
with different incipits). — Recipes and dietary rules, suprascription "Capitulo
de morsu canis," *inc.*: Cum canis utrum avis hominem. . ., ff. 10v-17r. — De
solucione continuitatis carni, *inc.*: Postque Deo Auxilio tractatu fuit. . ., ff. 17v-
18v. — Unidentified item, *inc.*: Si che poso lamore. . ., f. 19r. — Enplastra et
exempla, beginning with Epitima(!) cordiale, ff. 19v-20r (incl. portrait of
Mesue within initial E and Avicenna in another). — Ceroton, *inc.*: Ceroton
magistri Graciani comfortans stomacum. . ., together with Unguenta unguento-
rum, and "Chapitulo de la vena," ff. 20v-27v. — De vulneribus capitis et de eius
anatonomia(!), *inc.*: Dictis sub compendio his que circha primum huius libri
tractatus. . ., ff. 28r-31v. — De apostemantibus mamillarum, *inc.*: Postemata
mamillarum quedam sunt propria. . ., ff. 32r-33r, with De vulneribus coxarum
tibearum et pedum, ff. 33r ("Avicena ponitur" at end), De antidotis, cap. XVI,
Nota optimimum defensuum ("Berta Pallia" at end), De extractione ossium. . .,
De solucione continuitatis nervorum, ff. 33v-45v. — Pissis, achus, trepanum,

tenachula... (all caps.), ff. 70r-112r (ff. 75r and 76 in cipher). — Poem and notes on ff. 116r-117v. Dates on f. 91r (1521?), 91v (1525), 103v (1543), 104v, 105r, 106v (1545), 108r, 110r (1548), 117r (1530). In two or more hands? Water-stained toward the end. Gift of M.S. Wickersham.   *[10a/132]*

647. **Medical Prayer-Meeting.** Minutes, 1832-33 and minutes of its Committee on Prisons, 1828-29. *Philadelphia, 1828-33.*

1 v. 20 cm. Recorded by William Darrach, Secretary. Minutes begin at back of volume. Includes notes on epidemic cholera in Russia, ca. 1829-31. — Presented by Herbert Fox.   *[10a/246]*

648. **Medicinae Liber.** Collection of medical and household recipes in English, written in various hands over an extended period; a second sequence started at end of volume. *England, 17th-18th cent.*

[1], 242, [3] pp. (few leaves at the beginning and several between pp. 161 and 162 removed; a few inserts, incl. printed newspaper clipping, dated 1739). According to the dealer's note the volume had an inscription on a fly-leaf "Anne Layfielde, her Booke of Physicke and Surgery, 1640"; it is no longer extant. Many names appear at the end of prescriptions or recipes, at the beginning most frequently "Eliza Downing." Several medical doctors are mentioned, e.g. a Dr. Salvatica (p. 78), Dr. Meyhorne (p. 88), Dr. Marcelline (p. 233; same as Joannes Petrus Ayroldus Marcellinus?).   *[10a/214]*

649. **Medico-Chirurgical College of Philadelphia** [School]. Lists of students and graduates, lecture book. *Philadelphia, 1882-1917.*

3 v. ([54] ff., [54] ff., 128 pp.). 26-37 cm. List and updated list of College students and graduates, 1882-1917, arranged by year of graduation, including addresses and some death dates. Notebook, 1888-89, on the practice of medicine lectures delivered at the College by William F. Waugh.

[Z 10a/10, 10a/240]

————. See also nos. 20, 231, 622-3, 652, 784, 1069.

650. **Medico-Chirurgical College of Philadelphia** [Society]. Constitution and by-laws, minutes, membership lists, misc. correspondence, photos, etc. *Philadelphia, 1848-58, ca. 1970.*

153, 6, 6 pp. 33.5 cm. Minutes, 1848-58, of the Medico-Chirurgical College of Philadelphia (the name was changed in 1849, from College of Physicians and Surgeons of Philadelphia). At the end of the volume, as Appendix A, are the constitution and by-laws, ca. 1849, of the College, which was incorporated in 1850 as an association for the discussion of medical knowledge. Appendix B contains a list of original members, and some who were elected to the College later in 1848. Index, containing ca. 280 names mentioned in the minutes, prepared by donor Margaret E. Gee, great grand-niece of James

Bryan, College president 1848-58. Also some correspondence, ca. 1970, concerning the transmittal of the collection to the College of Physicians of Philadelphia, and some Bryan family photos and copies of pages from the family Bible.   *[ZZ 10/1]*

————. See also no. 225.

51. **Medico-Chirurgical Hospital.** Patients' records. *Philadelphia, August 1887-April 1888.*

250 ff. 36 cm. Cover title: Medical Clinic, Prof. Waugh. "Waugh per L.H.M." (i.e. L. Harrison Mettler) entered on several cases.   *[Z 10a/14]*

52. **Melnick, Theodore,** 1894-1965. Lecture notes. *Philadelphia and New York, 1913-15, 1918.*

1 envelope. 15, 24 cm (envelope, 31 cm). Extensive notes on lectures at the Medico-Chirurgical College (1913-15) by Drs. H.B. Mills, H. Lowenburg, L.N. Boston, S. Egbert, J.J. Gilbridge, W.L. Rodman, W.C. Hollopeter, H.S. Zulick, H.C. Wood, A. Morgan and H.J. Smith, and laboratory notes from the Rockefeller Institute (1918). Presented by Mrs. Theodore Melnick.
     [10a/495]

53. **Melvill, Thomas,** 1726-1753. Lexicon physicum, vel definitionum, quae ad veram spectant physicam. Ex operibus Newtoni, s'Gravezandii, Muschenbrockii, Whistoni aliorumque plurimorum collectio plenissima. *Scotland?, 1744.*

57 pp.; illus., table. 18 cm. Dictionary compiled while a student by an interesting Scottish scientist; see *D.S.B.* 9: 266-67.   *[10a/83]*

Method of Physick, *see* **Galen** (no. 324).

Methodus discurendi . . . morbus, *see* **Sixteenth-Century Lecture Notes.**

54. **Mettauer, John Peter,** 1787-1875. An essay on lithotomy. *Prince Edward Court House, Va., 1835.*

49 (vero 50) ff. 20.5 cm. Bound with his Notes on typhus or congestive fever, 1826-27. — Gift of George B. Johnston.   *[10a/192(1)]*

55. ————. An essay on scrofula, submitted to the examination of the Boylston Medical Committee for the Boylston Prize for 1839. . . . *Prince Edward Court House, Va., 1839?*

[2], 52 ff. 25 cm. Incomplete, f. 52 ends in mid-sentence. — Prel. f. 1 inscribed with names, evidently those of the Boylston Medical Committee.
     [10a/194(3)]

656. ―――――. Introductory address to a course of surgery in Washington Medical College of Baltimore. *Prince Edward Court House, Va., 1836.*

[1], 25 ff. 25 cm. Carbon copy of bibliography of Mettauer's publications at beginning of volume. Typewritten list of 41 contributions by Mettauer to various medical journals added, as gleaned from a survey of the journals themselves and from fragmentary lists in biographical notices of Mettauer (photocopies included). *[10a/194(1)]*

657. ―――――. Introductory address to the second series of lectures at Randolph Macon Medical College. *Prince Edward Court House, Va., 1839?*

36 ff. 25.5 cm. Incomplete; f. 36 ends in mid-sentence. *[10a/194(2)]*

658. ―――――. An introductory discourse delivered at the commencement of a course in the Medical Institute near Prince Edward Court House. *Prince Edward Court House, Va., 1837.*

[1], 27 ff. 25 cm. Two unnumbered ff. inserted between ff. 21 and 22. The Institute later became the Medical Department of Randolph Macon College. *[10a/194(5)]*

659. ―――――. Introductory lecture on the history of surgery. *Baltimore, 1835?*

24 ff. 25 cm. Mettauer describes himself on leaf 1, as "for the first time, a lecturer"; the unnamed institution appears to be the Washington Medical College, the year 1835, cf. Rucker, *Ann. Med. Hist.*, n.s., v. 10: 36 ff. (1938). *[10a/194(6)]*

660. ―――――. Lecture on chyle. *Prince Edward Court House, Va., ca. 1830.*

[4] ff. 25 cm. Fragment? *[10a/194(4)]*

661. ―――――. Memoir on lithotomy. *Prince Edward Court House, Va., 1844.*

[2], 69, [1 blank] ff. 24.5 cm. Laid in, in a different hand, notes on a classification of urinary calculi. *[10a/194(8)]*

662. ―――――. A memoir on strictures of the urethra. *Prince Edward Court House, Va., 1844.*

[iv], 113, [9 blank] ff. 24.5 cm. Published, with extensive deletions, rearrangement, and rewording, under title, *A Memoir on Stricture of the Urethra,...* (Farmville, Va., 1849). The printed version dedicated to T.D. Mütter; tne ms. dedicated to Thomas Robinson of Petersburg, Va. — Inscribed on t.-p.: From Dr. W.M. Holladay, Hampden Sidney, Va. *[10a/194(7)]*

663. —————. Notes on typhus or congestive fever. *Prince Edward Court House, Va., 1826-27.*

[4], 69 ff. (incl. a few blank). 20.5 cm. Incomplete, f. 69 ending in mid-sentence; f. 51 misbound after f. 69. — Presented by George B. Johnston.
[10a/192(2)]

664. —————. Treatise on surgery. *Prince Edward Court House, Va., 184—.*

22, 216 ff. 31.5 cm. According to George B. Johnston (donor), "Mettauer's surgery contains about 3,000 pages of ms., closely . . . written on blue legal cap paper. . . . I have the original . . . draft of this manuscript", cf. An address before the American Surgical Association, 1905 (p. 17). Introduction, entitled "Preliminary surgery," mentions chloroform as an anesthetic; this section evidently written after 1847. Pages 1-200 deal with diseases and injuries of the urinary organs, pp. 201-16 with diseases of the prostate gland. — Typewritten bibliography of Mettauer's publications tipped in at beginning of volume (3 ff.).
[Z 10/49]

665. **Mexico. Protomedicato.** Decree appointing Juan de Echavarria to investigate unqualified persons illegally practicing medicine, surgery, etc. *Mexico City, Oct. 3, 1717.*

4 ff., last blank. 31 cm (envelope, 37.5 cm). Signed by Juan de Brizuela, Juan Joseph de Brizuela, Marcos Joseph Salgado, F. Xavier Duxan. Transcribed, translated and discussed by Edith Armstrong Wright in *Eighteenth Century Medicine in Mexico* (Philadelphia, 1963?).
[Z 10/231]

666. —————. Examination of Juan Antonio de Avila for a license to practice medicine. *Mexico City, Nov. 8, 1715.*

4 ff. 31 cm (envelope, 37.5 cm). Signed by Juan de Brizuela, Juan Joseph de Brizuela, and Marcos Joseph Salgado. Transcribed, translated and discussed by Edith A. Wright, ibid.; carbon copy enclosed.
[Z 10/230]

667. **Miles, Deborah,** comp. Cholera in Philadelphia in 1832 and 1849. *Philadelphia, 1832, 1849.*

[90] pp. 44 cm. Scrapbook; broadsides and newspaper cuttings collected by Mrs. Deborah Miles. Presented by her grandson, Edward S. Miles, at the suggestion of Addinell Hewson.
[Z 10c/18]

668. **Miller, Adolphe William,** 1841-1923. Syllabus of the lectures in materia medica delivered to the medical class of '93 of the University of Pennsylvania by Adolphe G.[!] Miller. *Philadelphia, ca. 1891.*

Title page, 37 ff. text, blank ff. 21 cm. Notes and gift of John M. Swan.
[10a/336]

—————. See also no. 1080.

669. **Mills, Charles Karsner,** 1845-1931. Letters from American and foreign neurologists. *V.p., 1893-1929.*

3 v. 25-28 cm. Manuscript and typescript. Chiefly concerns Mills' book, *The Nervous System and Its Diseases* (Phila., 1898). Includes letters from: J. Babinski, Ramón Cajal, F.X. Dercum, C.A. Herter, Eduard Hitzig, Victor Horsley, J. Hughlings Jackson, W.W. Keen, S. Weir Mitchell, Wm. Osler, C.S. Sherrington, and D. Hack Tuke, etc. — Alphabetical index filed with collection. Gift of author.   *[10c/20]*

670. —————, comp. Notes regarding examinations of H.K. Thaw, by Mills, Adolf Meyer, and Frederick Peterson, March, 1912; by Peterson and Mills, April, 1912; by D.P. Hickling, November, 1913, also various memoranda relating to Thaw's trial, 1905, including photocopies and typewritten transcripts of letters used in evidence, etc. *V.p., 1905-13.*

1 box. 26.5 cm. Typewritten; some photocopies. — Presented by Charles K. Mills.   *[10d/24]*

—————. See also no. *185.632.*

671. **Mitchell, John,** d. 1768. Letter on the yellow fever. *N.p., 1748.*

49 pp. 23 cm. Silked and repaired, words and letters missing. At bottom of p. 49 undeciphered monogram and "scrip. 1748." P. Bond on p. [1]. Early manuscript copy of letter written in 1744 to Benjamin Franklin for the attention of the American Philosophical Society and referred to Cadwalader Colden for his commentary. Published in its entirety with the commentary and Mitchell's reply in *American Medical & Philosophical Register,* v. 4: 181-215, 378-87 (1814) as submitted by Benjamin Rush, and with deletions in the *Philadelphia Medical Museum,* v. 1: 1-20 (1805). — With typewritten transcript of F.R. Packard's speech at the College of Physicians of Philadelphia, Dec. 1933, at the presentation of letter by John Cadwalader and family.   *[10a/254]*

—————. See also no. 200.

672. **Mitchell, John Kearsley,** 1793-1858. Collection of prescriptions. *Philadelphia, 1850?*

1 v. 19 cm.   *[10a/86]*

673. —————. Lectures on various diseases. *Philadelphia, 1852-53.*

97 pp. 18.5 cm. Lectures discuss symptoms, treatment, etc.   *[10a/85]*

674. —————, comp. Likenesses of the insane, taken for Dr. Jn. K. Mitchell during his service at the Pennsylvania Hospital . . . *Philadelphia, 1827-34.*

22 sketches in volume, 15 × 12 cm. Without text, beyond title-page and biblical verse on a decorated oval, pasted inside front cover. − Gift of S.W. Mitchell.   *[10a/133]*

−−−−−. See also nos. 17, 141, 143, 147, 795, 825, 1050, 1112, 1128.

675. **[Mitchell, John Kearsley, 1859-1917].** Letters concerning his *Remote Consequences of Injuries of Nerves* (Philadelphia, 1895), etc. *Philadelphia, etc., 1892-1902.*

1 envelope. 31 cm. Letters on injuries of nerves (total of 12) incl. 2 by J.M. DaCosta, one each by W.W. Keen, William Osler and H.C. Wood; a list of correspondents is enclosed. Added: letters by Mitchell to John Ashhurst and C.P. Fisher; note on operation by a Dr. Morton (1892), and letter from T.J. Mitchell to W.W. Keen. Several letters are fragile.   *[n.c.]*

−−−−−. See also nos. 114, 346, 481, 765.

676. **Mitchell, Silas Weir, 1829-1914.** Address to the American Neurological Association. *Philadelphia, 1909.*

54 ff. 30 cm. Typewritten, with corrections in Mitchell's hand. Published in *Journal of Nervous and Mental Disease*, v. 36: 385-401 (1909). Presented by William G. Spiller.   *[10a/195, pam. 1]*

677. −−−−−. A case of uncomplicated hysteria in the male lasting thirty years with post-mortem examination, by S. Weir Mitchell and William G. Spiller. *Philadelphia, 1904.*

23 ff. 30 cm. Typewritten, with manuscript corrections in Mitchell's hand. Published, with corrections, in *Transactions of the Association of American Physicians*, v. 19: 433-45 (1904). Presented by William G. Spiller.
[10a/195, pam. 2]

678. −−−−−. Collection of miscellaneous items (reports, speeches, letters, poems, etc.). *Philadelphia, etc., 1853-1912.*

15 envelopes in 2 boxes. 39 cm. Arranged in chronological order: 1. 17 pieces of miscellany, incl. 1 letter by G.E. De Schweinitz of 1918 (1853-98). − 2. Speech at the College of Physicians of Philadelphia upon the presentation of a loving cup by "two gentlewomen" (Mrs. Conover and Mrs. S.W. Mitchell), 10 ff., autograph (1886). − 3. "A Doctor's Century;" autograph poem, 5 ff. (1887). − 4. Ms. index of the Gilbert Collection presented to the College of Physicians of Philadelphia by S.W. Mitchell, 8 ff. (1888). − 5. "The Physician;" autograph poem, 35 ff. (1899). − 6. Reports on acute fear of cats, response to questionnaire, published by M. as "Of Ailurophobia and the Power to Be Conscious of the Cat . . .", *American Medicine*, v. 9: 851-53 (1905); letters, photocopies, etc. (1902-03). − 7. Russell H. Chittenden to S.W.M. on sense of smell; letter of transmittal and 4-ff. report (1906). − 8. Letter on College of Physicians of Philadelphia business, etc., 6 pieces (1907). − 9. Letters to librarian of the College of Physicians of Philadelphia on acquisitions, etc., 7

pieces (1908-11). — 10.   Speech at the first dinner in the new building of the College of Physicians of Philadelphia; 20 ff. (1909). — 11.   Letters to Robert Abbé concerning Rush memorabilia; 6 letters (typed) and printed pamphlet on mementos in the College of Physicians of Philadelphia (1911). —12.   Poem by J. Levering Jones for S.W.M. and correspondence, 4 pieces (1912-15). — 13.   Miscellany; 5 pieces (n.d.). — 14.   Portrait of S.W.M. with clipping of his "Puzzle Verse" (n.d.). — 15.   Clipping on William Harvey (n.d.).

[10a/224]

679.   —————.   Correspondence (originals and photocopies).   *V.p., 1854-1912, 1915?, 1936.*

1 box.   39.5 cm.   Contents: I. *Originals.*   1.   Letters by S.W. Mitchell.   a.   Correspondence with A.P.C. Ashhurst, W.A. Hammond, Alfred Stillé, etc., and many to John Madison Taylor, the latter the gift of Mrs. J. Madison, with added letter from Mrs. S.W.M. to Dr. Guy Hinsdale (envelope, ca. 1880-1907, 1915?).   b.   Official correspondence on behalf of the College of Physicians of Philadelphia (env., 1876-94).   c.   S.W.M. to A.P.C. Ashhurst about proposed appointment of Wm. Osler to the Dept. of Medicine of the Univ. of Penna., written by Mrs. Mitchell; added B.A. Fife on M.'s puzzle verse, clipping attached (1 env., 1884?; 1936). — 2.   Letters to S.W. Mitchell.   a.   Correspondents include J.S. Billings, Henry Day, Dyce Duckworth, M.G. Echeverria, C.J. Finlay, J.H. Jackson, Wm. Osler, James Paget, D'Arcy Power and Jeffries Wyman (1 env., 75 letters, 1854-1912).   b.   Letters from B.F. Barker, Andrew Carnegie, J.C. Dalton and Samuel Lewis (1 env., 15 letters, 1874-1910).   c.   Letter from R.M. O'Reilly on the work of Walter Reed and W.C. Gorgas on yellow fever (1 folder, 1902).   II. *Photocopies* of correspondence and of poems in the Trent Collection, Duke Univ., and the Medical School of Yale Univ. — Partial lists of contents included.   *[autogr. coll.]*

680.   —————.   Correspondence between Dr. S. Weir Mitchell, Maj. R.S. Woodson, and General Leonard Wood on smallpox in Cuba in 1898.   *V.p., 1898-99, 1909.*

1 v. (33 ff.).   27.5 cm.   Tearsheets of S.G. Dixon's article, Smallpox as Found and Treated in Cuba during the Spanish-American War included. — Presented by Samuel G. Dixon.   *[10a/450]*

681.   —————.   Daily journal.   *Philadelphia, 1913.*

365 pp., [9] ff.   22.5 cm.   Printed journal with a variety of entries by S.W. Mitchell, in his shaky hand, some in another hand; many pages blank.   Incl. notes on physical condition, visits, invitations, literary matters.   The last entry in his hand entered on December 27, eight days before his death.   Few inserts. — Gift of Mrs. Macdonnough and Mrs. Freedley.   *[10c/64]*

682.   —————.   Nature of snake poisoning.   *Philadelphia?, between 1853 and 1860.*

1 v.   19 cm.   *[10a/87]*

683.   ─────. To Doctor Osler in regard to his book *Science and Immortality. Philadelphia, 1904?*

9 ff. 30 cm. Typewritten (5 ff., with manuscript corrections in Mitchell's hand), and manuscript.   *[10a/195, pam. 3]*

684.   ─────. Turner's Lane Hospital; case and follow-up studies of peripheral nerve disorders, including correspondence addressed to S.W. Mitchell. *Philadelphia, 1861-92.*

1 box. 39 cm. Incomplete but extensive notes of Civil War patients with gunshot wounds, principally taken by Mitchell; many used in *Reflex Paralysis* (Philadelphia, 1864) and *Gunshot Wounds and Other Injuries of Nerves* (Philadelphia, 1864), coauthored with George Morehouse and William Keen. Incl. correspondence and follow-up case notes.   *[Z 10/40]*

685.   ─────, comp. Collection of printed items and manuscript copies relating to Sanctorius Sanctorius, with English translations and notes. *Philadelphia?, ca. 1890-91.*

3 v. 25.5-32 cm. Probably brought together in preparation of M.'s "The Early History of Instrumental Precision in Medicine" (cf. *Transactions* of the 2nd Cong. of Amer. Phys. & Surg., v. 2: 159-98, repr. New Haven, 1892). Contents: *V. 1.* Arcadio Capello. De vita . . . Sanctorii Sanctorii; . . . sermo habitus Venetiis . . . MDCCXLIX (Venice, 1701[sic]; 8 ff.); . . . . Oratio ab eodem Sanctorio dum ipse primarium theoriae medicinae explicande munus auspicaretur. Venetiis, apud Jacobum Thomasinum, MDCCI (6 ff.); English translations with separate title-pages ([1], 20, [1], 12, [1], 16 ff.). — *V. 2.* Del Gaizo, Modestino. Ricerche storiche intorno a Santorio Santorio . . . (extract from *Resoconto*, Accad. Med.-Chir., Napoli, 1889; 60 printed pp., with few ms. annotations by Dr. Mitchell); Del Gaizo, M. Alcune conoscenze di Santorio Santorio intorno al fenomeni della visione ed il testamento di lui trovato per opera di Francesco Silvestre. Memoria letta all'Accademia Pontaniana . . . 1891 (Naples, 1891; 28 pp.); handwritten bibliography of Sanctorius, with additions (unnamed compiler, n.d.; 4 ff.); Zanetti, Joannes Hieronymus. De laudibus Sanctorii Sanctorii; oratio habita in Collegio medicorum . . . 1752, estratta dall'originale autografo esistenti da carte 121 a 128ᵛᵒ dal codice LVIII, Classe XI, mss. ital. Bibl. naz. S. Marco, Venezia (7 ff.; ms.); bound in letters concerning the mss. from Mario Girardi, libr., Regia Bibl. Univ., Padua (1 f.) and John Shaw Billings (1 f.). — *V. 3.* Gravisi, Girolamo. Memoir of Santorio, 1791 (Bibl. univ., Padua, Racc. Benvenisti, no. 2131, misc. v. 96; [1], 25 ff.); unnamed translator.   *[Z 10/20]*

686.   ─────, comp. Hospital tablets, battlefield Gettysburg. *V.p., 1912-14.*

1 v.; maps, photogr. 39.5 cm. Typewritten. The hospitals of Gettysburg, by S.W. Mitchell, correspondence (letters by J.P. Nicholson), record of Camp Letterman with list of medical officers, copy of resolution of the College of Physicians of Philadelphia, etc. Gift of S.W. Mitchell, Lt.-Col. J.P. Nicholson and F.R. Packard.   *[Z 10/53]*

687.   ────, comp. Miscellaneous letters about Harvey; notes, etc. — Letters relating to the supposed Janssen portrait of Harvey. — Correspondence in regard to the Harvey letters owned by Lord Denbigh. *V.p., 1659, 1880-1912.*

1 v.;illus., facs. 32.5 cm. Partial contents: Reprod. of portraits; letters by D'Arcy Power, John Venn, W.S. Thayer, Finch, Earl of Winchilsea, Harvey Cushing, etc.; photographic reproduction of Robert Grove's *Carmen de sanguinis circuitu* . . . (London, 1685); power of attorney Dr. Baldwin Hamey to Thomas Browne, witnessed and sealed (London, 1659); photogr. of Harvey's table in Biological Museum, Univ. of Toronto; coats of arms; anonymous poem (ca. 1675, copy). — Bequeathed by S.W. Mitchell.   *[Z 10/52]*

────. See also nos. 17, 100, *185.13, .235, .35, .51-2,* 213, 238, 253, 454, 466, 532, 589, 593, 669, 877, 918, 991, 1063, 1105.

688.   **Mitchell, Thomas Duché,** 1791-1865. The charge of falsehood against Dr. Rush refuted. *Philadelphia, after 1853?*

Ff. 272-88. 25.5 cm. Author identified by mention of his "son, B. Rush Mitchell," and by a printed clipping, pasted to the bottom of f. 286, listing the lectures heard by the Philadelphia Medical Society, session 1821-22, including Dr. Mitchell's "Medical Character and Theories of the Late Dr. Rush." Manuscript mentions several dates, chiefly in the 1820s and 1830s; on f. 277 is mentioned a yellow fever patient (presumably of 1793) who survived "nearly sixty years."   *[10a/127]*

────. See also nos. 52, 910.

689.   **Monro, Alexander,** 1697-1767. Course of publick lectures in anatomy, in the College of Edinburgh. Taken from him during the time of lecturing by John Redman, student of physic and surgery in the same college. In proprium usum A.D. 1746. Copied from original manuscript by B. Duffield. *N.p., 1769.*

[33] pp. 18 cm. Corresponds closely, often word-for-word, with the more complete photocopy of another manuscript (no. 690). — Gift of H.R. Wharton.   *[10a/137]*

690.   ────. The history of anatomy from the earliest ages of the world down to the present time. *Edinburgh, after 1732.*

166 pp. 28 cm. Photocopy. Original in possession (1972) of Charles S. Cole, Jr.; photocopy presented by him. Material corresponds closely, often word-for-word, with the incomplete transcription of Monro's lectures made by John Redman in 1746, and copied by Benjamin Duffield. The Duffield version ends at p. 35 of this manuscript.   *[10d/148]*

691.   **Monro, Alexander,** 1733-1817. A course of lectures on physiology. . . . *Edinburgh, 1792-93.*

[2] ff., 417 pp. 23.5 cm. "The following lectures were written in Edinburgh, by my father, during the winter of 1792 and 93 - He having accompanied . . . me during the first winter of my studying. . . . He was at that time 60 years of age. Saml Hughes Jun$^{r'''}$ (f. [2v]). Inside front-cover portrait of Monro "[John] Kay fecit 1790." "S.H. 1792" and "Dr. Jas. Darrach from his friend J.E.C[arter] . . . 1886" (on flyleaf).   *[10a/188]*

92.   —————. Lectures on anatomy and surgery. *Edinburgh, ca. 1770.*

6 v. 24 cm. Lectures on surgery begin with v. 5. Contents include the history of anatomy, diseases or disorders of each system, comparative anatomy, and observations with a microscope. Pencilled on flyleaf, v. 1: "Alex Munro the 2nd [known as 'Secundus'] Dr. Morton." — Gift of John Morgan.

[10a/91]

93.   —————. Notes of Dr. Monro's lectures on anatomy and surgery. *Edinburgh, 1784?*

3 v. 26 cm. 123 numbered lectures; each volume with partial index. V. 1 and 2 headed "Anatomy"; v. 3, "Surgery." — From Dr. Caspar Wistar's medical library, presented to the College of Physicians of Philadelphia in the name of Mifflin Wistar.   *[10a/90]*

94.   —————. Praelectiones anatomicae Alexand[ri] Monro . . . ex ejus ore captae in Acedemia Edenburgensis 1752 (corrected to 1762 in pencil). *Edinburgh, 1762.*

[70] ff. 21 cm. "The gift of Doctor John Morgan to the College of Physicians of Philadelphia 1788," on title. Not in Morgan's hand. According to W.J. Bell's biography of Morgan, the latter was not enrolled in Munro's course, but procured notes of the lectures.   *[10a/89]*

—————. See also nos. 111, 399.

95.   **Montaña, Luis José,** 1755-1820. D.O.M. magni Hippocratis in ussum[!] juventutis Mexicanae Aphorismorum analysis aphoristica, item dictione traddita[!] per Alloysium Montanna. . . . *Mexico, 1815.*

[1] f., 33 pp. 22 cm. Lecture notes taken by Joaquin Villa and certified by the lecturer (signed Luis José Montaña, cf. p. 33). A printed commentary on the Aphorisms by Montaña was published in Mexico in 1817 (see J.J. Izquierdo, *Montaña . . .*, Mexico, 1955, esp. pp. 332-33).   *[10a/222]*

96.   **Montgomery, Edward Emmet,** 1849-1927. Fifty years in the practice of medicine. *Philadelphia, 1925.*

[16] ff. 28 cm. Typescript. Read at the College of Physicians of Philadelphia, 1925. Published in *Medical Journal and Record*, v. 122: 41-43, 101-03 (1925).

[Z 10/152]

697.   **Montpellier, Université.** Institutiones medicae. *Montpellier, 1745.*

447, 72 pp. 22 cm. Probably a dissertation by unnamed person. Contents: Physiology (pp. 1-445, incl. index). — Pathology (pp. 1-70, incl. index; second sequence). "Phisiologia" divided in 36 chapters, incl. one on circulation of blood (pp. 55-115), nutrition (pp. 194-210), vision (pp. 368-79), etc.; "patalogia" in 3 parts, subdivided by chapters. Among the many authorities cited are H. Boerhaave, A. van Leeuwenhoek, G.B. Morgagni, G.A. Borelli, R. Vieussens, J. Swammerdam, M. Malpighi, and G.E. Stahl. — Gift of E.B. Krumbhaar.

[10a/359]

698.   **Morgagni, Giovanni Battista,** 1682-1771. [Epistola] Clarissimo viro D.D. Morando Joannes Baptista Morgagnus S.P.D., *inc.*: Post litteras tuas . . . 1747. *Padua, 1750.*

[1], 4 ff. (and blank f.). 25 cm. Original, Latin transcript and English translation. Refers to the 1745 volume of the Academie des Sciences, Paris, the *Connoissance des temps*, 1747, to six copies of his letters which had not appeared in his *Epistolae anatomicae*, to be distributed by Morand, and his *Nova institutionum medicarum idea*, a present to Morand. — Gift of John H. Musser, 1910.

[10c/17]

— — — — —. See also no. 697.

699.   **Morgan, Alonzo Richardson,** 1830-1903. Notes by A.R. Morgan, Homoeopathic Medical College. *Philadelphia, 1851.*

1 v. 20 cm. Notes on lectures by [Walter] Williamson on materia medica and therapeutics, [Francis] Sims on surgery, J.G. Loomis on obstetrics, [Charles] Neidhard on diseases of females, and [W.T.] Helmuth on practice.

[10a/431]

700.   **Morgan, Arthur Caradoc,** 1869-1940. Case records from the Philadelphia General Hospital. *Philadelphia, 1897-1904.*

489 pp. (and inserts); illus., charts. 27 cm. Extensive records, including diagnostic charts, reports from various doctors, photographs, clippings, forms, letters to the coroner, drawings by an insane patient, printed article by F.A. Packard, etc.; some pasted or bound in, others loosely inserted.   *[10a/497]*

701.   — — — — —. Reminiscences, and two letters to A.C. Morgan. Typewritten copies, presented by Margaret M. Harmon (Reminiscences prepared probably in the 1970s by Morgan's daughter M.M. Harmon in St. Petersburg, Fla.). *V.p., 1909-197—.*

8 folders. 28 cm. Contents: Reminiscences of Bp. Benjamin Tucker Tanner and family (3 ff.), Philadelphia Dental College (2 ff.), Dr. Harry Walter Albertson (1 f.), Dr. William Henry Pancoast (2 ff.), epilepsy (1 f.) and Old Blockley (Phila. General Hospital, 4 ff.). — Original letter by Dr. George Edward Pfahler, president of the American Roentgen Ray Society aspiring to

be named professor of roentgenology (1909, 2 ff.). — Original letter from State Police Officer H.A. Price to Captain A.C. Morgan on influenza epidemic in Pottsville and Minersville (1918, 1 f.).   *[n.c.]*

— — — — —. See also nos. 341, 652.

702.   **Morgan, John,** 1735-1789. A compendium of chemistry, historical theoretical and practical. Being the substance of a course of chemical lectures ... (compiled by) John Hodge. *Philadelphia, 1766.*

     225 pp.   19.5 cm.   Hodge graduated from Univ. of Penna. in 1769.
                                                   [10a/93]

703.   — — — — —. Diary; entries of May 21-22, 1764. *Rome, 1764.*

     12 ff.   17 cm.   Notes from "A course of antiquities which I have engaged to go through at Rome under the direction of M. Beyers" [i.e., Byers].   Entry for May 22 incomplete?   Published as "Fragment of a Journal Written at Rome, 1764," in *The Journal of Dr. John Morgan of Philadelphia from the City of Rome to the City of London, 1764,* ed. Julia M. Harding (Philadelphia, 1907), pp. 247-59. — Gift of S.W. Mitchell.   *[10c/15]*

704.   — — — — —. Lectures on chemistry, containing 1st the history of chemistry, 2^d an introduction; 3^d the objects of chemistry; 4th the chemical history of bodies, and the 5th operations of chemistry. *Philadelphia, ca. 1766.*

     1 v.   20 cm.   "Ex libris Jonath^n. Elmer." — Attributed to Morgan on the basis of textual similarity to no. 702.   *[10a/389]*

705.   — — — — —. Photocopies and microfilm of items by, or relating to, John Morgan, accompanied by correspondence and notes. *Philadelphia, (presented in) 1965.*

     1 box (ca. 350 pieces).   52 cm.   Material gathered by W.J. Bell for his book *John Morgan: Continental Doctor* (Phila., 1965). — Some Samuel Bard and Thomas Parke items included.   *[Z 10c/12]*

706.   [— — — — —]. Collection of nine letters addressed to John Morgan. *V.p., 1756-83.*

     9 folders.   21-39 cm.   Contents: 1. Provost William Smith to "my worthy pupil," expressing his friendship and referring to attacks on Smith's character (1756). — 2. Dr. John Fothergill on the teaching of medicine in Philadelphia (1768; contemporary copy). — 3. Williams Smibert on medical education, publications and politics (1769; top of letter torn; published by W.B. McDaniel in *Annals of Med. Hist.,* ser. 3, v. 1: 194-96 [1939]). — 4. James Finley subscribing \$40, presumably a contribution to the College, Academy and Charitable School of Philadelphia (later Univ. of Penna.; 1772). — 5. Edward Rutledge on the military situation in Carolina, etc. (1776). — 6. William(?) Eustice on the condition at the General Hospital in Norwalk (1776). —

7. Jonathan Trumbull on supply of medicine (1777). — 8. Benjamin Rush comparing American with British medical system (1777; contemporary copy). — 9. Aaron Burr on writ against a person (Blair) owing a debt to Morgan (1783). Most of these letters were mentioned by W. J. Bell, Jr., in his *John Morgan* (1965). *[10a/314]*

—————. See also nos. 114, 285, 694, 931, 1048-9.

707. **Morris, Caspar,** 1805-1884. Medical notebooks. *Philadelphia, ca. 1824-36.*

2 v. 23.5-25 cm. Volume 1 contains notes on occasional lectures by Chapman, some clinical histories, and some casual notes on medical topics. V. 2 consists chiefly of a long unfinished essay on fever; then, beginning at the other end of the book, a few entries in the journal of his visit to England in 1836, dated May 13-18. *[10a/367]*

—————. See also no. 965.

708. **Morris, Warder** (druggist). Recipt [sic] book, [of] Warder Morris. Incipit Sept. 4th, 1806. *Philadelphia, 1806-?*

52, [3] pp. 20 cm. Presented by Mrs. Marmaduke Tilden, through O.H. Perry Pepper, November 13, 1943. *[10a/345]*

709. **Morton, Samuel George,** 1799-1851. Two inaugural medical essays. . . . *Philadelphia, 1820, Edinburgh, 1823;* Introduction, *Philadelphia, 1829.*

[1] f., 39 pp., [10] ff., 37 pp. (interleaved), [5 blank] ff. 20.5 cm (envelope, 37 cm). Contents: Introduction (biographical); Popliteal aneurism (Univ. of Penna. thesis, 1820); De corporis dolore (printed Univ. of Edinburgh thesis, 1823). — Presented by Mrs. James Creese. *[10a/475]*

—————. See also nos. 773, 899.

710. **Morton, Thomas Story Kirkbride,** 1865-1930. Manuscript notes entered in syllabus of the Department of Medicine, University of Pennsylvania. *Philadelphia, 1884.*

2 v. 23 cm. Printed, interleaved text of vol. 1 with extensive notes on James Tyson's "General Pathological Anatomy" (pp. 189-249), scattered notes on D.H. Agnew's "Surgery" (pp. 341-450), the only two annotated items in this volume. Vol. 2 (pp. 251-339) is not interleaved and has few notes (R.A.F. Penrose's "Female Organs of Generation"). *[10b/64]*

711. **Mudd, Stuart,** comp., 1893-1975. Collection of materials by and about medical members of the Hodgen-Mudd family. *V.p., 1882-1930?*

1 envelope. 37.5 cm. Concerns: John Thompson Hodgen. Includes Memorial address by Ellsworth F. Smith, Sr., delivered at the opening of the 1882/83 session, St. Louis Medical College; "A Sketch of the Life of the Late

John T. Hodgen, M.D., by One Who Knew Him," reprinted from the *Medical Mirror*, Jan., 1890; Memorial exercises held under the auspices of the St. Louis Medical Society of Missouri, . . . April 28, 1907, publ. as Suppl. to the *St. Louis Medical Review*, May 11, 1907; "John Thompson Hodgen," by Harvey G. Mudd, repr. from *Surgery, Gynecology, and Obstetrics*, Apr. 1926: 579-81; "The Hodgen-Mudd Memorial," *Quincy Medical Bulletin*, Dec. 1928; Address of Harvey Gilmer Mudd (typewritten). — Henry Hodgen Mudd. "Modern medicine and modern surgery," an address read before the Round Table Club, by Henry H. Mudd, repr. from *Medical Mirror*, March, 1898; "In memoriam, Doctor Harvey Hodgen Mudd," by Ellsworth Smith, Jr., repr. from *St. Louis Courier of Medicine*, Nov. 1899; Untitled typescript, dated January 19, 1922, biogr. of H H. Hodgen; Henry Hodgen Mudd, M.D. [by H.G. Mudd?]; Typewritten copy "H.G. Mudd". — Harvey Gilmer Mudd, address at Livezey Hospital & St. Luke's, 1930, in honor of the graduating class of nurses, typescript and mimeographed copy.   *[Z 10/221]*

—————.   See also no. 1051.

712.   **Mühring, Peter.**   Artzney Buch, getheilet in fünf Bücher.   *Pennsylvania?, 1747.*

[2] ff. (first blank), 546 pp. (pp. 487-536 and 549-50 lacking).   16 cm.   The name Peter Mühring appears on p. 28.   Contents: Von des Menschen Gesundheit (pp. 1-28). — Von unterschiedlichen Kranckheiten zu heylen . . . nach der Ordnung des Alphabets (pp. 29-293). — Von zarter Kinder Kranckheiten (pp. 295-303). — Einiger destillirter Wässer Tugend und Kräffte und Würkung (pp. 322-32). — Einiger destillirter Öle Tugend (pp. 333-65). — Einiger Artzneyen Tugend (pp. 367-87). — Von einigen Artzneyen, welche ein Mensch allzeit um sich haben kan (pp. 389-94). — Die inwendige Beschaffenheit und Bewegung der Natur des menschlichen Leibes (pp. 395-425). — Sections on bees, cows, calves, sheep (pp. 427-43). — Haushaltungs Calender (pp. 445-83).   *[10a/268]*

713.   **Münz, Isak.**   The Jewish physicians of the Middle Ages; a contribution to the cultural history of the Middle Ages (published by J. Kaufmann Publications, Frankfurt a.M., 1922).   Personal translation by Samuel X Radbill.   *Philadelphia, 1933.*

86, [50] ff.   28 cm.   Typewritten.   Translation of *Die jüdischen Aerzte im Mittelalter*. — Gift of translator.   *[ZZ 10d/4]*

714.   **Mütter, Thomas Dent,** 1811-1859.   Lectures on surgery.   *Philadelphia, ca. 1847.*

105, [8 blank] pp., 1 quire missing, pp. 138-39, [7] blank ff.; illus.   20.5 cm (envelope, 27 cm).   Cover-title: Mütter's Syllabus.   Lectures given at Jefferson Medical College, recorded by unnamed student.   *[10b/8]*

—————.   See also nos. 112, *185.231, .63,* 338, 507, 765, 1105.

715. **Musser, John Herr,** 1856-1912. Notes on clinical medicine lectures. *Philadelphia, 1907-08.*

24 ff.; illus. 22 cm. Mainly on gastro-intestinal diseases. Several of the lectures given by Joseph Sailer. — Notes by, and gift of E.B. Krumbhaar.
[10a/421]

716. **Nägele, Franz Carl,** 1778-1851. System der Geburtshilfe (pars pathologica et diaetetica). Nach seinen Vorträgen geschrieben von K. Wilhelmi. *Heidelberg, 1835(-41).*

[1] f., 190 pp. 17.5 cm. Geburtshilfliche Dissertationen, pp. 184-86 (48 items, 1775-1841), and table of contents, pp. 187-90.   *[10a/94]*

717. **Nagle, Frank Orthmer.** Anomalies, 1878-79. *Philadelphia, 1879.*

[28] pp. 21.5 cm. Offered in competition for a student prize awarded at the Univ. of Pennsylvania, Department of Medicine by Hugh Lenox Hodge, who presented this ms. to the College of Physicians of Philadelphia.   *[10a/58]*

718. **Nassau, Charles Francis.** Decompression in cranial fractures. *Philadelphia, 1911.*

18 ff. 28 cm. Typewritten. Thomas Dent Mütter Lectureship at College of Physicians of Philadelphia, 1911.   *[10a/370]*

— — — — —. See also no. 837.

719. **Nock, Ebenezer.** Bio-bibliography of John Banester (or Banister; 1533-1610). *London, 1880.*

[8] pp. 19 cm.   *[10a/227]*

720. **Norris, George Washington,** 1808-1875. The early history of medicine in Philadelphia. *Philadelphia?, 187—.*

4 v. in 1 box. 33.5 cm. Partly rough notes, partly fair printer's copy. Published Philadelphia, Collins, 1886.   *[Z 10/75]*

721. — — — — —. Record of all capital operations and consultations on doubtful cases at the Pennsylvania Hospital. *Philadelphia, 1836-49.*

152 pp., blank ff., [2] pp. index at end of volume; illus. 31 cm. Incl. notes on patients attended to by staff surgeons George Fox, Thomas Harris, Edward Peace, and Jacob Randolph. With inserts, painted portrait at beginning; 2 engr. portraits and case report by Dr. A.M. White, transmitted to Dr. Norris by S. Caldwell, inserted. — Bookplate and gift of G.W. Norris.   *[Z 10/51]*

722.   —————. Record of private surgical practice and operations. *Philadelphia, 1835-43.*

37 pp., blank f., 1 p. index at end. 26 cm. Case histories. — Presented by G.W. Norris.   *[10b/29]*

723.   —————. Surgical notes and abstracts. *Philadelphia, 1842-74.*

1 v. 26 cm. Bibliographical references inscribed in commercial common-place book. Laid-in notes include abstracts of reviews of Norris' published works.   *[10b/30]*

724.   —————. Varioloid and vaccine diseases. *Philadelphia, 1830.*

[1], 21 ff. 25 cm. Thesis, M.D. — Univ. of Pennsylvania, 1830. Bound with W.F. Norris, *Generation and Development* (no. 731), and G.W. Norris, *The Moors in Spain* (no. 727). — Gift of George William Norris (with his bookplate).
[10a/248(1)]

—————. See also nos. 765, 1118.

725.   **Norris, George William,** 1875-1965. Diary, World War I. *Philadelphia, 1959.*

1 v.; ports., illus. 29.3 cm. Typewritten. Book plate of G.W. Norris inside front cover.   *[ZZ 10c/5]*

726.   —————. Medical memories. An account of events and personalities that I saw and heard as a medical student at the University of Pennsylvania, 1895-99. *Philadelphia, ca. 1897-99.*

1 v. (loose leaf); illus. (largely portraits). 29.5 cm. Typewritten, incl. clippings, etc. Some medical recollections by George W[ashington] Norris (ff. 3-8); Valedictory address . . . 1897 by William Fisher Norris, M.D. (ff. 66-unnumb. f. between ff. 73-74). Autograph letters by Francis R. Packard, his wife, William H. Good, Charles C. Norris, George H. Halberstadt, typewritten letters signed by Henry Norris and Julius L. Wilson, and letter by Alfred Stengel included.   *[ZZ 10c/13]*

727.   —————. The Moors in Spain. *Philadelphia, 1895.*

17, [1] ff. 25 cm. Typewritten thesis, A.B. — Univ. of Pennsylvania. Bound with nos. 724 and 731.   *[10a/248(3)]*

—————. See also no. 839.

728.   **Norris, William Fisher,** 1839-1901. Catalogue of medical books in his library. *Philadelphia?, 1881-87?*

2 v. 29 cm. Arrangement alphabetical by subject (in red), with author cross references. Compiled by Charles A. Oliver (cf. end fly leaves). Norris' library, now in the College of Physicians of Philadelphia, presented by his family.
[10a/155]

729.   — — — — —. Clinical notes on cases seen at the Douglas Hospital at Washington, D.C. during the Civil War. *Washington, 1864-65.*

[25] pp. 34.5 cm. In two hands, that of Norris, the other that of Henry Gibbons, Jr.   *[Z 10/70]*

730.   — — — — —. Collection of ophthalmological drawings made from cases in the practice of William Fisher Norris. *Philadelphia, 1874-1901.*

1 v.; portrait, col. illus., photogr. 33 cm. Binder's title: Atlas of ophthalmology. Case notes (largely not in Dr. Norris' hand) on interleaved paper; illustrations mounted, most signed or prepared by Margaretta Washington, some by Herman Faber, one signed M.L. Wood. Named patients, largely treated at Wills Eye Hospital and Hospital of the Univ. of Pennsylvania. — Gift of George W. Norris.   *[Z 10/37]*

731.   — — — — —. Generation and development. *Philadelphia, 1861.*

[2], 68 ff. 25 cm. Thesis, M.D. — Univ. of Pennsylvania, 1861. Bound with nos. 724 and 727.   *[10a/248(2)]*

732.   — — — — —. Letters. *Gettysburg, 1863.*

8 items. 20 cm. Norris' letters to his parents concerning his duties as assistant surgeon, U.S.A., at the Hospital of 3rd Division, 1st Army Corps and at the General Hospital, Gettysburg; also orders relieving him of duty at Gettysburg. One letter in typewritten copy. — Gift of George W. Norris.   *[10a/463]*

733.   — — — — —. Notes on the clinics and lectures on ophthalmology delivered to the medical class of the University of Pennsylvania. *Philadelphia, 1892-93.*

1 v. 21 cm. Notes taken by John M. Swan. Includes 27 case reports from University Hospital, 4 Oct. 1892 to 2 Feb. 1893. Three pages at end (dated 29 Oct.-5 Nov. 1920) appear to be clinical notes on five of Swan's later patients.   *[10a/327]*

— — — — —. See also nos. 36, 726, 747, 839, 1079-80.

734.   **Northern Dispensary** for the Medical Relief of the Poor, Philadelphia. Lying-In Department. Register of patients, 1836-1920, 1923-24. *Philadelphia, 1835-1924.*

291, 1 pp. 40 cm. Rules and regulations of the Lying-In Department, adopted by the Board of Managers November 4th, 1835 (p. 1). Pasted in at end a table, apparently comparing the number of prescriptions written by months for the years 1908-17.   *[Z 10c/15]*

735.   **Northern Medical Association** of Philadelphia. Constitution and by-laws, minutes, reports and addresses, membership lists, accounts, publications and clippings. *Philadelphia, 1846-1945.*

2 boxes, 7 v. 24-36.5 cm. Constitution and by-laws, located at the end of the first minute-book; minutes, 1846-69, 1888-1945, with some photographs, announcements, and clippings of the Northern Medical Association, organized to "cultivate the science of medicine, and to promote harmony among its members." Drafts of minutes; misc. reports and addresses to the association; lists of members, memoirs, biographies, and biographical data; account books, 1847-1933; contributions; misc. programs, publications, and reprints of association materials. *[Z 10/209-11]*

736. **Nurses' Beneficial Association,** Philadelphia. Account books, 1890-1917.

4 v. 35-40 cm. Various systems of bookkeeping used; records appear to overlap. *[Z 10c/24]*

737. ————. Correspondence (1890-93, 1908-22); minutes (1889-90); annual reports, 1891-92, 1893. *Philadelphia, 1889-93, 1908-22.*

1 box. 26 cm. Correspondence of Wharton Sinkler (president), Mrs. M.J. Lake (secretary), and Harriet H. Browne (secretary). *[Z 10c/28]*

738. ————. Members' register. *Philadelphia, 1889-191—?*

3 v. 40 cm. This set appears to be the index to volumes now missing, presumably having contained the record of dues to the association. *[Z 10c/26]*

739. **Obstetrical Society** of Philadelphia. Constitution and by-laws, minutes, correspondence, lists of officers and members, accounts, publications. *Philadelphia, 1868-1955.*

11 v. 21-41 cm. Constitution and by-laws, 1868; minute books, 1879-1946, with misc. related notes and correspondence, and rough drafts of minutes, 1879-94; correspondence, 1873-1920, acknowledging receipt of the society's *Transactions*, accepting honorary membership, responding to invitations, etc. Lists of officers, 1868-81, lists of members (incl. honorary, corresponding, and associate, among others Robert Barnes, James Matthews Duncan, Max Sänger, and Giovanni Battista Fabbri), 1868-1955; treasurer's accounts, 1868-77, 1896-1928, with index, incl. membership payments; reprints of L.C. Scheffey's "The Early Years of the Obstetrical Society of Philadelphia," *Trans. & Stud.*, ser. 4, v. 6: 125-47, 292-316 (1938). *[10a/347]*

————. See also nos. 401, 586, 609, 940.

740. ————. Library. List of books belonging to the Society. *Philadelphia, 1899.*

7 ff. 33 cm. *[Z 10c/6]*

741. **O'Hara, Michael,** 1832-1905. Medical journal. *V.p., 1854-57.*

2 v. 34 cm. Contents: V. 1. Medical journal of *U.S.S. Falmouth*, Home Squadron, Nov. 24, 1854-Aug. 23, 1855; Journal of *U.S.S. Saratoga*, Sept. 7, 1855-Oct. 5, 1856. — V. 2. Journal of *U.S.S. Saratoga*, Oct. 6, 1856-Apr. 28, 1857.

[Z 10a/6]

742. **[O'Hara, Michael,** 1869-1926]. Series of letters to Dr. O'Hara. *V.p., 1889-1903.*

1 envelope (3 folders). 37.5 cm. Contents: Folder 1. Eleven letters supporting his application for appointment as surgeon in the U.S. Army (1898). — 2. Seven letters (by his father [M. O'Hara, sen.], C.B. Penrose, etc.) on appointments to St. Agnes and the Gynecean Hospital, etc., and few misc. items (1889-1900). — 3. Twenty-five letters, or cards, concerning O'Hara's anastomosis forceps (1900-03). — Lists of correspondents enclosed.   *[n.c.]*

743. **Onderdonk, Henry Ustick,** bp., 1789-1858. Horae Londinenses; containing: 1. The surgical course of A. Cooper (pp. 1-258). — 2. The anatomical and surgical lectures of J. Abernethy (pp. 259-86). — 3. The surgical lectures of J. Abernethy (pp. 287-373). — 4. The anatomical &c. lectures of Messrs. Headington & Frampton at the London Hospital (pp. 375-459). — 5. Remarks and cases (pp. 461-83). *London, 1809-10.*

483 pp. 25 cm. Presented by Samuel Lewis.   *[10b/42]*

744. —————. On stone in the bladder. *New York, 1810?*

[3], 38 ff. 27 cm. Autograph, with numerous corrections and inserts between ff. 23-4. Thesis (Dr. Phys.) — Columbia College, New York, submitted Nov. 13, 1810. Obviously the copy sent to the printer, cf. slip addressed to Messrs. Swords, inserted before f. [1]. Bound with this is published version (New York, T. & J. Swords, 1810), 44 pp.   *[10a/139, no. 1]*

745. ———— —————. *New York, ca. 1810.*

32 ff. 26 cm. Another (earlier?) version, with many corrections and insert between ff. 28-9.   *[10a/139, no. 2]*

—————. See also nos. 111-2, 1129.

746. **Ophthalmic Club** of Philadelphia. Constitution (1922-23), program, acknowledgements of selection to membership, Executive Committee agenda, etc. *Philadelphia, etc., 1922-34, 1974-75.*

1 envelope (16 ff.). 31 cm.   *[n.c.]*

747. **Ophthalmological Society** of Philadelphia. Constitution, by-laws, minutes. *Philadelphia, 1870-75.*

2 v. (v. 1: 12 ff., 4 pp. — v. 2, unpaged). 24-32 cm. V. 1. Constitution and by-laws (1870) of Society to Promote the Study of Ophthalmology. — V.

2. Minute book (1870-72; 1874-75), concerning society's business, and incl. some discussion of papers presented at meetings. Contains the signatures of 14 early members in v. 1; v. 2 in the handwriting of the society's secretaries W.F. Norris and Douglas Hall. — Presented by Samuel D. Risley.

[v. 1: 10a/204; v. 2: Z 10/68]

748. **Oppenheim, Moritz,** b. 1876. Lectures on clinical dermatology. *Vienna, 1933.*

[2], 37, [5] ff. 20.5 cm (envelope, 26.5 cm). Typescript. Physical examination in dermatology (2 prel. ff.) inscribed Dr. Miskjian. With prescription blanks, clippings, and menu with names of American postgraduates and names of dermatologists. Includes index. Notes taken and presented by George W. Binkley.

[10a/469]

749. **The Organs of Sense.** N.p., ca. 1780?

33 pp. (pp. 1-2, presumably incl. title, missing). 20 cm (envelope, 27 cm). Pencilled note on margin of p. 3 indicates a connection with Abraham Chovet; the manuscript might be a transcript of his lecture, he may have been the author, or the note may be spurious.

[n.c.]

750. **Orme, David,** d. 1812. Heads of a course of lectures given by Drs. Orme & Lowder on the theory and practice of midwifery. *N.p., 1777.*

128 pp. 20 cm. Transcript of notes. Inscribed on flyleaf: "Wm. Dewees", "Isaac Hays."

[10a/95]

751. **Osborne, William,** 1736-1808. Notes from Drs. Osborne's & Clarke's lectures on midwifery, taken by T.C. James. *London, 1790-91.*

1 v. 24 cm. Signature of Tho. C. James on flyleaf. — After 1783 Osborne, with John Clarke, continued the annual lectures on midwifery founded by Thomas Denman. Topics and occasional passages show parallels to Denman's *An Introduction to the Practice of Midwifery*. Contents: Menstruation (42 pp.); diseases of the organs of generation in the female (26 pp.); generation (25 pp.); determination of pregnancy (15 pp.); difficult labours (22 pp.); praeternatural labours (53 pp.).

[10a/96]

752. **Osler, William,** bart., 1849-1919. Letters to Maude Abbott in Montreal. *Baltimore and Oxford, Sept. 1900-Aug. 18, 1906(-1918).*

1 envelope. 24 cm. Twenty-eight letters chiefly concerning the catalogue of the Medical Museum at McGill; incl. one to J.W. Croskey (Oxford, 1918), and two typewritten lists of books given by Osler to the Library of the College of Physicians of Philadelphia, with third combining the two earlier ones.

[10d/23]

753. ————. On erythromelalgia. — On Raynaud's disease. *Oxford?, 1909?*

[23, 27] ff.   26.5 cm.   Manuscript copy; interpolations and addenda in Osler's hand; sections of *Modern Medicine*, v. 6 (1909) include corrections and inserts for later edition, by Thomas McCrae. — Gift of N.B. Gwyn.   *[10a/458]*

754.   — — — — —.   Summary of the necropsies of Sir William Osler at Philadelphia General Hospital.   *Philadelphia, ca. 1940?*

1 envelope (1 half-sheet, 4, 6 ff.).   31 cm.   Compiled by, or under the direction of E.B. Krumbhaar.   *[n.c.]*

— — — — —.   See also nos. 29, 253, 346, 507, 552, 593, 669, 675, 679, 683, 801, 834, 1034, 1050, 1079-80, 1106.

755.   **Otto, John C.,** 1774-1844.   Paper on allergies and food poisoning. *Philadelphia, 1833.*

[12] pp.   25 cm.   Read at the College of Physicians of Philadelphia, Oct. 29, 1833.   *[n.c.]*

757.   **Paris. American Hospital.**   Case record of wounded.   *Paris, 1915.*

1 box; portr.; illus.   32 cm.   Typewritten and manuscript.   Extensive file of case records, largely or entirely by Daniel Josef McCarthy and unsigned, incomplete report of June 20, 1915 (9 ff.).   *[10a/487]*

758.   **[Paris, Hospitals].**   Case reports in English from the Hôpital de Charité, Hotel Dieu and Hôpital St. Louis, etc.   *Paris, 1819-20.*

296 pp.   25 cm.   Includes statistics on number of patients admitted, Dec. 1819-Feb. 1820, death, marriages, etc. (pp. 112-14, [in reverse] 262-257); Cours d'accouchemens of Paul Dubois (pp. 115-28); Phrenology (and psychology, pp. 129-224); Pathology-physiology (pp. 294-288, in reverse); Tourist notes, etc. — Bookplate of Hugh Lenox Hodge.   *[10a/121]*

759.   **Parke, Thomas,** 1749-1835.   Lecture before the American Medical Society, Nov. 17, 1770.   *Philadelphia, 1770.*

[8] ff.   25 cm.   Lecture found among the papers of the son of Dr. Parke; autograph.   Included the printed card of the American Medical Society, with motto "Spe uniti" beneath a decorative design, and "Philad*a*" on left, "1770" on right.   Lecture chiefly concerned with a case "of pleuropneumonia" in the Almshouse.   *[10a/451]*

— — — — —.   See also nos. *185.13*, 705, 1127.

760.   **Parrish, Joseph,** 1779-1840.   Lectures on practice of medicine. *Philadelphia, after 1820.*

1 v.   19 cm.   Lecturer identified by comparison with W.W. Gerhard's transcript of Parrish's lectures, 1827 (no. 761).   Ms. is incomplete, beginning with p. 53.   Notes taken by Joseph W. Paul, cf. inscription on front fly-leaf, and scribbles at the end.   *[10a/452]*

761. –––––. Notes of Doctor Parrish's lectures on the practice of medicine, taken by William W. Gerhard. *Philadelphia, 1827.*

116 ff. 26.5 cm. The first series of lectures (numbered I to [XVIII]) is principally concerned with fevers, the second (unnumbered) with certain gastrointestinal diseases, as dysentery, diarrhea, etc. Typewritten table of contents filed with volume.   *[10a/97]*

762. –––––. Surgical lectures n[umbers] 2, 3. Winter course 1824.5.6. *Philadelphia, 1824-26.*

[6] misnumbered ff., pp. 7-73, 51 ff. 18 × 22 cm (oblong). Notes taken by William Ashmead, part of lecture 2 by John Levering (cf. p. 42), and possibly by others. Misbound? Ashmead's signature found in several places.
                              [10b/26]

–––––. See also nos. 104, 791, 795, 804, 1107, 1115.

763. **Paschall, Elizabeth Coates,** b. 1702. Receipt book. *Philadelphia, 1749-66.*

90 pp. 21 cm. Presented by Mrs. Francis Strawbridge.   *[10a/352]*

–––––. See also no. 852.

764. **Paterson, George M.** Statement of phrenology in Calcutta, to the Phrenological Society, Philadelphia. *Calcutta, ca. 1830.*

[20] ff. (18-20 blank). 23 cm (envelope, 30.5 cm). Deals with the Phrenological Society of Calcutta and the Phrenological School of Munnunpaor(?), both established in 1825.   *[n.c.]*

765. **Pathological Society** of Philadelphia. Articles of incorporation; minutes. *Philadelphia, 1857-87.*

9 pp.; 2 v. 18.5 and 33 cm. Articles of incorporation, 1857 (9 pp.), signed by members of this society (incl. N. Chapman, C.D. Meigs, H.L. Hodge, W.E. Horner, G.B. Wood, W.W. Gerhard, G.W. Norris, W. Pepper, J. Carson, J.F. Meigs, T.D. Mütter, E. Hartshorne, and I. Parrish, established for the cultivation of general and special pathology, and the formation of a cabinet of specimens. – Minute books, 1857-87 (2 v.), recording society's bi-monthly business meetings; contain reports and discussions of cases brought before the members, written by secretaries (incl. J.M. Da Costa, J.H. Packard, J.H. Hutchinson, J.K. Kane, W.W. Keen, L. Starr, and J.K. Mitchell). – Cases also reported in the society's *Transactions*, beginning 1857.   *[10a/208; Z 10/34]*

–––––. See also nos. 299, 311, 523.

766. **Paul, John Marshall,** 1800-1879. Memoir of Dr. Thomas Hendry Ritchie. *Philadelphia, 1837.*

8 pp. 25.5 cm. Probably an earlier draft of Paul's memoir of Ritchie than that in the "Biographical Sketches and Memoirs of Members of the College of Physicians of Philadelphia," 1836-41, pp. 32-6.   *[n.c.]*

——————. See also nos. 142, 481.

767. **Paul, John Rodman,** 1893-1971. A pathological study of the pleural and pulmonary lesions in rheumatic fever, by J. Rodman Paul and William U. McClenahan. *New Haven?, 1928.*

118 ff.; 28 mounted, unnumb. illus., photogr. plates, table. 28 cm (envelope, 37 cm). Typescript (carbon copy). Alvarenga Prize Essay, no. 26, 1928. Twenty-eight case histories, pp. 80-107. Brief report of this study published in *Arch. of Pathology,* v. 8: 595-610 (1934).   *[10d/20]*

——————. See also no. 563.

768. **Peace, Edward,** 1811-1879. Medical notes. *Philadelphia, 1842.*

[28] ff. (irregularly numbered 47 pp.). 20 cm. Surgical case histories; list of cases at beginning of volume. Gift of the City of Philadelphia, originally in Phila. General Hospital.   *[10a/498]*

——————. See also nos. 721, 1118.

769. **Pediatric Society** of Philadelphia. Official records; correspondence; research papers, etc. *V.p., 1896-1958.*

13 v., 5 correspondence files; 3 boxes (27 folders correspondence, etc.); correspondence file and 1 large box (185 folders of research papers and discussions); 1 envelope, 1 spring binder, 1 drawer (membership file). 22-36 cm. Partial contents: By-laws, minutes and committee reports (1896-1947); ledgers (1908-41); papers of the Society's Milk Commission; presidential addresses; correspondence (partly indexed); research papers (indexed; among frequent authors are Rachel Ash, Harry Lowenburg, R.M. Tyson, I.J. Wolman); papers of 1956 Resident Price Award; S. X Radbill's address "The Philadelphia Pediatric Society; Historical Highlights" (1958).   *[10a/371]*

——————. See also no. 1081.

770. **Pelouze, Percy Starr,** 1876-1947. The gonophage by P.S. Pelouze . . . and Frederick S. Schofield. From the Department of Urology, University of Pennsylvania. *Philadelphia, 1926.*

[2], 57 ff.; tables, charts. 29 cm. Typewritten. Folio 36A and title of part 2 inserted between ff. 36 and 37. Alvarenga Prize Essay, no. 24, 1926. Published in *Journal of Urology,* v. 17: 407-38 (1927). Gift of authors.   *[10d/17]*

771. **Penington, John,** 1768-1793. On the phenomena, causes and effects of fermentation. *Philadelphia, 1790.*

[19] ff.   22 cm.   Penington's signature on cover and "John P" on bottom of f.
[19v].   Thesis, M.D. — Univ. of Penna.   Published Philadelphia, Joseph
James, 1790.   *[10a/225]*

772.   **Pennsylvania. Department of Health.** Committee of Public
Safety. Minutes . . . (of the meeting of the) Sub Committee on
Medicine, Sanitation and Red Cross. *Harrisburg?, April 26, 1917.*

73 ff. (f. 1, blank?, missing).   28 cm.   Typewritten (carbon copy), signed.   Includes "Report on Suggested Locations for Military Hospitals in Pennsylvania,"
by Samuel G. Dixon, commissioner of health, ff. 27-73.   *[10d/53]*

773.   **Pennsylvania College,** Gettysburg. Medical Department, Philadelphia. Five manuscript records. *Philadelphia, 1840-49.*

I.   An act authorizing the faculty of Pennsylvania College to confer the degree
of doctor of medicine.   Approved March 6, 1840 (1 p., 24 cm). — II.   Rules and
regulations of the dissecting rooms.   Oct., 1844 (1 p., 23 cm). — III.   Receipt to
Dr. William Robertson Grant, Oct. 27, 1846, signed Samuel George Morton (1
p., 20 cm). — IV.   Contract for building Pennsylvania Medical College.   [1849?]
(2 pp., 25 cm). — V.   Note from Dr. Morton to Dr. Grant, Nov. 20, 1849 (1 p., 20
cm).   *[10c/66]*

— — — — —.   See also no. 350.

774.   **Pennsylvania Hospital,** Philadelphia. Hospital gleanings —
Doct. Gerhard's term, July 1st, 1847. *Philadelphia, 1847.*

177, [10] pp.   25.5 cm.   Case records, presumably at the Pennsylvania
Hospital, by a student of Gerhard's. — Gift of William W. Gerhard.   *[10a/42]*

— — — — —.   See also nos. 83, *185.62*, 248, 331, 379, 439, 533, 553,
721, 926, 1047, 1112.

775.   **Pennsylvania Infirmary** for Diseases of the Eye and Ear,
Philadelphia. Board of Directors. Minute book, 1822-1829.
Philadelphia, 1822-29.

22 ff.   24 cm.   Secretaries Isaac Hay (donor of the ms., cf. presentation
inscription inside front cover), William H. Keating, and R. Eglesfeld Griffith.
This manuscript and the Infirmary were described by Charles A. Oliver, in "A
Brief Account of the Pennsylvania Infirmary," *Medical Library and Historical
Journal,* v. 1, April, 1903.   *[10a/98]*

776.   **Pennsylvania State Vaccination Commission.** Minutes of
meetings, including reports presented by proponents and oppo-
nents of vaccination in general, but especially against smallpox;
interrogations; discussions with a variety of documents. Sessions 2-35. *Philadelphia, 1912-13.*

6 boxes (containing 10 files). 30 cm. Typewritten (largely carbon copies), with handwritten corrections. Members of the Committee: Emil Rosenberger, chairman; Henry C. Lippincott, secretary; Edward A. Woods, William M. Welch, Jay F. Schamberg, John Pitcairn and Porter F. Cope. Reports and discussions deal with the history of vaccination and smallpox, their nature and symptoms, include statistics (U.S. and abroad), vaccination against typhus, also touches on tetanus and syphilis. Among persons reporting, testifying, or quoted extensively, are V.C. Vaughen, Adolf Vogt, Martin Friedrich, Robert N. Willson, Oscar Marcotte, C.M. Higgins, Benjamin Lee, and some members of the Committee. Considerably more extensive than the official printed report (Philadelphia, March 1913). Detailed index and corrections at end of last file in box 6.   *[ZZ 10d/1]*

777. **Penrose, Richard Alexander Fullerton,** 1827-1908. Notes taken on lectures delivered . . . by Dr. R.A.F. Penrose . . . during the winter of '64 and '65. *Philadelphia, 1864-65.*

1 v.; front. 17.5 cm. Book label of student Herbert M. Howe (verso front cover) and pencil drawing of Dr. Penrose by Howe.   *[10a/383]*

778. –––––. Notes taken [by H.M. Howe] upon lectures delivered by Prof. Jos. [?, R.A.F.] Penrose on the diseases of women and children. *Philadelphia, 186–.*

1 v. 17.5 cm.   *[10a/385]*

779. –––––. Obstetrics. *Philadelphia, 1876.*

135 pp. (followed by 202 blank pp.). 33 cm. Copy made by Charles Baum from shorthand notes taken by William Taylor (M.D. 1876, Univ. of Penna.). – Charles Baum's signature inside front cover; presented to the College by him. Table of contents tipped in.   *[Z 10/120]*

–––––. See also nos. 43, 226, 710, 1080.

780. **Pepper, Oliver Hazard Perry,** 1884-1962. Miscellaneous papers. *V.p., 1918-44[-47?].*

10 items. 28 cm. Partly typescript. Contents: Letters' (7), 1918-44, on various matters concerning the library of the College of Physicians of Philadelphia, to librarians (esp. W.B. McDaniel, 2d); letter to Francis R. Packard, 1947, responding to request for biographical material on William Pepper. – Speeches, remarks by toastmaster, 1st banquet, honorary consultants, Army Medical Library (1947?). – Address of welcome to Association of Military Surgeons as president of the College of Physicians of Philadelphia, 1943.   *[10d/89]*

–––––. See also nos. *185.13*, 551.

781. **Pepper, William,** 1810-1864. Notes on Prof. Wm. Pepper's lectures on principles & practice of medicine, University of Pennsylvania, 1863-64, taken by D.M. Cheston. *Philadelphia, 1863-64.*

115 pp. 18.5 cm. On the back flyleaf, a list of dates and topics of the lectures; on the end-paper, several lines of verse and a pencil sketch of an unidentified man. Lectures dated Jan. 14th to Feb. 15th, 1864.   *[10a/236]*

782.   —————. Notes taken [by] H.M. Howe upon lectures ... on the theory and practice of medicine, Oct. 13th 1863. *Philadelphia, 1863.*

1 v. 17.5 cm. Book label of Herbert M. Howe on verso of front cover.
                                                                [10a/380]

—————. See also nos. 114, 414, 965, 1112, 1118.

783.   **Pepper, William,** 1843-1898. Notes on the lectures on the theory and practice of medicine delivered to the medical class of the University of Pennsylvania. *Philadelphia, 1891-93.*

5 v. 21 cm. Lectures from 5 Oct. 1891 to 14 Feb. 1893. Vol. 5 largely blank. Notes taken by John M. Swan; his autograph in v. 2-5.   *[10a/326]*

—————. See also nos. 346, 765, 1010, 1035, 1079-80.

784.   **Percival, Milton Fraser,** 1882-1962, comp. Notes on medical subjects, from his student days at Medico-Chirurgical College, Philadelphia. *Philadelphia, 1891-1905.*

7 v. 26-30 cm. Contents: v. 1-2. Surgery, by Prof. William L. Rodman and Prof. E. Laplace (manuscript). — v. 3. Technique of operative surgery and bandaging as taught in the Surgical Laboratory of the Medico-Chirurgical College, Philadelphia, copyrighted 1901, by H.D. Jordan (typewritten, with manuscript index). — v. 4. Notes on Prof. John V. Shoemaker's lectures on therapeutics at the Medico-Chirurgical College, Part I, arranged by Aristoph Spare '98 (reproduced from typewritten copy, with manuscript index). — v. 5. Notes on obstetrics (reproduced from typewritten copy). — v. 6. Untitled, further notes on obstetrics and gynecology (reproduced from typewritten copy; second set of notes at end dated Oct. 7, 1891-April 18, 1892). — v. 7. Miscellaneous notes on anatomy, bacteriology, chemistry, and hygiene (manuscript).   *[10a/444]*

—————. See also no. 622.

785.   **Perkins, William Harvey,** 1894-1967. Anatomy drawings. *Philadelphia, ca. 1915-16.*

1 v.; col. illus. 22 cm. Prepared by Perkins while a student of J. Parsons Schaeffer at Jefferson Medical College. — Presented by Mrs. William Perkins.   *[10a/470]*

786.   **Petty, Elijah D.,** b. 1828. An inaugural essay on phthisis pulmonalis, presented to the faculty of the Philadelphia College of Medicine, for the degree of doctor in medicine, by Elijah D. Petty of . . . South Carolina. *Philadelphia, 1857.*

[1], 23, [3] ff. 25 cm.   *[n.c.]*

787. **Pharmacopoeia** of the United States of America. Draught of the Pharmacopoeia prepared by Drs. Hewson, Wood, & Bache as a committee of the College of Physicians — adopted by the College — transmitted to the Convention at Washington for 1830 — adopted by the Convention — referred by them to a revising & publishing committee — & after due revision, published at Philadelphia March 1831. *Philadelphia, 1828-29.*

> 2 v. (254 pp.). 20.5 cm. Paged consecutively. 1st revision. *[10a/99]*

788. — — — —. First revision. Manuscript draught. Prepared by Thomas T. Hewson, George B. Wood, and Franklin Bache, as a Committee of the College of Physicians of Philadelphia. *Philadelphia, 1828-29.*

> 380 pp. 19 cm. Presented by Hewson to Wood (cf. letter pasted on front flyleaf). — According to internal evidence, this revision may have been based upon the 2-vol. ms., but does not include the final revisions. The "Notes" (pp. 261-380) justifying changes proposed to USP 1820 correspond with those in "Notebooks to American Pharmacopoeia," cf. (unsigned) note by Glenn F. Sonnedecker. *[10a/84]*

789. — — — —. Committee of Revision. Circulars 1-351. *V.p., 1890-1900.*

> 2 v. (1500 ff., and inserts). 38-40.5 cm. Hectographed. Research reports (many signed), treasurers' reports, obituaries (some incl. bibliographies), reprints, etc. — Gift of H.C. Wood, who was a member of the committee. *[Z 10/19]*

790. — — — —. Journal of amendments by the Committee of Revision of the Philadelphia College of Pharmacy, on the United States Pharmacopoeia. *Philadelphia, ca. 1840-41.*

> v. 2 (232 ff. text). 20 cm. On the activities of the Philadelphia College of Pharmacy on the Committee of Revision and its membership, see *The First Century of the Philadelphia College of Pharmacy* (Philadelphia, 1922), p. 121. Its secretary was William Proctor. Undated letter, Proctor to George B. Wood enclosed. — Gift of H.L. Hodge. *[10a/118]*

791. **Philadelphia. Cholera Hospitals.** Case books. *Philadelphia, 1832.*

> 3 v. 20-55 cm. 1. Cholera Hospital No. 2. General case book, July 30-Oct. 25, 1832, containing description of admission, and summary information on 100 patients admitted to this hospital, at the City Carpenter Shop, Jones' Alley near Front; Joseph Parrish, physician-in-chief (gift of W.A. Schaeffer). — 2. Cholera Hospital No. 3. Case book, July 26-Aug. 21, 1832, with information on admission and description of symptoms and treatment of patients admitted to the hospital at No. 35 Dock St.; William E. Horner, physician-in-chief (gift of John M. Gelwix). — 3. Cholera Hospital No. 5. General case book, July 28-

Aug. 30, 1832, containing admission and descriptive information for 69 patients at the hospital, also known as the Sixth Street Hospital; Samuel Johnson, physician-in-chief.   *[Z 10/39; 10a/355; Z 10/32]*

792.   **Philadelphia. General Hospital.** Electrocardiograph records. *Philadelphia, 1909-15.*

1 envelope, large case of electrocardiograms. 31-70.5 cm. Incomplete records taken by various doctors at Blockley (Philadelphia General Hospital), marked A-K. Laid in letter of E.B. Krumbhaar with patient records and reproductions of printed items relating to the topic or to Dr. Krumbhaar.   *[Z 10/205]*

793.   — — — — —. Library catalogues. *Philadelphia, ca. 1890-1910.*

2 v. 36 cm. Catalogues, compiled ca. 1890-1910. Vol. 1 alphabetically listed by author (presented by E.B. Krumbhaar). — Vol. 2 arranged alphabetically by title or subject (received in exchange).   *[Z 10/74]*

794.   — — — — —. Ward for the Diseases of Women. Records of women's surgical cases. *Philadelphia, 1864-68.*

[1] f., 22 pp. 45 cm. Fifteen case histories. — Paper brittle.   *[Z 10c/40]*

— — — — —. See also nos. 211, 249-50, 525, 700-1, 754, 768, 798, 1010, 1014, 1112.

795.   **Philadelphia. Sanitary Committee.** Committee on Consultation. Minutes, resolutions, correspondence, etc. *Philadelphia, etc., 1832.*

1 v., 1 folder. 32 cm (envelope, 37.5 cm). Committee established "to assist . . . in divising the most prompt and efficient means to guard against the ravages of the spasmodic or asiatic cholera. . . ." The committee recommended the establishment in Philadelphia of a cholera hospital. Incl. two communications from the Special Medical Council of the Board of Health of the City of New York (A.H. Stevens, chairman). Among physicians involved are Dudley Atkins, George Fox, William E. Horner, Samuel Jackson, Charles D. Meigs, John K. Mitchell and Joseph Parrish.   *[Z 10/26]*

796.   **Philadelphia Academy of Surgery.** Constitution and by-laws, minutes, nominations and applications for membership, various memoranda, record of meetings, incl. a few printed items. *Philadelphia, etc., 1879-1982.*

2 v., 8 boxes. 26.5-37.5 cm. Contents: Draft of constitution and by-laws and act of incorporation (in the hand of S.D. Gross, 1879, with deletions, corrections and additions, incl. paste-ins; 3 sheets [1 a double-sheet, total 4 ff.], in box 8. — Constitution and by-laws as adopted, in formal hand (bound v., pp. 1-10) and signatures of members, 1879 to present (1982), with addresses (pp. 10-21, remainder blank, except p. 169); printed copy (1895, in box 7). — Minutes (1879-1909 in bound v.; 1909-54 in boxes 1-4; without 1949) incl. some secretaries' and treasurers' reports. — Nominations and applications for

membership (boxes 5-6), correspondence and memoranda relating to publication, etc. (in envelope). — Correspondence, attendance records, etc. of joint meetings with the New York Surgical Society, 1952, 1953, 1954 (3 folders in box 7), 75th anniversary celebration (1954, 1 folder, *ibid.*), investigation of Blue Shield Case involving the Wynnefield Hospital, several doctors and a number of chiropedists (1953-54; 1 folder, *ibid.*). — Deposited by the Academy.

[Z 10b/2]

— — — — —. See also nos. 239, 832, 1060.

797.   **Philadelphia College of Osteopathic Medicine.** Historic sketch. *Philadelphia, 1974?*

[1], 4 ff. 28 cm. Mimeographed. With letter of transmittal from Margaret F. Ferguson, director of public relations, to Dr. Radbill.   *[10c/134]*

798.   **Philadelphia Committee** for the Clinical Study of Opium Addiction. Case records and clinical studies. *Philadelphia, 1925-29.*

32 v. 29 cm. Case records, v. 1-21, list alphabetically 861 patients, most of whom lived in New York City, but also patients from Philadelphia and other cities, who were admitted to the narcotic wards of Pennsylvania General Hospital (1925-29). Includes admission record, ward notes, and primary history for each patient. Records of those patients who underwent psychiatric study contain in addition nurse's record, treatment sheet, and clinical laboratory record. Occasionally there is some correspondence from patients or their families along with the case history. Records of clinical studies, v. 22-28, include data on blood, circulation, respiration, water balance, etc., on each patient undergoing psychiatric study; v. 29 consists of psychological reports and summary; v. 30-31 contain condensed histories of patients admitted to the PGH Narcotic Wards (1927-29) and some statistical summaries of the patients (1925-29). Mostly typescript. — Gift of Arthur B. Light; used by him in his *Opium Addiction* (Chicago, 1929).   *[10d/26]*

799.   **Philadelphia County Medical Society.** Committee records and association accounts. *Philadelphia, 1878-1914.*

12 pp.; 2 v. 18.5-28 cm. 1. Committee on Hospital Efficiency. Correspondence (1914) of Edward Martin, chairman, concerning survey of Phila. area hospitals, and some comparative budget information. Printed report of committee (1913) to the society, with pencilled notes (12 pp.). — 2. Mutual Aid Association account books (1878-97) with accounts of individuals and organizations; cash book (1878-97). — Deposited by John B. Roberts.

[10c/42; 10d/79]

800.   — — — — —. Reports and correspondence by members of the Library and Archives Committee, dealing with the dissolution of the society's library, use of restricted funds, and liaison with the College of Physicians. *Philadelphia, 1957-65.*

1 box. 32 cm. Typewritten (incl. carbons), handwritten, few mimeographed items. Added: Appointment of S. X Radbill to the Committee (2 items, undated); resolutions (4, 1 ff.); letters to S. X Radbill on the "scientific and educational trust" (1964-65).   *[1h/715]*

—————. See also nos. 102, *185.2210*, 1025.

801. **Philadelphia Fellowship Commission.** Station WFIL, Philadelphia. "Within our gates" (radio plays). *Philadelphia, 1946.*

106 ff. 28 cm. Mimeographed, with manuscript corrections. Contents: No. 68, William Osler. — No. 69, A.W. Springs. — No. 70, Elizabeth Blackwell. — No. 71, E.B. Chain. — No. 72, Walter Reed.   *[Z 10/177]*

802. **Philadelphia Laryngological Society.** Constitution and by-laws, minutes, applications. *Philadelphia, 1911-69.*

6 v.; photographs. 26-35 cm. Constitution and by-laws, signed by the charter members (1911) and minute book (1911-25) of the society organized to stimulate and encourage the advancement of the science and technique of laryngology and rhinology. Applications (1914-69) for membership to the society. Photographic portraits of society's presidents, founders, and honorary members, and two vols. containing pictures of society's members. — Compiled and presented by the historian and librarian of the society, Herman Bernard Cohen.   *[Z 10/234]*

803. **Philadelphia Medical Book Club.** Accounts and scrapbook. *Philadelphia, 1865-92.*

2 v. 21-31 cm. Treasurer's accounts (1865-92) incl. subscriptions, fines, etc., taken by Robert P. Harris and John Ashhurst, Jr., and scrapbook (1865-86) incl. printed club rules, names and addresses of members, and catalogues (1867-69) of books and periodicals for sale with buyer and sale price written in, and invoices from booksellers and binders. — Presented by A.P.C. Ashhurst.   *[Z 10/41]*

804. **Philadelphia Medical Society.** Constitution, charter, by-laws, minutes, committee records, library catalogue, membership lists, essays, misc. printed forms and announcements. *Philadelphia, 1794-1868.*

7 v., 2 boxes, 1 envelope. 30-39 cm. Original manuscript of society constitution (1827); printed copies of charter and by-laws (1836-58). Minutes of weekly meetings, 1802-17 [(1826-45)-1868]. Minutes, 1827-40, of a committee concerned with quack medicines, patent trusses, and specifics and patents, with reports on Swaim's panacea and H. Chase's truss against hernia; letters, 1827, to the Committee on Patents, chaired by W.E. Horner, from J.F.D. Lobstein and S. Emlen, and 1839, from J. Warrington. Reports, 1841-60, of the Library Committee; library catalogue, ca. 1856 (largely books printed 1800-1856, but incl. some 16th-18th century items). Misc. committee minutes and

reports, and correspondence to the society [(1819-44)-1863]. Volume, listing members and honorary members, 1800-44, with residence, date of proposal and introduction; misc. notes on members, proposed, new, and honorary. Essays on variety of medical topics, 1794-1804. Misc. printed and engraved memberships, incl. engraved form of election of Samuel Jackson, in Latin, signed by Benjamin Rush, 1805 (on vellum, with seal), and engraved forms of election, in Latin, signed by P.S. Physick, J. Parrish, and S. Jackson, ca. 1830 (vellum); copper plate of invitation to membership; election and announcement materials. — Deposited by the society. Minutes, 1816-26, at the Historical Society of Penna.   *[Z 10c/38]*

— — — — —. See also no. *185.215.*

805. [— — — — —].   Papers read by candidates for membership.   *Philadelphia, etc., 1794-ca. 1810.*

20 pamphlets.   Various sizes, as follows:

a. Brockenbrough, Austin, Jr. Speculations on the modus operandi of digitalis in dropsies and consumptions. Ca. 1802. 1 f., 12 pp., 1 torn f. 20 cm. With references to William Cullen, Erasmus Darwin and Paul Ferrier.
(no. 7)

b. Brownley, Joseph. Treatise on intestinal fever . . . dysentery. Ca. 1804. 7 ff. (last blank). 20 cm. Second, i.e. repeated application for membership. No. 62 (f. 1r).   (no. 15)

c. Coke, Samuel. An essay on the deleterious effects of tobacco. 1803. [1], 8, 3 blank ff. 20 cm. Read Dec. 29.   (no. 13)

d. Cumming, John. On contagion. 8 Jan. 1794. 6 ff. 24 cm. Letter addressed to the president of the "American Medical Society of Philadelphia" in rebuttal of a "paper on the modus agendi of contagion by an unnamed author, read a few days ago in your hall." "No. 1 — 1794" and "84" entered in a contemporary hand.   (no. 1).

e. Douglas, Patrick. Observations on a billous inflammatory fever . . . in Loudoun & adjacent counties in 1804. 5 ff. 23 cm. Read Nov. 10.   (no. 14)

f. [Dysentery]. Causes and treatment. 1797. Pp. 5-20 only, 1 f. 24 cm. Read Feb. 4. By unidentified author.   (no. 3)

g. [Fermentation]. On the fermentation of vegetable substances. Ca. 1805. 11 ff. 25 cm. Numbered 66. With references to J.A. Chaptal. Unid. author.   (no. 19)

h. Gregg, Amos. On the medical properties of podophyllum foliis peltatis lobatis (may apple). Ca. 1802. 4 ff. 20 cm. No. 44 (f. 1r). Pencilled name of author on f. 4v. References to Dr. B.S. Barton.   (no. 5)

i. Harrison, John. Account of the autumnal epidemic, usually called in Maryland the bilious remitting & intermitting fever. 1803. 6 ff. (f. 1 blank). 25 cm. Read Dec. 3. Deals with the outbreak of malaria in Fredericktown, Md.   (no. 10)

j. Hernia; its symptoms, causes and cures. Philadelphia?, ca. 1810. 12 ff. 26 cm. Attributed to B.H. Coates on grounds of a letter by him found in the pamphlet; assignment almost certainly wrong, based on handwriting and date.   (no. 16)

k. [Inoculation]. Of inoculation for the small pox. Ca. 1810. 8 ff. 21 cm. Numbered 99. Unid. author.   (no. 20)

l. Jameson, Thomas. On mollugo verticillata virginiana, commonly called snake weed. 1802. 4 ff. 26 cm. Delivered Dec. 18th. Mollugo recommended as remedy against snake bites.   (no. 9)

m. McCall, Edwin LeRoy. On the power of some parts of the animal body to perform the function of other parts. Philadelphia?, ca. 1803. 4 ff. 26 cm.   (no. 8)

n. Martin, John S., d. 1844. Principle causes and methods of cures of cholera infantum. 1803. 8 ff. 24 cm. Read Dec. 10.   (no. 11)

o. North, Edward Washington, 1778-1843. On an uncommon case of suppression of urine, caused by a scrophulous tumor, at the hospital in Charleston, S.C. 1796. 6 ff. 21 cm. Read Nov. 19. Numbered 4.   (no. 2)

p. Parker, John. Paronychia or whilton. 1803. 14 ff., in contemp. paper cover. 24 cm.   (no. 12)

q. Pendleton, James. A dissertation on the systole & dyastole of the heart. 1799(-1800?). 16 ff. (f. 15 blank). 30.5 cm. "Commenced the 23rd of Novr anno domini 1799." No. 38 on title page. Signed by author on ff. 9r and 12r.   (no. 4)

r. Respiration. Ca. 1800. 8 pp. (end lacking). 23 cm. Numbered 22. Letter N (initial of author?) on p. 1.   (no. 17)

s. Stewart, (Samuel?). Essay on cholera infantum. Ca. 1805. 11 pp. 23 cm. Probably by Samuel or J.M. Stewart.   (no. 18)

t. Toles (or Towles), (John?). An essay on the advantages of vaccination. Ca. 1802. 8 ff. 24 cm. No. 45 (f. 1r). Name of author in two different spellings (f. 7r). References to E. Jenner, H.M. Hasson, J.R. Coxe and J.L. Moreau.   (no. 6)

[Z 10c/38; box 2]

06. ─────. Committee on Specifics (also called Committee on Patents or Committee on Quack Medicines). Correspondence, reports, resolutions, etc. *Philadelphia, etc., 1827-39.*

3 envelopes. 34 cm. Contents: a. Swain's panacea. Letters and reports by "Medicus" (i.e. W.E. Horner, chairman), others involving H.W. Harris, L.G. Wynn, J. Randolph, P.S. Physick, J. Rush, D.R. Beck, E. Cutbush, incl. unsigned letter reporting the case of Jacob Bush. Printed statement establishing the committee (these together 23 ff.). ─ b. Same topic with items by A.E. Kennedy, W.E. Horner, E.A. Attlee, C. Mifflin, T. Park, N. Chapman, G. Emerson, J. Bell, T. Harris (22 ff.); Resolutions concerning the publication of the committee's report in 2 medical journals as well as in the form of a pamphlet, incl. accounts on financing publication (6 ff.); printed "Ridgway's rob of l'Affecteur," reproducing the committee's condemnation of panaceas, advertisement signed R.S. Ridgway. ─ c. Heber Chase's truss against hernia; items by I. Parrish, committee report; Harris' resignation; resolutions against patents; index of papers issued March and June 1839 (12 ff.).

[Z 10c/38, in box 2]

07. ─────. Library. Annotated, descriptive catalogue, alphabetically arranged. *Philadelphia, ca. 1856.*

1 v. 30 cm. Largely books published 1800-56, also some 16th-18th century volumes. Reports on the library (1841 and 1843) enclosed.   *[Z 10c/38, v. 7]*

808.   **Philadelphia Neurological Society.** Constitution and by-laws; minutes; membership lists; speech text; scrapbook. *Philadelphia, 1883-1942.*

6 v.; 2 envelopes. 21-30 cm. Constitution and by-laws (1884) with amendments, signed by society's members; also includes lists of honorary members (1914-42), minutes (1883-1936), recording society's business, and some memorials. List of members (1945) with curriculum vitae, listing publications. Text (1935) of a speech by William G. Spiller, on the first fifty years of the society. Scrapbook (1923-26) containing responses to invitations to speak at the society's 40th anniversary celebration, and to notices of election as honorary members. W.G. Spiller's text presented by him.

[10a/315; ZZ 10c/16]

––––––. See also nos. 315, 985.

809.   **Philadelphia Orthopaedic Hospital** and Infirmary for Nervous Diseases. Constitution and by-laws; minutes; committee records; hospital and clinic records; case histories; financial records. *Philadelphia, 1867-1942.*

106 v. 20-60 cm. Constitution and by-laws, 1873. Minutes (1867-1920) of the Board of Managers, and rough drafts (1867-90) of reports; announcements and other printed matter laid in. Minutes (1884-1916) of the Executive Committee. Contributors' meeting minutes (1879-91); Property Committee minutes (1905-09); and Social Service Committee minutes (1911-20). Board of Patients account book (1889-92). – Record of patients treated in the hospital and clinic (1870-75); register of in-patients (1872-85), incl. name, residence, and age of patient, their physician and diagnosis. Hospital admission and discharge records (1885-1923). Register of clinical patients (1905-12) providing an index to patient case histories. Record of patients treated in the Department of Deformities (1876-1912). Record of patients treated in the Department of Nervous Diseases (1890-1900). Record of nervous clinic patients (1904-42) listing physician in charge, assistants, and the number of patients per day. Operations and apparatus record books (1890-1911) listing surgeon, patient, diagnosis and operation of hospital patients. Records of surgical clinic patients (1904-30) listing surgeon in charge, assistants, and the number of patients per day. Case histories (1872-1942) mostly divided by type of disease or problem.

Treasurer's correspondence and annual reports (1901-25). Voucher record books (1901-38) listing credits, debts, and accounts by department. Receipt books (1926-39). Patients' books (1887-1919, 1929-32) arranged by patient number, listing name of patient, length of stay, amount owed and amount received. Monthly payroll accounts (1922-40); weekly payroll record (1921-23, 1926-31); payroll book (1913-14) for masseurs. Register of employees, listing employees (1887-1940); dates of employment, salary, and occupation. Beginning in 1912, employees are listed by occupation. – Book of contributors (1869-1910); address books of contributors to the hospital (1890-1934). Contributors to the apparatus fund of the hospital (1891-1912). — Misc. printed annual reports (1869-81) and copy of the article of merger with the Univ. of Penna. in 1938.   *[ZDb/9, n.c.]*

Philadelphia Pediatric Society, *see* **Pediatric Society** of Philadelphia.

0.   **Philippe, V.** Observations de pratique chirurgicale. *Chartres (and Paris?), 1760-90.*

1 v. (18 pamphlets, ca. 620 pp. and 90 ff.); illus. 22 cm (in ill-fitting vellum binder, 24 cm). Philippe identified in the *Mémoires* of the Academy as "correspondant de l'Academie royale de chirurgie" and in pamphlets 8-9 as "Maître des arts et en chirurgie à Chartres." Contents: Pamphlet no. 1 (without cover) and cahiers 1-2, *Sur les abcès.* — Cahiers 3-6 and 7bis, *Sur les contrecoups.* — Cahier 5bis, *De lupiis dissertatio* (text in Latin). — 7, *Sur l'hidropisie de l'ovaire.* — 8, *Sur l'hysterotomie.* — 9, *Sur la luxation de la symphyse sacro-iliaque* (publ. in part in *Mémoires de l'Academie royale de chirurgie,* v. 4: 91-4 [1768]). — 10, *Sur le spasme sympathique des muscles du larinx, pharinx...* (title on last leaf: *Observations sur les convulsions...* with ms. notation "couronné"). — 11-13, *Observations de pratique.* — Unnumbered pamphlet without cover: *Observations sur quelques maladies des os.* Cahier 6 incomplete?, ends in midsentence. With manuscript corrections, additions and deletions, and references in the text and in footnotes to various authorities, incl. non-medical, e.g. Leibniz. Numbering of pamphlets not in chronological order.   *[10b/34]*

1.   **Philippus de Novellino,** D.O.M. Institutiones medicinae sive fundamenta maecanicis legibus innixa. *Naples, 1729.*

320 pp. 22 cm. No work by this author listed in the Surgeon General's Library or Hirsch, *Biog. Lex.* Index of chapters, pp. 317-20.   *[10a/275]*

2.   **Phillips, Thomas Wolden,** b. 1887. Practical points in anatomy. Sixth edition, revised for 1939-40. *Philadelphia, Hahnemann Medical College, 1938?*

[2], 209, xi, 4, [1] ff.; illus. 38 cm. Mimeographed. Manuscript annotations by Pomeroy Edward Polavey (student).   *[n.c.]*

3.   **[Physicians, U.S.].** Alphabetical list of names of physicians. *N.p., ca. 1836.*

1 v. 38 cm. Contains 1,444 names, with indication of places of residence. The purpose or use of this list has not been ascertained. Inscription inside front cover gives the date 1836.   *[Z 10/82]*

4.   **Physician's ledger.** *Oxford (Pa. or Md.?), 1827-32, 1837.*

[13], 117, [5] ff. 32 cm. Ledger of a Gideon Leeds(?) and possibly others. Two creditors frequently mentioned: C. Fitch and D. Side. Consists largely of entries for medical services, some entries for commodities.   *[n.c.]*

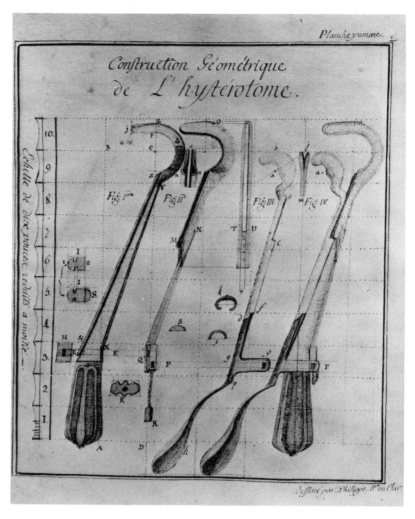

Plate 6. 810. V. Philippe. *Observations de practique chirurgicale.* 1760-90.

Note: *The lectures on surgery by Philip Syng Physick are arranged in approximate chronological order (instead of alphabetically by title).*

815. **Physick, Philip Syng,** 1768-1837. Lectures on surgery. Notes taken from the lectures of Philip Syng Physick on surgery by William Darlington . . . member of the American Linnean and Philadelphia Medical societies. Taken in the Winter of 1803-4. *Philadelphia, 1803-04.*

325, [iii] ff. 20 cm. Presented by the Chester County Medical Society. Darlington's presentation inscription to the society on flyleaf; his bookplate, "no. 17," inside front cover.   *[10b/9]*

16. ———— ————, etc. Notes of Richard Grier. *Philadelphia, 1806-07.*

1 v. (125 pp. text, [1] f., 23 pp., [3] ff. beginning at back of v.); illus. 20.5 cm. Various notes, incl. "Doctor Rush says there are 6 forms of diseases" and table of contents precede the lecture notes. Title "Diseases of the eyes" on p. 125, but without notes. At back of volume "Notes taken from Dr. Bartons lectures . . .", inscription of the notetaker R. Grier, and note about his death in 1808, supposedly after he completed his studies at the Univ. of Penna.; he is not listed among the university's alumni. Gift of Messrs. R.W. Foster, S. X Radbill and F.C. Wood.   *[10b/60]*

17. ———— ————, November 1807 to February 19, 1808. *Philadelphia, 1807-08.*

2 v. ([279] pp.). 23.5 cm. Headings and page numbers elaborately decorated. Lecture on scirrus and cancer in v. 2, pp. 73ff., by John Syng Dorsey. — Gift of William Ashmead Schaeffer.   *[10b/25]*

18. ———— ————. Notes of the lectures on surgery delivered by Philip S. Physick . . . taken in 1808-9 by John P. Betton. *Philadelphia, 1808-09.*

1 v. 28 cm. Bookplate of Thos. Forrest Betton. Portions damaged; ink bled.   *[10b/10]*

9. ———— ————. Notes on surgery, taken from the lectures of Philip Syng Physick . . . by William Elmer . . . during the Winters of 1808-9-10. *Philadelphia, 1808-10.*

509 pp. 24.5 cm. Ms. verse eulogizing Rush inside front cover. — Gift of Walter G. Elmer.   *[10b/51]*

0. ———— ———— taken by A.B. Tucker in the years 1809 and 1810 and 1811, enlarged in 1811 & 12. *Philadelphia, 1809-12.*

232, [v] pp. 25.5 cm. Presented by W.H. Pancoast.   *[10b/14]*

821.   ———— ————, by Philip S. Physick and John S. Dorsey, taken by J.R. Butler in the sessions of 1809, 1810, 1811, and copied by Wm. F. Irwin. *Philadelphia, 1809-11.*

> 1 v.; illus. 26.5 cm. Dorsey served as adjunct prof. to his uncle Philip Syng Physick. Contains drawings of Physick's and Hutchinson's improvements on Desault's splint and Physick's fracture box. — Presented to the Lewis Library by John Keating. Inscribed on flyleaf "Presented to Dr. J.M. Keating by his friend, J.J. Barker, Phila., Aug. 1, 1889."   *[10b/40]*

822.   ———— ————. Notes on surgery from the lectures of Philip S. Physick. Vol. 2nd. *Philadelphia, 181—?*

> [4], 132 pp. 20 cm. Presented by James Darrach. May be the notes of his father, William Darrach, M.D., Univ. of Penna., 1819, Physick's last year of teaching surgery. — Contains lectures 20-34, on fractures, dislocations, sprains, and injuries of the head.   *[10b/28]*

823.   ———— ————. Notes on lectures by P.S. Physick on surgery, taken by Francis Julius Le Moyne. *Philadelphia, 1820?*

> [6] ff., 271 pp. (unnumbered blank ff. between pp. 24-5, 66-7, 178-79), [4] ff., 243 pp., 16 blank ff. 25 cm. "These notes were taken by Dr. F. Julius Le Moyne at the University of Pennsylvania during 1822-'23," entered by W.L. Wills in presenting the volume to V.L. Ellicott in 1927 (f. [1]). The fact that the lectures are by Dr. Physick was established by comparison with other students' notes; but Dr. Physick resigned the chair of surgery in 1819 (to fill the chair of anatomy vacated by the death of his nephew J.S. Dorsey) and was succeeded by William Gibson, appointed prof. of surgery in Sept. 1819. Eight matriculation and admission cards kept with the manuscript also present complicating evidence: admission ticket of Le Moyne (1) for lectures on surgery by Gibson, and (2) for the lectures in "practical anatomy" by Physick, both dated Nov. 1820. Either Physick continued to teach surgery beyond 1819, or, more likely, Gibson used Physick's text during the first years following his appointment. — Presented to the College of Physicians by V.L. Ellicott in 1977 (f. [2]). Bookplate of F.J. Le Moyne.   *[10b/61]*

824.   ———— ————. Notes on the lectures on surgery. *Philadelphia, 18——.*

> 3 v. 19.5 cm. No title-page or statement of authorship; identified by comparison with lectures known to be by Physick. — Presented by Leonardo S. Clark.   *[10b/21]*

825.   ————. Questions on surgery from the lectures of Philip Syng Physick ... delivered in the Winter of 1818-19. *Philadelphia, 1818-19.*

> 150 pp. 34.5 cm. "Members of the Club: materia medica, Wm. L. Powell; anatomy, Wm. Moseley; practice, J. McCraa [sic; i.e., Macrae]; chemistry, J.P.

Harrison; midwifery, Wallace; surgery, J.K. Mitchell." All these "members," class of 1819 (Univ. of Penna.), came from Virginia. — Presented by S. Weir Mitchell.   *[Z 10/7]*

—————. See also nos. 52, 82, 114, 171, 259, 269, 294, 329, 361, 459, 471, 804, 806, 899.

826. **Picard, Jean Baptiste,** b. 1796. Manuscrit sur la médecine et la chirurgie. *Paris, 1823-31.*

125 [i.e. 127] pp. 20.5 cm. Commonplace book containing student notes on lectures, notes on books and journal articles, remedies, copies of personal petitions for professional appointments, etc.   *[10a/209]*

827. **Piersol, George Arthur,** 1856-1924. Examination papers (i.e., questions) in anatomy, 1901-08, for dental and medical students at the University of Pennsylvania. *Philadelphia, 1901-08.*

1 v. (38 cm) and 1 envelope (25 cm). Handwritten and typewritten examination questions. — Gift of the Piersol Anatomy Library, Univ. of Penna., 1971.   *[Z 10c/35]*

828. —————. Notes on histology from the lectures delivered to the Class of '93, Medical Department, University of Pennsylvania. *Philadelphia, 1890-92.*

1 v. 24 cm. Notes taken by John Mumford Swan. Histology notes dated 10 Oct. 1890-25 Mar. 1891 (21 pp.); notes headed "Embryology" 6 Oct. 1891-8 April 1892 (48 pp.).   *[10a/325]*

—————. See also nos. 540, 592.

829. **Pike, Anne Hollingsworth,** b. 1920. Notes of lectures on gynecology, July 1944-March 1945. *Philadelphia, 1944-45.*

1 box ([304] pp. in 8 folders). 28 cm (box, 32 cm). Lecturer at Woman's Medical College of Pennsylvania unidentified. With forms from the College's hospital.   *[10a/478]*

830. **Poffenberger, Joseph C.** Report of two obstetric cases of Out-Patient Department of Jefferson Maternity Hospital. *Philadelphia, 1911-12.*

18 ff. 28 cm. Typescript. — Presented by Edward Davis.   *[Z 10/54]*

831. **Polyclinic Hospital.** Ladies' Aid Society. List of contributing and active members. *Philadelphia, 1910?*

100 pp. (mostly blank). 17 cm. Gift of Mrs. S. Solis Cohen.   *[10c/22]*

832. **Pomeroy, Lawrence Alson,** 1883-1955. Carcinoma of the cervix uteri. *Cleveland, 1954.*

[2], 12 ff. (numbered 1-11B). 28 cm. Typescript. Submitted 1954 in the competition for the Samuel D. Gross Prize of the Philadelphia Academy of Surgery. *[n.c.]*

833. **Poor Mans** [man's] **Treasure.** *N.p., 18th cent.*

176, [5] pp. 17 cm. Contains remedies and receipts. — Inscription: "Job Lousley's book. Hampstead, Norris, Berks; purchased in 1845." *[10a/100]*

834. **Potts, Charles Sower,** 1864-1930. An essay on arsenic in glass and the caustic alkalies. *Philadelphia, 1885.*

[1], 25, [1] ff. 26 cm. Essay submitted for the degree of doctor of medicine in the University of Pennsylvania, with pencilled corrections (by the preceptor, John M. Keating?). "Dr. M.", H.C. Wood, Leidy, and Osler signatures on verso of second flyleaf. — Presented by the City of Philadelphia from the Philadelphia General Hospital. *[10c/139]*

835. **Powell, Lester Lovett,** 1875-1939. Diary, August 27, 1917-May 8, 1918. — Field messages, Oct.-Nov. 1918, etc. *France and U.S.A., 1917-[20?].*

2 v.; envelopes; illus. 12-31 cm (box, 32 × 23 cm). Contents: World War I diary, many entries in form of letters to Dr. Powell's wife, incl. reports on poison gas attacks, casualties, etc. — Booklet with field messages (12 cm) incl. at end loose-leaf diary entries (July 1917). Misc.: letter in French, 2 photographs, clippings, paper on old age (typed and handwritten). *[10a/494]*

836. **Pratt, Henry Charles.** A dissertation on the origin, nature and cure of venereal diseases . . . *Philadelphia, 1826.*

41, [3] ff. 20 cm. Tipped in after f. [44] "A case history of George Biddle seaman, aet. 36, dated June 1st, 1827." — Inscribed on cover: "Henry Charles Pratt, July 5th, 1826." Inscribed at bottom of f. 41: "Finis. July 15th, 1826. Dr Chapmans study." *[10a/101]*

837. **Presbyterian Hospital,** Philadelphia. Surgical case records. *Philadelphia, 1892-94.*

1 box (8 folders). 31.5 cm. Written on printed forms. Reports by Drs. C.F. Nassau, J.M. Swan, H.J. Rhett, J.W. White(?) and few others, for Drs. H.R. Wharton and O.H. Allis. *[10a/324]*

—————. See also nos. 1009, 1025.

838. **Price, Eli Kirk,** 1797-1884. Ledger containing legal and financial statements concerning the estate of Jonas Preston. *Philadelphia, 1836-39.*

1 v. 32 cm. Contents: Copy of the will of Jonas Preston, M.D. (1835), witnessed and probated in 1836 (with seal), pp. 1-11. — Inventory and appraisement of goods and chattels, rights and credits, 1836, pp. 13-14. — Dr. Eli K. Price, one of the executors . . . in account with the estate, 1836-39, pp. 16-27. — Request for legal opinion by E.K. Price and answer by John Sergeant, 1836, pp. 257-63. — Application by Preston Retreat, 1836 (with signatures of J. Sergeant, Jane Preston, John R. Thomas and E.K. Price), pp. 264-70. — Letters concerning the estate by E.K. Price, John Sergeant, Jane Preston, to John S. Adams, George Thomas, Building Committee of the Preston Retreat, etc., 1836-37, pp. 307-(26). — Receipts, Dr. Preston's estate, 1836-39 (incl. printed forms, signed), pp. 401-(23).   *[Z 10c/1]*

39. **Proud, Robert,** 1728-1813. Observations in Philadelphia on yellow fever. *Philadelphia, 1799-1804.*

38 pp. 21 cm. Contents: On part of a publication in Fenno's paper . . . 1799, respecting what is there called the yellow fever, by Nerax. Of the plague of Athens, from the Greek of Thucydides by R.P. 1802, with Creech's translation from Lucretius on the same. Of the great pestilence . . . in the 6th century, &c, by R.P. 1804. — Part of Proud's library was bought by Dr. William Norris and sold by Dr. George Norris, at which time this manuscript was bought by Dr. William Pepper, Jr., who presented it to the College of Physicians of Philadelphia; with his bookplate.   *[10a/311]*

40. **Pusey, William Allen,** 1865-1940. Dermatological notes and illustrations. *Chicago, ca. 1900.*

2 v.; illus. 20-36 cm (in envelope, 31 cm). Contents: V. 1. Brief notes on staining techniques; drawings of skin lesions, pp. 1-32, 176-85 (the remainder blank). — V. 2. Dermatological drawings of syphilitic conditions (10 ff.). German terms and remarks interspersed. References to Paul Ehrlich on pp. 22, 177 and 182. Authorship established by letter of transmittal from donor Samuel M. Bluefarb.   *[10a/464]*

41. – – – – –. Notes from Hospital St. Louis in Paris and various hospitals in London. *Paris and London, 1892.*

[54] and [3] laid in ff.; illus. 18 cm. Contains notes on cases of skin diseases of Drs. E.H. Besnier, J.B. Hillairet (in Paris), J.J. Pringle, H.R. Crocker and Sir M.A. Morris. — Gift of S.M. Bluefarb.   *[10a/507]*

42. **Radbill, Samuel X,** b. 1901. The case of Mary Green. *Philadelphia, 195—?*

5 ff. 28 cm (envelope, 37.5 cm). A case of scrofula taken to court in Ipswich, Mass. in 1660 in dispute over the payment of fees. — Gift of the author.   *[n.c.]*

43. – – – – –. John Eberle, a Pennsylvania Dutch pioneer in American medical education. *Philadelphia, 1935.*

13 ff. 28 cm. Typescript. Inscribed on last page: "Read before the 2d annual meeting of the Residents Association of the Lancaster General Hospital . . . June 27, 1935." Published in *Bull. Inst. Hist. Med.*, v. 4: 121-36 (1936). — Gift of the author.   *[10c/127]*

844.   — — — — —.   Thomas Jefferson and medical education.   *Philadelphia, 1969.*

> 15 ff. 28 cm. Typescript; manuscript corrections throughout. Read before the Hobart Amory Hare Honor Society and the Alpha Omega Honorary Society at Thomas Jefferson University, Medical College, Dec. 3, 1969. — Gift of the author.   *[10c/126]*

— — — — —.   See also nos. 81, 104, 270, 275, 334, 713, 769, 797, 800, 1043-4.

845.   **Radzinsky, L.D.**   Miscellaneous records (invoices, receipts, reports) by, or relating to, the acting assistant surgeon Radzinky, U.S. Army.   *Washington and camps in Virginia, 1862.*

> 1 envelope (9 items). 39 cm. Contents: Invoice of medical supplies, Feb. 27, 1862, signed C.H. Laub and countersigned Radzinsky. — Two receipts for medical supplies, Camp California, Va., March 2, 1862. — Report of sick and wounded, Camp Winfield Scott, Va., April 1862. — Requisition of medical supplies, April 23, 1862, *ibid.* — Muster roll of the Hospital Dept., Harrison's Landing, April-June, 1862. — Three smaller misc. items, June-July, 1862.
> *[10c/142]*

846.   **Randall, Burton Alexander,** 1858-1932.   An experimental study of reparatory inflammation in arteries after ligation.   *Philadelphia?, 1880.*

> 36 ff.; 14 drawings on 11 ff. 25 cm. Thesis (M.D.) — Univ. of Penna., 1880. Tipped in ms. note: "Awarded to share . . . the thesis prize of the Alumni Society of the Medical Department of the Univ. of Penna., March 15th 1880." Note on flyleaf: "Examined by Leidy [and] Ashhurst." — Gift of B.A. Randall.   *[10b/54]*

847.   — — — — —.   A record of the anomalies found in the dissecting rooms of the University of Pennsylvania during the years 1878-79.   *Philadelphia, 1879.*

> 1 v.; col. illus. 22 cm. Offered in competition for a student prize awarded by Hugh Lenox Hodge, who presented this ms.   *[10a/55]*

— — — — —.   See also no. 1079.

848.   **Randolph, Robert Lee,** 1860-1919.   The regeneration of the crystalline lens, an experimental study.   *Baltimore, 1899.*

> 40 ff.; 6 figures. 27 cm. Typescript. Awarded the Alvarenga Prize, 1899. Published in *Contributions to the Science of Medicine, Dedicated by His Pupils to William Henry Welch* . . . (Baltimore, 1900), pp. 237-63.   *[10a/144]*

49. **Reading, John Herbert,** 1889-1945. Pediatric therapeutics. *Philadelphia, 1924.*

> 20 ff. 28.5 cm. Typewritten. – Delivered before the Tri-County Medical Society (homeopathic), October 14, 1924; with the minutes of the society.
>
> *[10a/449]*

Note: *Collection of recipes, in chronological order, items nos. 850-853.*

50. **Recipe book** "for John H. Mundall." *Pennsylvania, 1745 to late 18th cent.*

> [1] f., 89 pp. 23 cm (envelope, 30 cm). Recipes, as far as identified, by private individuals, doctors, or copied from magazines, letters, etc. Dated recipes range from 1745 to 1785. – Gift of Emily Daniel through M.L. Kauffman.
>
> *[10a/405]*

51. **Recipes.** *N.p., ca. 1790(-1815)?*

> [548] pp. 20 cm. Medical and household recipes, with index. Attributed to Robert Johnson (?, d. 1793), surgeon in the American Revolution. Inscribed in front: "J. Boggs." Notes at back in different hands dated 1813, 1815. – Presented by H.R. Wharton.
>
> *[10a/303]*

52. **Receipt book.** *N.p., 1790 to early 19th cent.*

> 171 (vero 182) pp. (pp. 158-82, and some others, blank). 20 cm. Based in part on the receipt book of Elizabeth Coates Paschall. Source of recipes given for many entries. Tipped-in newspaper clippings and handwritten copies from a variety of newspapers, 1790-1805, in latter part of the volume. Incomplete table of contents on flyleaf. – Presented by Mrs. Francis Strawbridge through Samuel Bradbury.
>
> *[10a/351]*

53. **Recipes** of medical remedies, cosmetic and household items. *Pennsylvania?, late 19th cent.*

> 236 (and blank) pp. 19.5 cm. The manuscript was erroneously assigned to Edgar M. Hewish whose prescription is pasted inside front cover. It was probably compiled mainly by a pharmacist whose name started with M (cf. frequent initials following the prescriptions). Some of the remedies were extracted from journals, dated 1865 to 1888. With additions in a later hand, and two partial indexes. Few inserts.
>
> *[10a/434]*

54. **Redman, John,** 1722-1808. An account of the yellow fever of 1762. *Philadelphia, 1793.*

> 12 pp. 25 cm. Fragile. Printed, with slight editorial alterations, as *An Account of the Yellow Fever as it Prevailed in Philadelphia in the Autumn of 1762; a Paper Presented to the College of Physicians of Philadelphia at its Stated Meeting, September 7, 1793, by John Redman. . .,* Philadelphia, 1865. Pasted on flyleaf engraved portrait of Redman (oval, 14.5 × 11 cm) similar to the College of Physicians of Philadelphia's pastel portrait.
>
> *[10a/126]*

855.   ─────. Letter to the Reverend Ashbell Green, Princeton, referring to the yellow fever epidemic in and around Philadelphia. *Philadelphia, Sept. 14, 1798.*

1 f.   37.5 cm.   Presented by William Pepper, January 7, 1912.   Silked and bound.   *[Z 10/47]*

─────. See also nos. 13, 114, *185.13, .211*, 200, 285, 689.

856.   **Reed, James W.** Interview with Emily Hartshorne Mudd. *Cambridge, Mass., Schlesinger Library, Radcliffe College, ca. 1976.*

1 v.; ports. (original photographs).   28 cm.   Photocopy of typewritten transcript taken from interviews taped by J.W.R. at home of E.H.M. at Haverford, Pa., May 21-23 and August 13, 1974; part of the Schlesinger-Rockefeller Oral History Project.   Concerns Dr. Mudd's background, education, and activities in establishing and directing the Marriage Council of Philadelphia, and as director, Division of Family Study and professor in the Department of Psychiatry, University of Pennsylvania. ─ Gift of Schlesinger Library.
                                                                          [ZZ 10d/20]

857.   **Reichert, Edward Tyson,** 1855-1931.   Notes on the lectures on physiology delivered to the medical class of the University of Pennsylvania. *Philadelphia, 1890-91.*

3 v.   21-23 cm.   Notes taken by John M. Swan from 3 Oct. 1890 to 6 April 1891.   Additions tipped in.   *[10a/332]*

858.   ─────. Physiology notes, Univ. of Penna. Dept. of Medicine ... October 2d, 1911 through Fri. January 26th, 1912 ... Taken by Emlen Wood. *Philadelphia, 1911-12.*

1 v.   26 cm.   *[Z 10/217]*

859.   **Reina Mercedes** (Spanish Cruiser).   Single leaf of surgeon's log book, one of many salvaged by William Griscom Coxe, with typed letter of transmittal, W.G. Coxe to Richard H. Harte, pencilled note, and 2 photographs. *Santiago and Wilmington, 1897-1909.*

1 v.   21 × 32 cm (oblong).   Gift of R.H. Harte.   *[10b/27]*

860.   **Rhazes** (Abu Bekr Muhammad ben Zakhariah Abrazi), 852-932.   A chapter on remedies for very young children, translated from the Arabic of Rhazes in 1453, from Latin in 1966 by Maria Wilkins Smith. *Gladwyne, Pa., 1966.*

[1], 15 ff.   28.5 cm.   Translated from the Milan 1481 edition of the *Liber ad Almansorem.*   *[10c/151]*

861. **Rhett, William B.** Account book of patient fees. *Beaufort, S.C., 1798-99.*

1 v. 41 × 17 cm. "From Dr. A. De Markley to Dr. J.B. Dunlap taken from the residence of Wm. B. Rhett" pencilled inside front cover. Title page and several leaves torn or missing. — Presented by S. Weir Mitchell.   *[Z 10/31]*

862. **Richards, Alfred Newton,** 1876-1966. The John Morgan Society of the Hospital and Medical School of the University of Pennsylvania. *Philadelphia, 1957.*

[1], 15 ff. 28 cm. Mimeographed. Origin and early history of the society, founded Apr. 17, 1907. — Presented by Francis C. Wood.   *[10d/143]*

863. — — — — —. Survey of medical affairs, University of Pennsylvania, by A.N. Richards and T. Grier Miller. Prepared for President Gates [Univ. of Penna.] and submitted to him on March 5, 1931. *Philadelphia, 1931.*

6, 144, 72, 2 ff.; tables. 28 cm. Photocopy of typewritten original, on which was inscribed, "This is one of 3 copies." Presented by the American Philosophical Society. Appendices include comparisons with non-university hospitals, clinics, etc., and recommendations for improvements in certain university medical departments.   *[ZZ 10c/15]*

864. **Richardson, Joseph Gibbons,** 1836-1886. Correspondence, notebooks, reports, lecture notes, etc. *Philadelphia, etc., 1860-86.*

3 boxes. 32-39 cm. Autograph, typewritten and printed. Boxes 1-2 contain recipes, items relating to Civil War service, notebooks, and letters, among these several by Asst. Adj. General J.R. Freese (1862), J.H. Salisbury (1868) and J.J. Woodward (1868-69). — Autograph poem "The new Esculapiad" (marked "No. 7, Semper ego auditor tantum," 19 ff.); fragment "Molecules in blood and severity of symptoms of rheumatic and neuralgic diseases" (ff. 3-4, 6-13, 20; n.d.); Construction of eye and mechanics of vision (21 pp., 4 ff.; n.d.); condolences upon R's death; printed forms, abstracts, obituaries, etc. — Box 3 contains irregularly paginated or foliated lecture notes, as follows: a-b. Two different sets of lectures on hygiene, both undated (1884-86?, 68 ff. and 113 ff.); c. Lecture on electricity (28 ff., 1886); d. Conclusion of epidemic infection; lessons of Memphis contagion (29 ff., 1884?; with printed report from *Trans. & Stud.*, ser. 3, v. 7: 41-50 [1884; icplt.] with pencilled note on p. 41); e. The germ theory, chiefly from Soc. Sci. Lect[ures?]; Pasteur's inoculation of 50 sheep with anthrax; Ziegler's *Pathological Anatomy* (33 ff., 1884); f. End of germ theory; graft theory; race as far as raw composite in U.S. (60 ff., + 1 f. list of [female] students, 1884-86?). — Letter of transmittal, Mrs. Francis R. Packard to W.B. McDaniel on behalf of Josephine Howell, filed in box 1.   *[10a/338]*

865. **Roberts, Algernon Sydney,** 1855-1896. Club-foot. *N.p., 1885?*

33 ff. 26 cm. Typewritten, with manuscript corrections and additions to the bibliography (f. 33). Bound with galley proofs of Roberts' and Samuel Ketch's article on club-foot in the *Reference Handbook of the Medical Sciences* (1885-93), pp. 196-[214]. — Bookplate of A. Sydney Roberts inside front cover.   *[10d/92]*

866.   **Roberts, John Bingham,** 1852-1924, comp. Collection of newspaper cuttings, letters, postcards and publicity materials, relating to medical licensure legislation for Pennsylvania. *Philadelphia, 1884?-93.*

> 1 v. 40 cm. Scrapbook. Includes some clippings on local quacks, especially John Buchanan.   *[Z 10c/16]*

867.   —————. Correspondence, largely letters to Dr. Roberts. *V.p., 1871-1922.*

> 1 box (9 folders). 39.5 cm. Relating to the Board of Medical Examiners (1884-1907), the American Surgical Association (1887-1920), the Pan American Congress of 1892, various other medical associations or groups; with acknowledgements of his publications (1877-1913), matters of consultation (1876-1906), etc.   *[n.c.]*

868.   —————. Notes of life in a hospital, by a resident physician. *Philadelphia, 1877.*

> 17 ff. 27 cm. Presented by the author.   *[10a/164]*

869.   [—————]. Report on surgical clinics, at the Woman's Hospital of Philadelphia . . . reported by Mary Alice Schively. *Philadelphia, 1894-95.*

> 1 v. 26 cm.   *[10b/19]*

870.   [—————] —————, submitted by Mary Wenzel. *Ibid., 1896-97.*

> [4], 171 ff.; illus. 27 cm. Typescript.   *[10b/20]*

871.   [—————] —————, reported by S. Edith Ives. *Ibid., 1897-98.*

> [5], 75 ff.; illus. 27 cm. Typescript.   *[10b/17]*

872.   [—————] —————, compiled by Lily G.H. Pridgeon. *Ibid., 1897-98.*

> [7], 130 ff.; illus. 27 cm.   *[10b/18]*

873.   [—————] —————, reported by Katrina Freudenberger. *Ibid., 1897-98.*

> [13], 172 ff.; illus. 28 cm.   *[10b/15]*

74. [– – – – –] – – – – –, [reported] by Rose Hirschler. *Ibid., 1899.*

xxiv, 160 ff.; col. illus. 29 cm. Typescript. [10b/16]

Note: *Titles of this and the 5 preceding items vary. All 6 are the gift of J.B. Roberts.*

– – – – –. See also nos. 149, 799, 876.

75. **Robertson, Francis Marion,** 1806-1892. Controversy over obstetrical statistics between Robertson and Henry A. Ramsey. *Charleston and Philadelphia, 1851-52.*

1 envelope ([6, 4, 2, 1 pp., statistical table], 3 printed items). 31 cm. Mostly (or entirely) copies of correspondence. Involves also John Barclay Biddle, Joseph Carson, the American Medical Association and the *Medical News,* etc. [n.c.]

76. **Robertson, William Egbert,** 1869-1956. Memoir of John B. Roberts. *Philadelphia, 1926-27.*

9 (vero 10) ff. 28 cm. Typewritten. Read Jan. 10, 1927 at the College of Physicians of Philadelphia and published in *Trans. & Stud.* ser. 3, v. 49: lxxvii-lxxxii (1927). – Presented by Dr. Emlen Wood. [10d/36]

77. **Robins, Robert Patterson,** comp. & transl., 1857-1905. De pulsilogio et thermometro; notes on the pulsimeter and thermometer, extracted and translated out of Sanctorius, G.B.C. Nelli and Viviani on Galileo, Fludd, etc., compiled for S.W. Mitchell. *N.p., 1891.*

2 v. (185 pp., pp. 41-2 removed without affecting text); illus. 20 cm. Contents: Sanctorius, *Commentaria in primam fen primi libri Canonis Avicennae* (pp. 5-51). – B.B.C. Nelli, *Vita . . . di Galileo Galilei* (pp. 59-127). – Vincenzio Viviani, "Vita di Galileo Galilei," in G.'s *Opere,* 1718 (pp. 127-29). – Mario Giardi, Letter re Sanctorius (pp. 131-37). – Extracts from Joh. Kepler, communicated by A. Hall (pp. 139-45). – Robert Fludd, *Philosophia moysiaca* (pp. 149-71). – R.P. Robins and S.W. Mitchell, Outline for the construction of a short biography of Sanctorius (pp. 173-85). – Used by Dr. Mitchell in "The Early History of Instrumental Precision in Medicine." [10a/88]

78. **Roesler, Hugo,** b. 1899. Pre-Harveian concepts of the circulation. *Philadelphia, 1936.*

8 ff. 28 cm. Typewritten (carbon copy). Delivered at the Section of Medical History of the College of Physicians of Philadelphia. [n.c.]

79. **Rogers, Fred Baker,** b. 1926. Basic science lectures, Graduate School of Medicine, University of Pennsylvania. *Philadelphia, 1949-50.*

262 pp.   28 cm.   Manuscript notes, drawings, etc., interspersed with mimeographed schedules, outlines, etc.   Lectures on pathology, physiological chemistry, physiology, pharmacology, bacteriology, immunology and human development, by Julius H. Comroe, David L. Drabkin, Seymour S. Kety, and William Ernst Ehrich. — Gift of F.B. Rogers.   [ZZ 10a/23]

880.   ─────.   Notes on basic studies of internal medicine, University of Pennsylvania, Graduate School of Medicine.   *Philadelphia, 1949-50.*

1 v.   28 cm.   Manuscript notes, drawings, etc., interspersed with mimeographed schedules, outlines, notes, etc.   Lectures, ward rounds, etc., given by over 30 members of faculty and staff. — Gift of F.B. Rogers.   [ZZ 10a/22]

881.   ─────.   Painless myocardial infarction.   *Philadelphia, 1951.*

[1], 29, [2], 10 ff.; tables.   28.5 cm.   Typescript.   Thesis — M.Sc. (Med.) — Univ. of Penna.   Includes carbon copy of related text on the same topic (10 ff.). — Letter from E.F. Evans inserted. — Gift of F.B. Rogers.   [n.c.]

882.   ─────.   Personal log, *U.S.N.S. General S.D. Sturgis,* (T-AP 137) MSTSA, 21 July 1952 . . . to 8 January 53.   *At sea, 1952-53.*

1 v.; illus.   26.5 cm.   Printed and mimeographed inserts included.
                    [ZZ 10c/6]

─────.   See also no. 502.

883.   **Rogers, John,** 1866-1939.   Thyroidism and its treatment by a specific antiserum.   *New York, 1907.*

60 ff.   27 cm.   The article entitled "The Treatment of Thyroidism by a Specific Cytotoxic Serum," by Rogers and S.P. Beebe (*Arch. Int. Med.,* v. 2: 297-329 [1908]), has note "This article represents the Mütter Lecture, which was delivered before the College of Physicians in Philadelphia, Dec. 13, 1907." Manuscript and the printed version are dissimilar in structure and wording.
                    [10a/369]

884.   **Rogers, Theophilus,** 1731-1801.   Recipes, prescriptions, etc.   *Norwich, Conn., 1779-1801.*

78 pp.   19 cm.   Letter inside front cover gives brief biographical information about Rogers; Dr. Rogers prepared the book for his daughter's use.   Tipped in: Bill for medical services to William Backus of Windham, 1727 [sic] — Presented by Mrs. Howland Wood through Dr. Russell Richardson.
                    [10a/296]

885.   **Rubin, Rose Sylvia,** 1879-1948.   Manuscript notes in syllabus on pathology, probably by Aloysius O.J. Kelly.   *Philadelphia, 1907.*

85 ff.   27 cm.   Mimeographed syllabus, interleaved for ms. notes, with interlinear and marginal additions.   Typed list of drugs (10 ff.) enclosed.   Issued for students at Woman's Medical College.   [10a/499]

886. **Ruffell, Charles Einwechter.** b. 1879.   Scrap book containing prescriptions, medical advice, various notices of interest to physicians (e.g. "The advantages of medical history," p. 61), etc. *Philadelphia, 1900-12.*

[3] ff., 203, [26] pp.; illus. 29 cm. Handwritten notes on pathology (1900) on preliminary 3 ff., alphabetical index A-J on 10 pp. toward end of volume. Includes also clippings, a letter from the Bayer Co., New York (undated), pamphlet on synthetic Hydra-stinin-Bayer, prescription by Dr. William C. Posey for Mrs. Ruffell, few typed items and manuscript annotations, household hints, etc.   *[10a/479]*

887. **Ruschenberger, William Samuel Waithman,** 1807-1895.   Common place book, commenced November 25th, 1828. *Pacific Ocean, 1828-29.*

1 v. 26 cm. Contains poems, prose quotations, an early recollection of the writer, a few medical observations, etc.   *[10c/75]*

888. ─────. A trip from the East (notes abroad); or, Letters from Brazil, Arabia, Hindostan, Ceylon, Java, Siam, Cochin China, Canton, Bonin Sandwitch & Society Islands, Peru, Chile and the West Indies, in the years 1835-37 . . . Observations on climate & nautical hygiene and the diseases of seamen and marines . . . *On board ship, etc., 1835-37.*

1 v. 33 cm. Manuscript draft of his *Voyage Around the World* (1838).
                                                  [Z 10c/2]

─────. See also nos. 112, *185.13.*

889. **Rush, Benjamin,** 1745-1813.   Apprentices to Dr. Rush. *Philadelphia, 1770-1812?*

[6] ff. 25 cm. Photocopy of manuscript list "included . . . in a notebook indexed under 'Facts and Observations'," in Rush's handwriting, among the Rush manuscripts at the Library Company of Philadelphia; also photocopy of James E. Gibson's article, "Benjamin Rush's Apprenticed Students," *Trans. & Stud.,* ser. 4, v. 14: 127-32 (1946-47), incl. lists rearranged alphabetically and geographically.   *[10a/340]*

890. ─────. Corrected proof of pp. 330 and 335 for volume IV of *Medical Inquiries and Observations,* 2nd revised and enlarged edition, Philadelphia, 1805; manuscript additions on both lower margins, and on verso of p. 335 (21 lines). *Philadelphia, 1804 or 05.*

1 conjugate leaf. 28.5 × 23 cm. Autograph corrections (correctly entered in the edition of 1805). The extensive additions in Rush's hand were not printed in the edition of 1805; the extension on the lower margin of p. 330 was largely adopted in the 1809 reprint, but not the other additions (cf. pp. 347-53 of the 1809 edition). Photo reproduction from the edition of 1805 enclosed.
                                              [10a/250, no. 8]

891.   –––––. A course of lectures on the theory and practice of chemistry. *Philadelphia, 1771.*

> 2 v. (294; 213 pp.). 27.5 cm. Signature "F. Alison" on title-pages of v. 1 and 2. The earliest extant manuscript of Rush's chemistry lectures given at the University of Pennsylvania. On the characteristics of the text see H.S. Klickstein in *Bull. Hist. Med.*, v. 27: 52-3 (1953) and W. Miles in *Chymia*, v. 4: 46-7 (1953).   *[10a/176]*

892.   –––––. Draft of agreement between Rush and Edward Earle disposing of the copyright of Rush's edition of John Pringle's *Observations Upon the Diseases of the Army. Philadelphia, ca. 1810.*

> 1 f. 19 cm. Autograph. Writing on recto only. Undated. Transfer of right for 14 years at a remuneration of $100 in books and $100 in cash, plus 12 free copies of each edition.   *[10a/250, no. 9]*

893.   –––––. Excretions of the body, C. 1[-4]. *Philadelphia, ca. 1800.*

> 46 pp. 18-20 cm (unbound). Followed on p. 44 by The influence of weather on the living system (incomplete). Authorship uncertain; not in Rush's handwriting.   *[10a/250, no. 4]*

894.   –––––. Few thoughts upon political science. *Philadelphia?, 1805.*

> 15 pp., [2] blank ff. 21 cm. Autograph. "An oration &c. for James Montgomery 1805" (p. 1, line 1), repeated on the verso of last blank f. Possibly draft of a paper to be delivered not by Rush, but by his son's friend James Montgomery before Clio, one of two literary and debating societies of Princeton University. Term used in the text: science of government. Corrections, in the hand of Rush, throughout.   *[10a/250, no. 1]*

895.   –––––. Five letters to Dr. John McClellan, 1794-1812; copies. *Philadelphia?, ca. 1889.*

> [5] ff. 32 cm. McClelland (should be Mclellan) spelled McCleland in letters of 1797-98. Concerns medical as well as personal matters. Added: Letter of transmittal from Dr. J.H. Musser; note about possession of originals (n.d., icplt.); copy of letter from Elbridge Gerry to ex-president John Adams, with reference to Rush (facs. reproduction).   *[10a/250, no. 15]*

896.   –––––. Fragment of the manuscript of *An Account of the Life and Character of Christopher Ludwick* (published Philadelphia, 1801). *Philadelphia, n.d.*

> Ff. 25-28. 20.5 cm. Autograph. Numerous corrections. The Library Company of Philadelphia owns the text in manuscript (Commonplace Book, 1789-91).   *[10a/250, no. 16]*

897.   —————. Fragmentary notes, largely extracts from the Bible,
relating to mental states and disorders. *Philadelphia, ca. 1809-10.*

pp. 131 (misnumbered 130) -138, 163-[164]. 33 cm. Autograph. Pp. 163-
[164], torn; consists of short statements on government, religion and discovery
of electricity.   *[10a/250, no. 12]*

898.   ————   —————, primarily pertaining to nervous disorders.
Philadelphia, early 19th cent.

[30] ff. Various sizes (average ca. 20 cm). Autograph. Leaves numbered in
the 200s, 400s and 500s. Like the preceding item (with lower numbers) these
are notes, presumably for articles, books, or lectures, probably related to his
Medical Inquiries and Observations Upon Diseases of the Mind.   *[10a/250, no. 3]*

899.   ————   ————— on miscellaneous topics. *Philadelphia, 1795-
1809?*

[76] ff. Various sizes (average ca. 20 cm). Autograph. Many leaves numbered; numbers repeated. Presumably likewise notes for articles, books, or
lectures. Among topics are yellow fever, dropsy, consumption, apoplexy,
nervous disorders; references to authors include Harvey, Sydenham, Morton,
Pringle and Physick. On verso of f. 20: "Vexations of a medical life from a
physicians brethren[!] omitted as a peace offering to those of them who had
injured me. Nov. 4. 1803."   *[10a/250, no. 2]*

900.   —————. From Lind; brief notes on James Lind's *Essay on
Diseases Incidental to Europeans in Hot Climates. Philadelphia, ca.
1810.*

6 ff. (ff. 4-6 blank). 17 cm. Presumably composed in connection with the
forthcoming publication of the American edition (1811) of Lind; these "brief
notes" were not included.   *[10a/250, no. 7]*

Note: *Rush's Lectures on institutes and practice of medicine, notes on
these, and parts of the Lectures are listed in chronological order, rather
than alphabetically by title.*

901.   —————. Lectures on institutes and practice of medicine.
Notes from a course of lectures on the practice of physic..., taken
by Thomas C. James. *Philadelphia, 1786.*

[178] pp. (and blank ff.). 17 cm. Signature of James on preliminary f. and
his stamp on title page. Covers 9 lectures. — Gift of H. Lenox Hodge, with his
bookplate.   *[10a/107]*

902.   ————   —————. Lectures. *Philadelphia, 179—.*

2 v. 20.5 cm. Note-taker unidentified. Volume 1 begins with physiology,
then goes into practice. Vol. 2 continues the study of specific diseases. No
therapeutics, but "cures" given for each disease with its description. Between

pp. 82 and 83 of v. 1, 60 unnumbered pp. interpolated, concerned with the theory of medicine and disease. These are in a different hand; glosses in both volumes in this hand. − Gift of G.H. Arrow.   *[10a/356]*

903.   −−−− −−−−−. Extract from Dr. Rush's lectures. *Phila-delphia, after 1793.*

3 v. 19 cm. Note-taker unidentified. Notes on course on institutes and practice of medicine.   *[10a/111]*

904.   −−−− −−−−−. Notes from Rush's Lectures on institutes and practice of medicine, taken by John Archer(?). *Philadelphia, 1796-97.*

2 v. 19 cm. Covers first year of a two-year course.   *[10a/453]*

905.   −−−− −−−−−, taken by Elijah Griffiths. *Philadelphia, 1797-98.*

194 pp. 20 cm. Second-year course.   *[10a/106]*

906.   −−−− −−−−−. Notes from Doctor B. Rush's lectures delivered in the University of Pennsylvania, commenced 27 Nov. 1797. *Philadelphia, 1797-98.*

1 v. 21 cm. Facsimile reprint of ms. in Welch Medical Library, Baltimore.   *[10a/374]*

907.   −−−− −−−−−, taken by William Darlington. *Philadelphia, 1802-04.*

3 v. 21 cm. More complete than the 1796-97 and 1797-98 lectures (1st & 2nd year?); v. 3 incl. appendix, lecture on the pulse. − Gift of Chester County Medical Society.   *[10a/105]*

908.   −−−− −−−−−, taken by Benjamin Archer. *Philadelphia, 1804.*

2 v. 16.5-20 cm. Found among Archer's effects by Anna R. Craven and presented by her.   *[10a/136]*

909.   −−−− −−−−−, taken by Joseph G. Shippen(?). *Philadel-phia, 1807/8-08/9?*

3 v. 20.5 cm. Covers only part of the course. − Gift of Edward Shippen and Edward Shippen Morris.   *[10a/108]*

910.   −−−− −−−−−, taken by Thomas D. Mitchell. *Philadelphia, 1809-11.*

2 v. 20 cm. Volume 1 begins with syllabus of sections on therapeutics and practice; then proceeds with the text of these two sections. − V. 2 completes section on practice; final 28 pp. consist of index and list of recipes for

remedies. Four stanzas in praise of Rush, 1st and 2d on fly-leaf of each
volume; 3d and 4th stanzas after t.-p. of vol. 2. — T.D. Mitchell's bookplate in v.
2.　　　　　　　　　　　　　　　　　　　　　　　　　　*[10a/177]*

911.　───── ─────, taken by John Sommer(?). *Philadelphia,
1810.*

2 v.　25 cm.　Covers part of the course.　　　　　　*[10a/104]*

912.　───── ─────, by unidentified person. *Philadelphia, 1810?*

340 ff.　20 cm.　Part of course only. — Gift of G.E. de Schweinitz.　　*[10a/199]*

913.　───── ─────, by unidentified person. *Philadelphia, 1810?*

2 v.　20 cm.　Part of course only. — Gift of Leonardo S. Clark.　　*[10a/148]*

914.　───── ─────. Notes... *Philadelphia, ca. 1810.*

2 v. (224 ff.; 451 pp.).　24 cm.　Title on spines: Rush's lectures.　Labels of
"John P. Betton", presumably owner, but not the scribe, on front cover.　Subti-
tles in volume 1: Pathology (f. 1), Therapeutics (f. 102), The Practice of
Medicine (f. 150; continued in v. 2).　John P. Betton is not listed among the
graduates of the Univ. of Penna. — Bookplate of Thomas Forrest Betton and
Bibliotheca Bettoniana, Coll. Med. Philadelphia.　　　　　*[10a/103]*

15.　───── ─────, taken by George F. Lehman (?). *Philadelphia, 1810-11.*

3 v.　19.5 cm.　Part of course only.　Prov.: Augustus Muhlenberg. — Gift of
John Bernard Flick.　　　　　　　　　　　　　　　　*[10a/239]*

16.　───── ─────. Notes on physiology from Rush's Lectures on institutes and practice of medicine, taken by William
Horner. *Philadelphia, 1813.*

457 pp.　25 cm.　Contains the first of four sections of the course on institutes
and practice, including lectures on the mind. — Bookplate of St. Joseph's
Hospital Library.　Gift of E.E. Montgomery.　　　　　*[10a/283]*

17.　─────. Lectures upon the mind. *Philadelphia, n.d.*

245 ff., and [44] ff., numbered 434-77.　22 cm.　Autograph, with typewritten
title-page.　Heavily edited: rewritten, interlined, and crossed out.　Much of
this material, condensed and somewhat rephrased, was used in his lectures on
physiology.　Section "Of pleasure: Lect: 20th," ff. 473-77, corresponds word-
for-word with some parts of "Two Lectures upon the Pleasures of the Senses
and of the Mind," at the end of his *Sixteen Introductory Lectures* (Philadelphia,
1811).　Not otherwise published, except briefly, as Rush echoes definitions,
etc., under headings similar to those above, in his *Medical Inquiries and
Observations on the Diseases of the Mind* (Philadelphia, 1812).　This manuscript is
briefly mentioned by Prof. Shryock (*Jour. Amer. Psychiat.*, v. 100: 429 ff. [1945]);
and at somewhat greater length by Farr (*ibid.*, v. 100: 10 ff. [1944]); both
describe it as "early."　Listed by Goodman among the manuscripts of Rush

(*Benj. Rush, Physician and Citizen, 1746-1813*; Phila., 1934, p. 380), but erroneously described as 954 pp. More fully discussed by P.S. Noel and E.T. Carlson (*Jour. Hist. Behav. Sci.*, v. 9: 369-77 [1973]).   *[10a/102]*

918.   — — — — —. Letter to Dr. Elisha Hall, Fredericksburg, Va., with report on the condition of Mary Washington, suffering from breast cancer. *Philadelphia, 6 July 1789.*

2 ff.   23 cm.   Letter of transmittal to the College of Physicians of Philadelphia, by Hunter McGuire (1887) through S. Weir Mitchell, tipped in.   *[10a/190]*

919.   — — — — —. Letter to John Nicholson on behalf of the officers of the African Church. *Philadelphia, Nov. 28, 1792.*

1 p. (11 lines text).   23.5 cm (mounted).   "Letter from Doctr Benjᵃ Rush Decʳ. 5. 1792 presented by Absalom Jones & Wᵐ. Gray persons of color," on verso of letter.   *[10a/250, no. 13]*

920.   — — — — —. Medical bills, accounts, payments. *Philadelphia, 1781-1813.*

29 pieces.   Various sizes.   Handwritten, some autograph (one torn, few fragile).   Partial contents: To the estate of Ann Maria Clifton, services rendered 1781-1811 (£152.15.0). — 22 payments of bills for medical services (1794-1813) made to the estate of Rush.   *[10a/250, no. 11]*

921.   — — — — —. Notes on physiology taken from lectures delivered in the University of Pennsylvania . . .; notes enlarged by M[icajah] Clark. *Philadelphia, 1809-11.*

233 ff.   20 cm.   Volume 1 of Rush's Physiology, "taken at Charleston, S.C., immediately after the evacuation . . . by the Rebel Army. I found it in the house opposite Gov. Aikin's dwelling. . . .   Samuel Cuskaden, Co.D., 52d Regt. P.V.V." (note tipped in at beginning of volume).   Contains first of four sections of the course on institutes and practice, including lectures on the mind.   Has table of contents. — Gift of Samuel Lewis.   *[10a/300]*

922.   — — — — —. Obstruction in the viscera; sketches of the Brunonian system of medicine. *Philadelphia, 1807-09, and later.*

5 pieces of paper (torn and brittle).   Various sizes.   Autograph.   Part of sketch (in form of a chart) has patient's report on verso.   *[10a/250, no. 6]*

923.   — — — — —. On the liver; draft. *Philadelphia, ca. 1800.*

4 ff.   19 cm.   Autograph.   Contains references to yellow fever.

[10a/250, no. 5]

924.   — — — — —. Prescriptions. *Philadelphia, 1799-1813.*

[8] ff.   18-19.5 cm.   Contents: 1. 1799.   "Directions for Mr. Eyre" before sailing to the West Indies; copies (one with water mark dated 1889, a second by the donor, Dr. A.P.C. Ashhurst [2 + 2 ff.]). — 2. 1809.   "Prescription for

Jacob Broom," autograph (2 ff.). — 3. 1813. "Dr. Rush for Richard Hancock,"
autograph (2 ff.), presented by John V. Craven. Added, an envelope with
broken seal, addressed to Rush; "Done" in Rush's handwriting.

[10a/250, no. 10]

925.   — — — — —.   Practice of physic; notes on his lectures. *Philadelphia,
after 1794.*

178 ff. 21 cm. Previously attributed to Chapman (in spite of references in
text to Rush as the lecturer); if entry (Rush) is correct, these notes, written by
Robert Alison (M.D. 1819, Univ. of Penna.), were presumably copied from
another person's manuscript.   *[10a/180]*

926.   — — — — —.   Three printed forms signed by Rush. *Philadelphia,
1796-1810.*

20, 10 × 17, 10 × 24 cm. Contents: 1. 1796. Admission to the Pennsylvania
Hospital for madness. — 2. 1809. Referral to the Pennsylvania Hospital, case
of fever. — 3. 1810. Certificate of internment, disease: madness.

[10a/250, no. 18]

927.   [— — — — —].   Bills (some receipted) for materials or services
rendered to Benjamin Rush and his heirs between 1798 and
1817. *V.p., ca. 1800-17.*

31 pieces. Various sizes. Added: Summons to appear as witnesses in a case
involving "Rush" (no first name), Sept. 29, 1817, City of Philadelphia. —
Unpaid bill for plastering, unopened (summons?), May 25, 1815.

[10a/250, no. 17]

— — — — —.   See also nos. 42, 114, *185.11-12*, 200, 242, 269, 291,
294, 344, 394, 446, 450, 559, 573, 623, 671, 678, 688, 706, 804,
806, 816, 1004, 1107.

928.   **Rush, James,** 1786-1869.   Essence of Dr. Rush's lectures . . .
Philadelphia, 1817.

[6] ff., 317 (vero 318) pp., blank and [2] ff. 24.5 cm. Full title: "Essence of Dr.
Rush's lectures from notes taken by me in the Winters of 1815 and 1816. Elias
Boudinot Stockton, Philada. May 1817." Elias Boudinot Stockton, a relative
of Benjamin Rush's wife, studied at the Univ. of Penna. from 1813 to 1816,
when he received his M.D. Index inside front cover and on the flyleaf. Read-
ing list at end of vol. (2 ff. bound in, 1 loose f.). Some inserts, incl. Dr. Dorsey,
Feb. 4, 1818. Rubefacients; Dr. Ferriar on arsenical solution in the last stage of
typhus, and Rush on impotence. The notes appear to follow the sequence of
Benjamin Rush's *Syllabus on the Institutes and Practice of Medicine*, beginning with
Section II, Hygiene, and continuing on to the end of Practice. Whitfield Bell,
Jr. mentions in his article on James Rush (*J. Hist. Med. & Allied Sci.*, v. 19: 419-21
[1964]) that the younger Rush read his father's lectures to private classes for
four years after Benjamin's death in 1813. — Presented to the Lewis Library by
W.F. Atlee.   *[10a/301]*

929. **Rush Medical Club.** Minutes, committee records, financial accounts, etc. *Philadelphia, 1865-1907.*

1 v., 2 envelopes in box. 34-37 cm. Minutes (1865-98) of annual meetings, and of Book Committee meetings; treasurer's account book (1865-1902); misc. related materials (1891-1907) of medical book club, formed in 1865, with membership limited to fifteen. — Presented by Stricker Coles.   *[Z 10/42]*

930. **Rush Society.** Correspondence and accounts. *Philadelphia, 1912-28.*

1 box. 26 cm. Correspondence (1912-15, 1924-28) about founding and lecture arrangements of the Rush Society (later, Rush Society for the Correlation and Support of Medical and Biological Lectures in Philadelphia), organized, largely as the result of activities of Richard M. Pearce, at the University of Pennsylvania in 1912 with the aim to diffuse knowledge concerning recent advances in medical and biological sciences, methods and problems of education, public hygiene, and later, to correlate and occasionally make arrangements for medical lectures in Philadelphia. — Account book (1912-16) containing paid subscriptions and society's disbursements; lecture notices (1913-17). — Presented by E.B. Krumbhaar.   *[Z 10/178]*

931. **Ruston, Thomas,** ca. 1740-1804. Papers, etc., 1764-65, 1771, 1779, 1782, 1784, 1786-96, 1790, 1794, 1797, 1802 and 6 undated items. *Edinburgh, London and Philadelphia, 1764-ca. 1802.*

[35] ff. Various sizes (in box, 37.5 cm). Incl. printed forms. Partial contents: Remonstrance of medical student concerning the standards of education at Edinburgh (April-May, 1764; 2 ff.), incl. the names of Americans Arthur Lee, Samuel Bard, Corbin Griffin, Thomas Ruston and Samuel Martin. — Clinical lectures (I-II) by Dr. Cullen used on versos by Ruston to draft letters to his father (?, Job Ruston, Sept. 1764), to Mr.(?) Westly, undated; and to Dennys De Berdt (August 1765); with references to Dr. M (John Morgan), Dr. S (Wm. Smibert or Wm. Shippen?) and De Berdt (on 8 pp.). — Letter from John Hope (Prof. of materia medica, Nov. 1765, 2 ff.). — Epigram on the marriage of Dr. Ruston to Mary Fisher, by Sir William Brown (July 1771). — Election to Medical Society of Edinburgh (1779, printed, 1 f.). — Appointment to Devon and Exeter Hospital (1779, 1 f.). — 2 printed forms, Society for the Improvement of Medical Knowledge, London (1782). — Maxims by John Peter Craft showing that the will constitutes the power in man to do anything (n.d., 2 ff.). — Prescriptions (n.d.). — Bailey's *Pocket Almanac*, 1800 (with annotations and newspaper clippings, 10 cm). — Bill to the estate of Rob't. Aitken, Bookbinder, Philadelphia (ca. 1802).   *[n.c.]*

932. **St. Joseph's Hospital,** Philadelphia. Miscellaneous papers. *Philadelphia, 1859-93.*

[5, 1, 5] ff. 25-34 cm (envelope, 37.5 cm). Contents: 1. Copies of contract with the Sisters of Charity of St. Joseph's, leasing them land and buildings for use as a hospital, July 29, 1859. — 2. Copy of letter from W.S. King to John Moore, 1862, notifying hospital of termination of government contract. —

3. Typescript of two letters protesting admission or treatment of charity patients, Philip Fitzpatrick to E.J. Heraty, and E.J. Heraty to Robert B. Cruice, both dated 1893.   [10c/101]

————. See also no. 214.

933. **Sajous, Charles Euchariste de Médicis,** 1852-1929. The endocrine system as a fundamental factor in the vital process. *Philadelphia, 1924?*

28 ff. 28 cm. Typewritten. Folio 28 torn (xerox copy enclosed). "Emphasizing . . . closer community of thought between physiology and the various departments of medicine."   [ZZ 10a/29]

934. ————. Papers, correspondence, reports, etc. *V.p., 1891-1929.*

13 boxes. 26.5 × 39 cm. Autograph, typewritten (incl. carbons) and printed materials. Contains financial and legal papers (1891-1929); dealings with the publishing firm F.A. Davis (1892-1923); working material for the *Analytical Cyclopaedia of Practical Medicine, Monthly Cyclopaedia,* etc. (1893-1927); naval matters (1894-5); general correspondence (1896-1928), miscellaneous correspondence and working papers (1895-1924), incl. reports on patients, on the American Congress of Internal Medicine, the American College of Physicians; correspondence and other items concerning the Medical School of Temple University, incl. especially the Laboratory Committee and the Committee on the Library, involving in parts Dean Hammond (1908-29); correspondence relating to the *New York Medical Journal* (1911-17[-24]); items concerning his son Louis Theo de Médicis Sajous (1914-15). — Handwritten index of contents by boxes, typed index by subject, and *Fugitive Leaf,* n.s. no. 59, reproducing correspondence with Temple University's Dean Hammond (*et al.*) filed in box I. — Partly gift of Samuel Moyerman.   [10c/99]

935. **Sargent, John H.** Hypertrophy of the heart. *Philadelphia, 1876.*

[1], 27 ff. (24-27 blank). 26 cm (in box, 39 cm). Thesis — Jefferson Medical College, 1876. Boxed with family scrapbook centered on the singer Iranetta Sargent, of no or slight medical interest, except for an advertisement of Dr. J.H. Sargent's improved spectacles. — Gift of R.W. Foster.   [10c/147]

936. **Sartain, Paul Judd,** 1861-1944. Papers. *V.p., 1875-90, 1940.*

1 box. 26 cm. Partial contents: Letters from Vienna, Innsbruck and Heidelberg, to his family in Philadelphia (1886-89); letters of recommendation from German and English physicians, chiefly in photocopy (1887-90); medical notes, taken at the Medical School of the Univ. of Penna.: chemistry (T.G. Wormley) 1883/84; 2 v., physiology (Harrison Allen) 1883/84; theory and practice of medicine (lecturer unidentified), 1885; pathology (Formad's quiz lectures), n.d.; case-book, 1887 (in German).   [Z 10/174]

937. **Say, Benjamin,** 1755-1813. Ledger: accounts with his patients for attendance & medicines. *Philadelphia, 1796-1804.*

416 pp. 33.5 cm. Some bills, etc., laid in; pasted on flyleaf, a list of Say's memberships and degrees. – Gift of Francis Fisher Kane.   *[Z 10/78]*

938.   **Sayre, Francis Bowes,** 1766?-1798. Case of arthropuosis. *Philadelphia, 1788.*

[13] pp. 20.5 cm. Inscription on t.-p.: "The American Medical Society requested a copy of this essay which was afterwards published by their particular order." Commentary by W.B. McDaniel, 2d. on author and the essay published in *Fugitive Leaves*, n.s. no. 31, Sept. 1959.   *[10a/414]*

939.   – – – – –. Water. *Philadelphia?, ca. 1790.*

[18] pp. 25.5 cm. Apparently prepared for the American Medical Society (cf. *Fugitive Leaves, ibid.*). – Presented by descendant Francis B. Sayre (1959).
     [10c/82]

940.   **Scheffey, Lewis Cass,** 1893-1969. Discussions relating to the history of the Obstetrical Society of Philadelphia, by E.J. Morris, D.C. Longaker, G.M. Boyd, Alexander Macalister, W.E. Parke and Addinell Hewson, read by Dr. Scheffey. *Philadelphia, 1938.*

[15] ff. 28 cm. Typewritten. Partial list of subjects beyond the main topic: women in medicine and science; smallpox at time of delivery.   *[10d/56]*

– – – – –. See also nos. *185.13*, 739.

941.   **Schéle, Sune.** Anatomy. *Stockholm, 1963.*

16 ff. 30 cm. Typescript (carbon). Cornelis Bos as an anatomical iconographer. Preliminary to the author's book *Cornelis Bos; a Study of the Origins of the Netherlands Grotesque* (Stockholm, 1965). Incl. survey of anatomical illustrations and their relation to those of Bos, among these W. Ryff, *Omnium humani corporis partium descriptio* (Paris, 1545; only known copy in the library of the College of Physicians of Philadelphia).   *[n.c.]*

942.   **Scheller, Otto,** b. 1881. Petitions for justice concerning the (actual or imagined) property of O. Scheller and his family. *Philadelphia (Byberry), 1918-28.*

3 boxes. 38 cm. Petitions to various governmental agencies and the Republic of Czechoslovakia (never delivered?). Includes ward notes from Drs. Joseph McIver and Thomas Butterworth (diagnosis: paranoia). – Presented by J. McIver.   *[10a/289]*

943.   **Schweinitz, George Edmund de,** 1858-1938. Letters to and from Dr. de Schweinitz, reports, essays, etc. *V.p., 1901-18, 1933.*

4 boxes. 32 cm. Xerox copy of typed list of letters (boxes 1-3), and handwritten list with index of reports and essays filed with the collection. Beyond items thus recorded are included a. Bibliography of his writings, 1887-1907 with notes; b. Address (primarily on the Ambulance Hospital, Paris, 1915), in Box 2; c. Report of ophthalmological clinics held at Jefferson

Medical College Hospital . . . 1899-1900, reported by R.B. Hayes (1 v.) and
d. Records of the results of the examination of the eyes of patients at the Univ.
of Penna., 1904-12 (3 v.), in Box 3. Box 4 contains correspondence to de
Schweinitz, largely on matters of consultation, incl. extensive correspondence
with Edward Jackson, editor of the *Ophthalmic Year Book* and F. Park Lewis of
the Committee on Prevention of Blindness of the AMA. — Bequest of G.E. de
Schweinitz.   *[10d/3]*

944.   — — — — —. . . . Painful tumors, with special reference to neuro-
mata. *Philadelphia, 1881.*

115 ff.; 6 plates.   25.5 cm.   Thesis (M.D.) — Univ. of Penna., 1881.   *[10b/53]*

945.   — — — — —. Reminiscences from the time he was prosector of
Dr. Joseph Leidy; address before the Historical Club of the
Medical School of the University of Pennsylvania. *Philadelphia,*
1917.

13 ff.   28 cm (envelope, 31 cm).   Typewritten (carbon).   Fragile; photocopies
enclosed.   Without "references to Dr. Leidy's achievements in science . . . ably
described this evening by Dr. Rohrer."   *[n.c.]*

946.   — — — — —. The toxic amblyopias; their symptoms, pathology
and treatment. *Philadelphia, 1894.*

276 ff.; illus.   28 cm.   Typewritten and manuscript.   Alvarenga Prize Essay
no. 4, 1894.   Published, with revisions, under title *The Toxic Amblyopias; Their*
Classification, History, Symptoms, Pathology, and Treatment (Philadelphia, Lea,
1896).   *[10a/112]*

— — — — —. See also nos. 8, *185.13*, *.237*, 253, 346, 678, 1050.

947.   **Secreti medici, ed altri:** 1. Libro de medixine anomenado
bonsecorso, *inc.:* [I]n lo nome de deo e della santa trinitade . . .
Elle vera cosa, che naturalmente tuti omini e femine, che
nasseno al mondo siconveno . . . (ff. 2r-19v). — 2. Libro molte
experientie anominado cara cosa, *inc.:* [C]ocio sia cosa, che
insuxo questo picolo volume . . . (ff. 1r-22v, and 2 unnumb. ff.).
— 3. Secrete per la salude . . . et experimenti, *inc.:* Qui sinotera
molti zecrete . . . (line 8, text): Inquit noster autor cum esset in
babilonia . . . (ff. 1-61). *Italy (Venetian territory?), 14th-15th cent.*

3 texts in 1 vol.   23.5 cm.   Nos. 1-2 on vellum, 3 on paper.   First leaf of no. 1
missing.   Nos. 1 and 2 in the same 14th-cent. hand, 1 with 15th-cent. addition
(Cap. 130), 2. with additions in 15th-cent. and 18th-cent. hands. — 3. Except
for the introduction, the recipes are in Italian. — The collective title "Secreti" is
in a 17th- or 18th-cent. hand. — Gift of M.S. Wickersham.   *[10a/131]*

948.   **Sennert, Daniel,** 1572-1637. Medicinarum usitatissimarum
materia, usus, et dosis, ex Sennerto, *inc.:* Manna est nox[?] in
terram deridit (pp. 1-329). — With an appendix relating to "ye

former work by way of astrology. . ." (pp. 330-74), and "Index or table" (pp. 374-83). *England, 2nd half 17th cent.*

8 ff., 384 pp., 2 ff.   10.5 cm.   *[10a/213]*

949.   **Shaffer, Newton Melman,** 1847-1928. Clinical lectures on orthopedic surgery, delivered at the Cornell University Medical College, reported by L.W. Hubbard. *New York, 1882-83.*

177, [5] pp.   26 cm.   Typewritten. — Bookplate of Sydney Roberts.   *[10d/19]*

950.   **Shamburger, William F.,** b. 1834. An inaugural essay on cynanche laryngea, presented to the faculty of the Philadelphia College of Medicine, for the degree of doctor in medicine, by William F. Shamburger of Mississippi. *Philadelphia, 1857.*

[2], 32 ff.   25 cm.   *[n.c.]*

951.   **Shaw, Joseph B.,** 1861-1936. Essay on diphtheria. *Philadelphia, 1885.*

27 ff.   26 cm.   Thesis, M.D. — Univ. of Penna., 1885. — Gift of Sir William Osler.   *[10a/130]*

952.   **Shaw-Mackenzie, John Alexander,** b. 1857. Letters to Frederick L. Hoffman on cancer and immunity. *London, 1931.*

17 ff. (carbon copies of 4 letters; incl. 2 copies of letter 3).   26 cm (envelope, 36 cm).   Letter 2 refers to G.E. Deatherage.   Clippings and articles (the latter by Shaw-Mackenzie) are included with letters 1, 2 and 4.   *[10a/439]*

953.   **Shay, Harry,** 1898-1963. Experimental studies in gastric physiology in man. II. Phyloric function; role of the duodenum in its control; effect of acid and alkali, by Harry Shay and J. Gershon-Cohen. *Philadelphia, 1933.*

[2], 38 ff.   28 cm.   Typescript (carbon copy).   Alvarenga Prize Essay no. 30, 1933.   *[10d/38]*

954.   **Shippen, William,** 1712-1801. Letter to George Washington upon his retirement to his family. *N.p., 1783.*

1 f.   28 cm (binding 35 cm).   Gift of William Pepper.   *[Z 10/48]*

— — — — —. See also no. 931.

955.   **Shippen, William,** 1736-1808. Anatomical lectures. . . . *Philadelphia, 1777?*

171 pp.   21 cm.   Inscribed on flyleaf: William McWilliam's, 1777; Wm. McWilliam not listed as a graduate of the Univ. of Penna. — Presented by J.R. Bahl.   *[10b/49]*

956. — — — — —. Recommendations for an army medical corps in the Revolutionary War. *Philadelphia, 1777.*

[6] ff. 35.5 cm. Photocopy of original in the Library of Congress. Gift of E.B. Krumbhaar.   *[Z 10/83]*

— — — — —. See also nos. *185.13,* 1049.

957. **Shuman, Jesse Elmer,** b. 1869. Notebook, consisting largely of prescriptions. *Philadelphia, 1889-1900.*

15 ff. (2 ff. removed between ff. 9-10 and 11-12), 35 blank ff., 4 ff. addresses. 9 × 15 cm. (oblong). Probably notes taken at the Dept. of Medicine, Univ. of Penna where J.E. Shuman received his M.D. in 1891.   *[n.c.]*

958. **Signirkunst, Signirwissenschaft, ars signata** . . . Anatomie der Arzneimittel. *Germany, first half 19th cent.?*

38 (i.e. 40), 78, 22 pp. 21 cm. Original manuscript, with corrections. Learned historical survey, seemingly influenced by the iatrochemical writings of Paracelsus, with references to ancient (e.g. Hippocrates, Galen, Pliny), Renaissance and later writers (e.g. van Helmont, A. Kircher).   *[n.c.]*

959. **[Sixteenth-Century Lecture Notes].** 1. Methodus discurendi circa quosvis morbos et symptomata proposita, *inc.:* Nihil utilius . . . medico, ff. 1r-6v. — 2. Curatio morborum malae temperaturae absque materia, *inc.:* Morborum malis[?] tempus . . . , ff. 8r-16v (dated at end 24 Jan. [15]82). — 3. Bottoni, Albertino. De febribus, ff. 23r-183v (with a number of subsections, one entitled De curatione febris tertianae, f. 105r). — 4. Idem. De morbis, ff. 190r-247r (begins with De morbis summi ventris which is not listed in the index of diseases on f. 190v). — 5. Idem. Tractatus de semine et sanguine menstruo (ff. 254r-87v, dated 1581). — 6. Mercurialis, Hieronymus. Tractatus . . . de affectibus mamillarum muliebrium et primo De defectu lactis, ff. 290r-325v (with index on f. 290r). — 7. Idem. De morbis puerorum internis, ff. 326-63. *Padua?, ca. 1581-82.*

3 blank ff. (the first with table of contents), 366 ff. (ff. 7, 17-22, 78, 184-89, 212, 248-53, 266, 273-74, 288-89, 364-66 blank; 3 ff. removed between ff. 100 and 102, a few slips laid in). 21 cm. Written in two or more hands.   *[10a/154]*

960. **Slack, Horace George Bewick.** Parenteral treatment of iron deficiency anaemias with special reference to the use of an intravenous iron preparation. *Manchester, 1948.*

[2], 176 ff.; tables, graphs. 34 cm. Photostat copy of typescript. Thesis (M.D.) — Manchester. — Gift of Smith, Kline & French.   *[n.c.]*

961. **Smith, Albert Holmes,** 1835-1885.   Notes taken by Herbert M. Howe on lectures by Dr. A.H. Smith, delivered at the Nurses' Home.   *Philadelphia, 1864.*

    1 v.   16.5 cm.   Book label of Herbert M. Howe in back of front cover.
                                                                    [10a/382]

    — — — — —.   See also nos. 226, 993.

962. **Smith, Allen John,** 1863-1926.   Notes on lectures on pathology. *Philadelphia, 1915-16.*

    173 ff.   29 cm.   Typescript (hectographed).   Provenience: W.C. Hausheer (M.D. 1918 — Univ. of Penna.).   Includes Dr. Kolmer's last lecture, Feb. 15, 1916.   *[ZZ 10a/28]*

    — — — — —.   See also no. 540.

963. **Smith, Francis Gurney,** 1818-1878.   Lectures on physiology. *Philadelphia, 1874.*

    33 ff.   20 cm.   Notes taken by Frederick P. Henry.   Includes notes on (Protestant) Episcopal Hospital cases by F.P. Henry (ff. 27-30) and Henry's report on a case of extra-uterine pregnancy (ff. 31-33) with laid-in report on autopsy (1 f.), brief summary (2 ff.), and pulse chart (1 f.).   Pencilled notes on back fly-leaves. — 1 f. between leaves 30 and 31 removed.   *[10a/501]*

964.   — — — — —.   Notes on lectures.   *Philadelphia, 1874-75.*

    2 v.   24 cm.   Notes in the form of questions and answers. — Presented by Frederick Porteous Henry.   *[10a/269]*

965.   — — — — —.   Notes on . . . lectures on physiology & the institutes of medicine, University of Pennsylvania.   *Philadelphia, 1863-64.*

    2 v.   19.5 cm.   Title-page of v. 2 inscribed D.M. Cheston.   From the back of v. 2 are 74 pp. entitled "Notes on Prof. Wm. Pepper's Lectures on the theory & practice of medicine, University of Pennsylvania, 1863-64.   D.M.C."   Various miscellaneous notes and lists include (v. 1, p. 119) a list of topics in Smith's examination; (v. 2, p. 29) list of "Drs. in the family": Dr. James Cheston, Dr. James Murray, Dr. Caspar Morris, Dr. Robert Murray, Dr. J. Cheston Morris, Dr. D. Murray Cheston, "Dr. in embryo, C. Morris Cheston. . . ."   *[10a/238]*

966.   — — — — —.   Notes taken upon lectures . . . on the institutes of medicine [by] H.M. Howe.   *Philadelphia, 1864-65.*

    [96] ff.; illus.   18 cm.   H.M. Howe received his M.D. at the Univ. of Penna. in 1865.   *[10a/379]*

    — — — — —.   See also nos. 414, 439.

967. **Smith, Franklin Buchanan,** 1856-1912.   Record of anomalies for year 1877-78.   *Philadelphia, 1878.*

146 (incl. blank) ff.; illus., part col. 21.5 cm. Offered in competition for a student prize at the Univ. of Penna., awarded by Hugh Lenox Hodge, who presented this manuscript.   *[10a/59]*

968. **Smith, Henry Hollingsworth,** 1815-1890. Notes taken by H.M. Howe upon lectures delivered by Prof. H.H. Smith on surgery. *Philadelphia, 1863.*

1 v. 17.5 cm (envelope, 26.5 cm). H.M. Howe received the M.D. at the Univ. of Penna. in 1865. Pencil portrait on recto of last f.   *[10b/50]*

— — — — —. See also nos. 114, 1112.

969. **Smith, Nathan,** 1762-1829. Lectures on the theory of physic... [Yale]. Vol. III. [Notes] taken by A.F. Warner. *New Haven, 1815-16.*

1 v. (177 pp., first blank; 4 ff. on points of midwifery; 1 f. prescriptions, blank ff., 2 ff. literary quotations towards end). 19 cm. Table of contents of main text on pp. 3-4. — Gift of William Helfand.   *[n.c.]*

970. **Smith, Sidney Irving,** 1843-1926. Lecture notes on comparative anatomy (pp. 1-25). — With **Russel Henry Chittenden,** Lecture notes on microscopy (pp. 119-64). Both recorded by Henry Howard Whitehouse. *New Haven, 1885(?).*

232 pp. (pp. 26-118, 165-232 blank); illus. (partly colored). 21 cm.
[10a/480]

971. — — — — —. Physiology of animals: the frog, cat, and rabbit. — R.H. Chittenden. Microscopic examination of yeast, etc. *New Haven, 1885?*

[1] f., 231 pp. (pp. 26-118, 166-231 blank); illus. 20.5 cm. Part of lectures, recorded by H.H. Whitehouse (names of Smith, Chittenden and Whitehouse on prel. f.).   *[n.c.]*

972. **Snodgrass, Leeman Espy,** b. 1899. G[wilym]. G[eorge]. Davis, anatomist, surgeon and teacher; life and work. *Philadelphia, after 1918.*

117, [16] ff. 30 cm. Typewritten. Presented by the author.   *[Z 10/212]*

973. **Société Médicale Américaine** de Paris. Constitution and by-laws. *Paris, 1894.*

7 ff. 31 cm (envelope, 37.5 cm).   *[n.c.]*

974. **Society of Neurological Surgeons.** Correspondence and records. *St. Louis, etc., 1920-25, 1931.*

1 box (13 folders). 32 cm. Handwritten and typed (incl. carbons). Much of the correspondence deals with meetings and proposals for membership; incl. membership lists, case histories (1921), mimeographed constitution, and bank deposit book with cancelled checks.   *[Z 10b/1]*

975. **Solis-Cohen, Jacob da Silva,** 1838-1927.   Diseases of the throat and nasal passages. *Philadelphia, 188—?*

2 boxes. 26 cm. Manuscript and typescript. Incomplete manuscript draft of portions of a 3d ed., never published. Contains parts of chapters 3-9, 11, and 14. Box 2 contains duplicates.   *[10d/32]*

976. ————. Index rerum of medical science chiefly relating to throat and nose affections, tracheotomy and foreign bodies in the air passages. *Philadelphia, 1869-78?*

2 v. 26.5-36 cm. Vol. 1 inscribed in a copy of John Todd's *Index rerum: or, Index of Subjects* (Northampton, Mass., Bridgman & Childs, 1867); a book of blank pages, indexed alphabetically. — Gift of author.   *[Z 10/79]*

977. ————, comp. Index to medical literature. *Philadelphia, late 19th-early 20th cent.?*

2 v. 28.5 cm. Two separate indexes by subject, roughly alphabetized, covering the general range of medical literature, incl. a few 18th- and some early 19th-century references, the first written into a copy of *Burr's Library Index . . .* (Hartford, J.B. Burr Publ. Co., 1881), the second into a blank book, thumb-indexed. — Gift of the compiler.   *[Z 10/38]*

978. ————. Injuries and diseases of the esophagus. *Philadelphia, 1886.*

1 box (12 folders). 32-34 cm (folders, 37 cm, box 39 cm). Twelve sections, each present in manuscript and typewritten copy with corrections (except 5, ms. only and 12, typewritten only): apnoea, esophagotomy, gastrostomy, stomach tube, dilatation and sacculation, paralysis, morbid growths, stricture, malformation, foreign bodies, wounds and ruptures, spasm. Published in *International Encyclopedia of Surgery*, v. 6: 1-43 (1886).   *[10d/4]*

979. ————. Note-book. *Philadelphia, 1860.*

1 v. 16 cm. Pencilled notes, some in shorthand, on many subjects, including obstetrics, blood, chemistry. Mentions Dr. Jackson and Dr. Hodge, instructors at Univ. of Penna. — Presented by the author.   *[10a/267]*

980. ————. Notes on the lectures of Samuel D. Gross, Robley Dunglison, and Franklin Bache, at Jefferson Medical College. *Philadelphia, 1856-57.*

4 v. 19 cm. Contents: V. 1-2, continued in v. 3; Gross' Lectures on surgery (417 pp., complete). — V. 3. Dunglison's Lectures on institutes of medicine

(91 pp.) and continuations of Gross and Bache. — V. 4. Bache's Lectures on chemistry (continued at the back of v. 3; 239 pp., complete). — Gift of Dr. Solis-Cohen.	*[10a/266]*

81.	— — — — —. Two cases of laryngectomy for adeno-carcinoma of the larynx . . . read before the American Laryngological Association at its Fourteenth Annual Congress. *Philadelphia, 1892.*

12 ff. 27 cm (envelope, 37.5 cm). Typewritten with corrections. Printer's copy (*New York Med. Jour.*, v. 56: 533-35 [1892]). Added: Commentary on Felix Semon's "Discussion on Cancer of the Larynx," (1 f., 1904) and "Progress in the Treatment of Laryngeal Carcinoma Since the Organization of the American Laryngological Assoc." (3 ff., 1911?).	*[n.c.]*

82.	— — — — —. The use of compressed and rarified air, as a substitute for change of climate, in the treatment of pulmonary diseases. *Philadelphia?, 1884.*

5 ff. 36 cm. Typescript. Read before the American Climatological Association, May 5, 1884, and published in the *New York Med. Jour.*, v. 40: 422-24 (1884).	*[n.c.]*

83.	[— — — — —]. Correspondence comprising 71 letters and 6 cards. *V.p., 1869-1914.*

3 folders. 30 cm. Letters addressed to Dr. Solis-Cohen, largely pertaining to laryngology and tuberculosis.	*[n.c.]*

— — — — —. See also nos. 474, 1120, 1138.

84.	**Speed, William M.,** b. 1834? An inaugural essay on marasmus, presented to the faculty of the Philadelphia College of Medicine, for the degree of doctor in medicine, by William M. Speed of South Carolina. *Philadelphia, 1857.*

1 blank, 12, 1 blank ff. 25 cm.	*[n.c.]*

85.	**Spiller, William Gibson,** 1863-1940. The first fifty years of the Philadelphia Neurological Society. Read before the . . . Society at the College of Physicians, January 25, 1935. *Philadelphia, 1935.*

21 pp. 28 cm. Typewritten. Published in the *Proceedings* of the Philadelphia Neurological Society (*Arch. Neurol. & Psychiat.*, v. 34: 899-906 [1935]). — Gift of the author.	*[ZZ 10c/16]*

— — — — —. See also nos. 677, 808.

986. **[Stall, Sylvanus**, 1847-1915]. Correspondence and documents, concerning the Rev. Stall and his Vir Publishing Company. *V.p., 1899-1911.*

121 ff. 36 cm. Includes 3 letters from Emma Frances Angell Drake, Denver (1906).   *[10c/81]*

987. **Starr Center Association.** Blood pressure books, etc. *Philadelphia, 1918-22.*

2 v.; 2 charts. 39 × 32 cm, oblong (envelope, 38 cm). Contents: Pregnancy and blood pressure readings (handwritten). – 35 cases under 20 years of age, 69 cases 25-29 years, 42 cases 30-34 years, 21 cases 30-39 years, 12 cases 40 years old and older (16 sheets typed tabulation). – Memoranda regarding blood pressure reading of 35, 24 and 49 prenatal cases under 20 years of age (typewritten, partly in multiple copies, together 45 ff.). – Postnatal blood pressure (2 and 6 handwritten ff.). – Comparative prenatal and postnatal pressure, revised tabulation, May 1, 1922 (typewritten, 5 ff.).   *[ZZ 10a/4]*

988. **Steiner, Paul Eby,** b. 1902. Medical history of a Civil War regiment. *Philadelphia?, 197—.*

2 bundles. 28 cm. Material consists of largely handwritten preliminary matter, chapters I-III, V-VI and carbon copy of the entire text (283, [6] ff.). Fragmentary correspondence in folder. Published in Clayton, Miss., 1977.   *[n.c.]*

989. **Stengel, Alfred,** 1868-1939. Lectures on clinical medicine. *Philadelphia, 1907-08.*

[26] ff. 22 cm. Notes taken by E.B. Krumbhaar at the Univ. of Penna.
                                                                              [10a/424]

990. — — — —. Notes on the clinical lectures of Dr. Alfred Stengel and Dr. John Herr Musser, taken by Robert H. Ivy. *Philadelphia, 1906-07.*

75, 45, 71 pp. 21-28 cm. With explanatory note and typescript copy of notes by Ivy, with list of contents. – Presented by R.H. Ivy.   *[10a/401]*

— — — —. See also nos. *185.13*, 356, 756.

991. **Steward, Clayton Milton,** b. 1911. S. Weir Mitchell, another Philadelphia genius? *Saranac Lake, N.Y., 1960.*

[1], 19, [1] ff. 28 cm. Typewritten (carbon copy). Author's presentation inscription on title-page. Presented before the Osler Club, Saranac Lake Medical Society, February 3, 1960.   *[10c/132]*

992. **Stillé, Alfred,** 1813-1900. Farewell address to his medical classes at the University of Pennsylvania, delivered April 10th, 1884. *Philadelphia, 1884.*

Title, [42] ff. 26 cm. Autograph. Published in *Medical News*, v. 44 (1884). Presented by I. Minis Hays.   *[10a/113]*

93. — — — — —. Lectures. *Philadelphia, 1868.*

315 pp. 31 cm (in folder). All except the last lecture autograph. Contents: 1. Rheumatic paraplegia (9 pp.). − 2. Diseases of the nervous system (152 pp.). − 3. Myelitis, etc. (19 pp.). − 4. Erysipelas, etc. (13 pp.). − 5. Chronic pneumonia, etc. (12 pp.). − 6. Vampoid-clubbed fingers, etc. (8 pp.). − 7. Signs of tuberculosis of the lungs (8 pp.). − [7bis]. Phthysis (2 pp.). − 8. Clinical umbilical hernia, etc. (10 pp.). − 9. Action of iodide potassium, etc. (16 pp.). − 10. Rheumatism of the walls of the chest, etc. (6 pp.). − 11. Chorea (17 pp.). − 12. Theory and practice of medicine; diseases of the blood (28 pp.). − 13. Spinal affections, etc., in shorthand signed [Jacob Mendez] Da Costa. Practice report... under the direction of A.H. Smith, 1866-1867 laid in.   *[Z 10/137]*

94. — — — — —. Notes from lectures. Vol. IV [of Theory and practice of medicine], sessions 1872-73-73/74, taken by J.M. Keating. *Philadelphia, 1872-74.*

1 v. ([1] f., 156 pp., [1] f.). 21 cm. Table of contents, pp. 153 to end. Main topics of this volume: cardiology and neurology. Front cover missing. − Gift of Mark Willcox, Jr. − Cf. no. 997.   *[n.c.]*

95. — — — — —. Notes on therapeutics. *Philadelphia, 1854?-91.*

5 v. 27 cm. Bibliographic references on therapeutics entered in various commercially-published commonplace books. − Presented by the author.   *[10a/149]*

96. — — — — —. Pathological (clinical, historical, biographical, etc.) index. *Philadelphia, 1855-90?*

4 v. 26.5 cm. Index to journals, monographs and pamphlets as listed on prel. ff. of v. 1. Alphabetical listing of all subjects on pp. [vii]-xxxi of v. 4. Entered in commercial commonplace books, publ. by Carlton & Porter in New York. − Presented by the author.   *[10a/150]*

97. — — — — —. Practice of medicine (vol. II of Theory and practice of medicine). *Philadelphia, ca. 1880.*

1 v. (pp. 203-376, [1] f.). 31 cm. Hectographed. Presented by J.K. Mitchell.   *[Z 10/9]*

98. — — — — —. Truth in medicine and truth in life inseparable. *Philadelphia, 1885.*

8 pp. 35.5 cm. Presented by Edward H. Goodman.   *[Z 10a/13]*

— — — — —. See also nos. 37, 44, 114, *185.13*, 225, 253, 346, 589, 623, 679, 1037.

999.   **Stoddart, Gideon.** Apis mellifica; an essay on the common honey bee. *Rydal, Pa., ca. 1910?*

26, [1] ff. 23 cm (envelope, 31 cm). [10c/136]

1000.   **Stöhr, Philipp,** 1849-1911. Diagrams of the nervous system. *Würzburg, 1887.*

12 ff.; 50 (mostly colored) illus. 23 cm (envelope, 26.5 cm). Numbers and outlines hectographed; descriptions and details of illus. entered by unnamed English-speaking student. [10a/492]

1001.   **Stoerk, Oskar,** 1870-1926. Pathology; lecture notes on specimens. *Vienna, 1906.*

1 v. (book I); illus. 19 cm (envelope, 31 cm). Description of 256 specimens, those beginning with no. 157 under the heading pigmentation. Note taker not identified. [10a/466]

1002.   **Stokes, John Hinchman,** 1885-1961. The fundamentals of everyday dermatology; diagnosis and treatment. *Philadelphia, 1931.*

3 envelopes (133, [4] ff.). 27 cm. Mimeographed. Fourth revision of the guide distributed to students of the Univ. of Penna. Medical School, keyed to Stokes' *Modern Clinical Syphilology.* [10d/34c]

1003.   **Strahan, John,** 1852-1896. The diagnosis and treatment of extra-uterine pregnancy. *Philadelphia, 1889.*

6, [118] ff. 35 cm. Awarded the William F. Jenks Memorial Prize of the College of Physicians of Philadelphia, 1889. Published in *Trans. & Stud.,* ser. 3, v. 11 (1889), and separately (Philadelphia, Blakiston, 1889) with table of contents, index, bibliography. Manuscript has index and pencilled notes keyed to published version. — Fragile. [10a/307]

1004.   **Strictures on the doctrine of diseases** taught at present by B. Rush. *Philadelphia?, after 1798.*

27 ff. 20 cm. Criticism of Rush's theory of disease and other specifics of practice by unidentified author. [10a/110]

1005.   **Sturgis, Katharine Rosenbaum Guest Boucot,** b. 1903. Correspondence, awards, diplomas, photographs, etc. *V.p., 1953-73.*

5 boxes. 30-53 cm. Partly material used for an exhibit at the College of Physicians of Philadelphia, honoring Dr. Sturgis (1972). Gift of Dr. Sturgis. [Z 10c/32]

— — — — —. See also nos. 184, *185.13.*

006.   **Sturgis, Margaret Castex,** 1885-1962.   Accounts with patients. *Philadelphia and Ardmore, 1940-47.*

    2 v.   20.5 cm.   Presented by Samuel Booth Sturgis.   *[Z 10c/31]*

    — — — — —.   See also no. 1008.

007.   **Sturgis, Samuel Booth,** b. 1891, donor.   Collection of death certificates, signed by early Philadelphia physicians. *Philadelphia, 1806-15.*

    29 pieces.   Various sizes.   Presented to S.B. Sturgis by Douglas Macfarland, and then to the College of Physicians of Philadelphia.   *[10c/125]*

008.   — — — — —.   Papers.   *V.p., 1917-19.*

    3 v. (loose-leaf).   28 cm.   Manuscript and typewritten.   Letters, photographs, orders, clippings, pamphlets, and other memorabilia of his service in U.S. Army Medical Reserve Corps in the U.S. and France during World War I.   Principal correspondents include Margaret Castex Sturgis (his wife) and Major John Wesley Long, MRC, USA.   Detailed inventory with the collection.
    — Gift of author.   *[ZZ 10a/21]*

009.   **Swan, John Mumford,** 1870-1949.   Case notes on etherizations, Presbyterian Hospital.   *Philadelphia, 1893-99.*

    1 v.   21 cm.   Notes on 119 operations performed.   *[10a/330]*

010.   — — — — —.   Case reports on a great variety of ailments observed at Philadelphia General Hospital and University Hospital.   *Philadelphia, 1890-93.*

    2 v.   23 × 15 and 21 cm.   Reports of 126 cases (with gaps) from 24 Sept. 1890 to 6 April 1893, attended to by at least 8 different doctors, but the largest number by Drs. William Pepper and James Tyson.   *[10a/337]*

011.   — — — — —.   Curriculum vitae.   Rochester, N.Y., 1941-42.

    11 ff.   28.5 cm (envelope, 30 cm).   Typescript.   Includes extensive bibliography, letter of transmittal and acknowledgment by W.B. McDaniel.   *[10d/84]*

012.   — — — — —.   Dominican Republic sanitary survey collection. *V.p., 1901-20.*

    3 boxes.   39 cm.   Materials gathered while Dr. Swan was Red Cross commissioner, including correspondence, transcripts of his observations, meteorological and demographic reports, photographs, financial records, health laws, maps, memorabilia, clippings, and material on Haiti, Puerto Rico and the Virgin Islands.   Partial table of contents filed with the manuscript.
                                             [Z 10/165]

1013.   —————. Lecture notes taken at the Department of Medicine of the University of Pennsylvania. *Philadelphia, 1892-93.*

[63] ff., incl. blank ff. (first f. torn out). 21 cm. Contents: Notes from the Pathological Laboratory of Henry Formad (ff. 2-17r). — Notes on the lectures on bacteriology . . . by Joseph McFarland and John Guitéras (ff. 17v-30r). — Ehrlich's Solution of the blood, etc. (ff. 31-2). — Notes on the demonstrations on morbid anatomy by H.W. Cattell (ff. 38v-51r). — Formulae (ff. 52v-5v). — Loosely added 7 ff.   *[10a/335]*

1014.   —————. Notes on gynaecological clinics held at the Philadelphia Hospital and the University Hospital. Notes on didactic gynaecology by B.C. Hirst. Diseases of children by J.P. Crozier (—Griffith). *Philadelphia, 1891-93.*

1 v. 21 cm. Notes on 44 cases from gynecological clinics of Drs. Edward P. Davis, William Goodell, and from Dr. J.P. Crozier-Griffith's clinic on diseases of children. Interspersed are notes on gynecology, apparently from the lectures of Dr. Hirst.   *[10a/328]*

1015.   **Taylor, John,** 1703-1772. Detail de la maladie singulière et du succés, que j'ai eu par ma manière de traiter la Freule de Nariskin . . . (transl.:) An exact description of the singular disorder and recovery of sight of the illustrious Lady Nariskin, of the imperial family of Russia. *London?, 1753 or 54? [photostat, ca. 1923-30].*

30 ff. 20 cm. Photostat facsimile of manuscript belonging to the Royal College of Surgeons of England, presented by Sir D'Arcy Power to Burton Chance, and by him to the College of Physicians of Philadelphia.   *[10a/287]*

1016.   **Taylor, John Madison,** 1855-1931. Collection of papers (lecture notes, drafts, correspondence), clippings, reprints, etc. *Philadelphia, etc., 1880-1930.*

6 boxes. 26 cm. Includes notes for, and drafts of, his published books, papers on convalescence, foods, chronic diseases, posture, aging, body shape, relaxation, nervousness, diet, citizenship, etc., largely typewritten. Parts are on fragile paper.   *[Z 10/136]*

—————. See also no. 697.

1017.   **Taylor, William Johnson,** 1861-1936. Correspondence. *V.p., 1887-1933.*

1 envelope. 37 cm. Contents: 1. Letters by Dr. Taylor. 2. Letters to Taylor in 3 parts: a. 10 letters, at least in part concerned with the College of Physicians of Philadelphia. — b. 18 letters primarily on medical topics (cancer of the uterus, prostatectomy, etc.) — c. 8 miscellaneous items.   *[n.c.]*

—————. See also no. *185.13.*

18. **Tendeloo, Nicholaas Philip,** b. 1864. General pathology (outline and explanations of his course). *Holland, 1927.*

8 numbered (and blank) ff. 22 cm. Manuscript with notes of E.B. Krumbhaar. [10c/89]

—————. See also nos. 507, 545.

19. **Thaw, Harry Kendall,** d. 1947. Testimony of Harry K. Thaw before the commission appointed to examine into the mental condition of the said Harry K. Thaw, beginning on Thursday, March 28, 1907, at 2 P.M. in the City of New York. *New York, 1907.*

pp. 30-226; 589-600. 27 cm. Typewritten. With this is bound Testimony of Harry K. Thaw at White Plains, N.Y., July 29, 30 and August 6, 1909 (365 pp.). [10d/141]

—————. See also no. 670.

20. **Thébault, Emmanuel Alexandre,** d. 1868. L'Examen des organes . . . du cadavre de François Jouenne . . . apporté à Avranches. *Avranches, 1847.*

1 blank f., 5, [1] pp. 26.5 cm (envelope, 30.5 cm). Autopsy conducted by Drs. Thébault and Auguste Bouret, and pharmacists Pierre Louis Pinel and Victor Porrée, finding arsenic poisoning. [10a/407]

21. **Thomas, Theodore Gaillard,** 1832-1903. Notes of Prof. Thomas' lectures on obstetrics, delivered at the College of Physicians and Surgeons, New York during the Winter of 1867-'68, by Frederick P. Henry. *New York, 1867-68.*

[84] pp. 21 cm. [10a/174]

22. **Thomson, Adam,** d. 1767. Discourse on the preparation of the body for the small-pox: and the manner of receiving the infection. As it was delivered at the public hall of the Academy, before the Trustees and others, on Wednesday, the 21st of November, 1750. *Philadelphia, Franklin & Hall, 1750; copied Washington, 1906.*

[2], 29, [2] ff. 28 cm. Typewritten copy of the original; presented by Henry Lee Smith. — Donor's handwritten biographical notes on title-page. [10d/15]

23. **Thomson, William,** 1833-1907. Case books. *Philadelphia, 1869-91.*

17 v. incl. 2 v. indexes. 21-33.5 cm. Extensive record of Dr. Thomson's practice of ophthalmology, 1869-71, 1873, 1875-84, 1887-91; with inserts. — Gift of Burton Chance. [10a/372]

1024.   — — — — —. Letters. *Philadelphia, 1875-99.*

> 9 pieces in envelope (30 cm). Autograph, typewritten and hectograph. Contents: 4 letters to "My dear kinsman," presumably Cornelius R. Agnew, on ophthalmologic matters, with family references (incl. 4 typewritten copies). Other correspondents include A.P.C. Ashhurst, W.W. Keen, and C.A. Oliver. — Presented by H.D. Barnshaw.   *[10b/59]*

1025.   **Thorington, James,** 1858-1944. Papers. *V.p., 1889-1941.*

> 1 box. 32 cm. Typescript and printed. Contents: Scrapbooks of clippings, advertisements, etc., relating to optometry bill before Pennsylvania Legislature, 1909, collected by Thorington (2 v.). — Album of photographs of patients before and after surgery on eye muscles, performed at Presbyterian Hospital, 1921-35. — Envelopes 1-2. Correspondence, incl. ophthalmologic examination records and related correspondence of Will Rogers and William H. Welch. — Env. 3. Typewritten letter to W.C. Gorgas, Canal Zone, XII-15-1910 (10 ff.), describing mortality and morbidity from yellow fever in the Canal Zone, July, 1882 to August, 1889 and two letters from Gorgas. — Env. 4. Documents concerning Thorington's election to Philadelphia County Medical Society, 1893; receipt for New Jersey licensure examination, 1893; notices of election to Faculty of Philadelphia Polyclinic (instructor, Oct. 19, 1893, adjunct professor, Nov. 29, 1895). — Printed notice of special post-graduate study week on muscular anomalies and squint, beginning Nov. 19th, 1894. — Gift of J. Monroe Thorington.   *[Z 10/164]*

— — — — —. See also no. 1137.

1026.   **Tilghman, William,** 1756-1827. Letters containing information respecting the life of Caspar Wistar, received by William Tilghman in 1818. *Philadelphia, 1818.*

> 1 v.; 2 ports. 30 cm. Presented by the heirs of Joseph Carson.   *[Z 10c/11]*

— — — — —. See also no. 112.

1027.   **Tissot, Samuel Auguste André David,** 1728-1797. Observationes practicae in Nosocomio ticinensi habitae auspice celeberrimo. *[Pavia? and] Venice, 1783?* (cf. p. 115)*-89.*

> 163 pp., [24] ff. (incl. some blank). 31.5 cm. Largely case histories with prescriptions. Main text ends on p. [164] with the explicit "Finem imposui Venetiis die 10 Juni anno 1789 ex labore[?] F.A. GVB." Several cases with names (of Tissot's assistants?) on margins, among them Giacomo Locatelli (p. 137) and Angelo Zulatti (p. 104). "Opinione del Sig^re Tissot e di Sig^re Borsieri" (pp. 163-64). "Remedies from Dr. Rowley's Female diseases" (ff. [18-24], in English). Writing faint in many places. — Bookplate of C. Percy La Roche, gift of Montgomery Harris.   *[Z 10/58]*

1028.   **Trenton Municipal Colony Hospitals.** Constitution and bylaws, minutes, reports, etc. *Trenton, N.J., 1915-54.*

1 envelope. 28.5 cm. Constitution, by-laws, and incomplete run of minutes (1915-34; 1954) of the medical board and staff of the hospitals (established 1910), incl. reports, staff assignments, and hospital pamphlets. The hospitals were renamed F.W. Donnelly Memorial Hospitals, ca. 1935.   *[10c/84]*

029. **Tri-County Medical Society** (Chester, Delaware, and Montgomery Counties, Pa.). Minutes, Oct. 14, 1919 to June 23, 1942. Incl. other papers, lists, etc. *V.p., 1919-42.*

2 v. (loose-leaf), 1 envelope. 29-37.5 cm. Typewritten. Presented by Horace Darlington, through Dorothy I. Lansing, 1970. Added: photocopy of Dr. Lansing's article on the society, in *Chester County Medicine*, v. 7, no. 8 (Oct., 1970).   *[Z 10a/12]*

030. **Trousseau, Armand,** 1801-1867. Article aphasie, de ma seconde edition, consacré à l'étude de l'intelligence chez les aphaseges. *Paris, 1864.*

[1], 22 ff. 27 cm. Addressed to "mon cher Edouard"; originally joined with an autograph of the Duc de Noailles (leaf [1]). With additions, deletions and corrections.   *[n.c.]*

031. **Trudeau, Edward Livingston,** 1848-1915. History of the tuberculosis work at Saranac Lake. *Saranac Lake, N.Y., 1903.*

32 pp. 26.5 cm. Typewritten, with ms. corrections. Published, with illustrations, in the *Annual Report of the Henry Phipps Institute*, v. 1: 121-40 (1903).   *[10d/13]*

032. **Tryon, James Rufus,** 1837-1912. Manuscript notes on lectures by Joseph Carson, Hugh L. Hodge, Samuel Jackson, Joseph Leidy, Robert E. Rogers and George B. Wood. *Philadelphia, ca. 1859.*

1 v. 24 cm.   *[10a/364]*

033. **[Typhus].** Of Typhus, etc. *N.p., ca. 1800.*

[10, 6, 4, 8, 8] ff. 17 cm. Fragmentary, except for the item on typhus; the rest deals with venereal diseases, the last 3 items numbered 17, 133, 149.   *[n.c.]*

034. **Tyson, James,** 1841-1919. Addresses, papers, reports, etc. *Philadelphia, 1898-1914.*

1 box (26 folders). 32 cm. Contains brief autobiography (no. 21; 8 ff.); eulogy of J.A. Packard (no. 3; 3 ff.); preparations for the complimentary dinner for William Osler (nos. 4-5; 6 ff.); College of Physicians of Philadelphia (nos. 10-11, 16; 25 ff.); Dept. of Medicine, Univ. of Penna. (nos. 7, 13, 15, 26; 31 ff.); black physicians and the black community, cf. Frederick Douglas Memorial Hospital and Training School (no. 14; 2 ff.); uric acid (no. 2; 24 ff.); inflammation of the gall bladder (no. 23; 10 ff.); Niemeyer's pill (no. 19; 2 ff.); general practitioners (no. 1; 24 ff.); training of nurses (no. 8; 13 ff.), and a few miscellaneous items.   *[10c/30]*

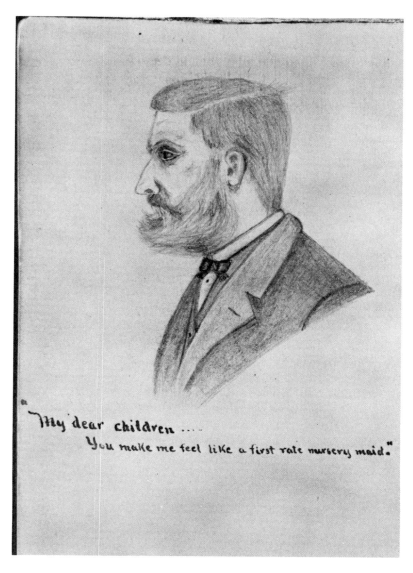

"*My dear children* ....
You make me feel like a first rate nursery maid."

Plate 7. 1038. Sketch of James Tyson from the student notes of Joseph McFarland,1888.

1035.   —————. Notes on lectures on pathology by J. Tyson and H.F.
Formad. *Philadelphia, 1885.*

> 1 v. 23 cm. Notes taken by Thompson Seiser Westcott, 3rd-year student,
> Dept. of Medicine, Univ. of Penna. Beginning in reverse William Pepper's
> lectures, October-Nov. 1885, with occasional assistance from others. Large
> part of these lectures crossed out.   *[10a/445]*

1036.   —————. Papers. *V.p., 1889-1915.*

> 1 box. 26.5 cm. Correspondence, incl. letters from relatives with general
> information; folder with material on genealogy of the Tyson family; letters,
> etc., relating to the Rush Hospital for Consumption; handwritten and typed
> addresses (incl. presidential address, College of Physicians of Philadelphia,
> 1908, and one to the Berks Co. Medical Society), testimonials, paper on
> diabetes mellitus, etc.; clippings.   *[10c/44]*

1037.   —————. Pathology (107 pp., [1] f.). — H.F. Formad. Bill of
fare (4 ff.). — D.H. Agnew. Surgery (222 pp., [1] f.). — A.
Stillé. Theory and practice of medicine (v. 2, 376 pp., [1]
f.). *Philadelphia, ca. 1883.*

> 2 v. 30.5 cm. Hectographed, with handwritten additions (e.g. Formad) and
> corrections, presumably by J.C. Mewhinney (Class of '83, Univ. of Penna.). —
> Property stamp of Dr. Mewhinney; gift of William Pepper and E.B. Krumbhaar.
>   *[Z 10/97]*

1038.   —————. Pathology; lecture notes taken by Joseph McFarland.
Philadelphia, 1888-89.

> 1 v.; illus. 23 cm. Forty-seven numbered lectures, dated Oct. 1888-April
> 1889. 5 pp., listing demonstrations, Nov.-Dec. 1888, at end of volume. —
> Pencil sketch of Tyson (professor of clinical medicine, Univ. of Penna.) at front
> of volume.   *[10a/353]*

1039.   —————. Review of the progress of medicine during the last
half century. *Philadelphia, 1912.*

> 60 ff. 28 cm. Typewritten, with ms. corrections. Published, with additions,
> in *Pennsylvania Med. Jour.* v. 16: [1]-24 (1912-13) under title "President's
> Address: Review of the Progress. . . ." Delivered at the meeting of the Medical
> Society of the State of Pennsylvania, September 24, 1912.   *[10d/10]*

—————. See also nos. 43, *185.13*, 589, 710, 1010, 1080, 1082.

1040.   **United States. Army. General Hospital. B.E.F. France. Pathological Laboratory 16, Philadelphia.** Post-mortem and surgical pathology, May 1917-Feb. 1919, compiled by E.B. Krumbhaar.
V.p., 1917-19.

> 2 v. 32 cm. In several hands, but largely Dr. Krumbhaar's.   *[Z 10/197]*

1041.   —————.   —————.   **General Hospital, Philadelphia.** Ward
C. Medical case book, kept by H.M. Bellows. *Philadelphia,
1863-64.*

> 32 (and blank) ff. 34 cm. Cover title: U.S.A. Medical Department. Blank
> book.   *[Z 10/233]*

1042.   —————.   —————.   **Medical Department.** Morning report
of the sick and wounded, various regiments, 1st Army Corps,
March 1, 2, 28-May 4, 1865, and U.S. 6th Veteran Volunteers,
June 1, 1865-March 30, 1866. *Washington, D.C. and Harrisburg,
Pa., 1865-66.*

> 1 v. 46 cm. Printed report forms filled in by hand, showing statistical
> summaries according to company, of those reporting sick, etc. Entries for 1st
> regiment, 1st Army Corps, Camp Stoneman, D.C., 3d-7th regiment, and 6th
> regiment U.S. Veteran Volunteers, Camp Stoneman, D.C., Harrisburg, Pa.
> (Camp Return), Capitol Hill, D.C., Camp Fry Barracks, Washington, D.C. Week-
> ly summaries interspersed; "Remarks" column contains brief miscellaneous
> notes. — Reports signed by A. Wm. McDowell (whose bookplate is inside front
> cover) as surgeon, 6th Vet. Volunteers, D.C., Lloyd, ass't. surg., and Geo. Upton,
> also ass't. surg.   *[Z 10/11]*

—————. See also nos. 456, 593, 1041.

1043.   —————.   —————.   **Medical Field Service School.** Administrative and training papers, incl. insect pest control, map
reading, etc. *Carlisle Barracks, Pa., 1942.*

> 1 box. 39 cm. Mimeographed, with marginalia and notes by Dr. S. X
> Radbill.   *[Z 10/184]*

—————. See also no. 1046.

1044.   —————.   —————.   **Station Hospital, Fort Crockett, Texas.**
Hospital regulations; boards of officers; professional standing
orders; miscellaneous papers. *Fort Crockett, Texas, 1941-45.*

> 1 box. 39 cm. Mimeographed, carbon copies, and manuscript notes by S. X
> Radbill.   *[Z 10/182]*

1045.   ———— —————.   **Surgeon General's Office.** List of medical cadets who obtained rank of assistant sugeon and surgeon of
volunteer regiments, &c. during the Civil War, with the ranks
and the names of their regiments. *Washington, ca. 1910?*

> [i, 1], 4, [9] ff. 33 cm. Typewritten. Apparently unpublished. Incl. 1 p. on
> confederate losses in the Civil War; and 9 ff. containing alphabetical "List of
> medical cadets in service during the War of the Rebellion," with dates of
> enlistment and discharge. The two lists are not identical. — Gift of S. Weir
> Mitchell.   *[Z 10a/8]*

046. ———— ————. **Surgeon General's Office. Army Service Forces.** Circular letters, nos. 8-252 (incomplete), administrative papers, course outline, disease control, etc., some (or all)
issued for and by the Medical Field Service School. *Carlisle
Barracks, Pa., 1941-45.*

> 1 box. 39 cm. Mimeographed and carbon copies; with notes by Dr. S. X
> Radbill.   *[Z 10/183]*

————. See also nos. 91, 178.

047. ————. **Public Health Service.** Reports, records, certificates,
bills and packing lists. *Philadelphia, etc., 1864-1934.*

> 1 box (12 folders, 1 envelope). 39 cm. Mainly covering the years 1877-
> 82. Includes monthly reports from Pennsylvania Hospital and Jefferson
> Medical College Hospital.   *[10a/406]*

048. **University of Pennsylvania.** [Authorization] To all charitable
persons, patrons of literature and friends of useful knowledge
the trustees of the College, Academy and Charitable School of
Philadelphia . . . given to John Morgan, to solicit funds in the
West India Islands. *Philadelphia, 1772.*

> 1 f. (vellum). 57 × 44 cm. With seal. Signed by James Hamilton, president
> of the trustees, and countersigned by Joseph Shippen, Jr., secretary to Richard
> Penn, governor of Pennsylvania.   *[n.c.]*

049. ———— **Department (School) of Medicine.** Collection of
lectures on various medical topics. *Philadelphia, last quarter 18th
cent.?*

> 1 v. 24.5 cm. No t.-p., but with pencilled table of contents in a hand different
> from the uniform hand used in the text. Contents: 1. Lectures on physiology,
> icplt. at beginning, ending with lecture 41 (331 pp.); probably transcription of
> the lectures of William Shippen, since occasional passages correspond word
> for word with his lectures as transcribed by Wm. McWilliam in 1777. —
> 2. Lectures on midwifery (59 pp.); pp. 357-61 at end may be continuation of
> no. 1. — 3. Lectures on materia medica by Adam Kuhn (157 pp.). —
> 4. Lectures on physiology by John Morgan (65 pp.). — 5. Lectures on the
> practice of physic by John Morgan (78 ff.). — 6. Introduction to natural
> philosophy, Dec. 27, 1769 (60 pp.); concerned chiefly with matter, motion and
> mechanics.   *[10a/92]*

050. ———— ————. Correspondence and lists concerning the
dedication of the new medical laboratories, 1904. *Philadelphia,
1903-04.*

> Table of contents (typed, 1 f.), 6 hectographed, 14 typewritten ff. (several with
> signatures or handwritten annotations). 38 cm (envelope). Concerns the

Entertainment Committee (John K. Mitchell, chairman) and the Invitation Committee (George E. de Schweinitz, chairman); with lists of acceptances (e.g. John S. Billings, Sir William Osler) and declinations. [n.c.]

1051. ―――― ――――. **Committee on Bacteriology.** Correspondence, documents, memoranda and minutes relating to the selection of a head of the Department of Bacteriology. *V.p., 1930-31.*

1 folder. 30 cm. Dr. E.B. Krumbhaar, chairman of the committee. Includes bibliography of some candidates (Stuart Mudd, K.E. Birkhaug, E.E. Ecker, Lloyd Felton, H.K. Ward [partial], Charles Weiss). [n.c.]

1052. ―――― ――――. **Department of Anatomy.** Accounts of the anatomical chair, Oct. 1, 1839 to Feb. 1, 1853 in the handwriting of Wm. E. Horner, professor of anatomy. *Philadelphia, 1839-53.*

1 v. 20 cm. Some pencilled entries in another hand continue the accounts to June 6, 1853. − Presented by O.V. Batson. [10c/112]

1053. ―――― ――――. **Department of Pathology.** General pathological histology; demonstrations to second year students, first term. Technique of preparation of tissues for microscopic examination. Experimental (pathology). *Philadelphia, 193—?*

41, 30 ff.; illus. 28 cm. Mimeographed, with E.B. Krumbhaar's pencilled notes and drawings on the verso of some leaves. At head of title of *Experimental pathology*: Part III[?]. [ZZ Ai/12]

1054. ―――― ――――. **Laboratory of Dermatological Research.** Guest register. *Philadelphia, 1937-52.*

1 v. 14 × 19 cm (oblong). Business cards and notes laid in. − Presented by Walter B. Shelley. [10c/62]

――――. See also nos. 20, 45, 70, 101, 110, 114, 116, 122, 130, *185.14*, *.614*, 204, 240, 260, 262, 279, 293, 309, 319, 329, 357, 403, 409, 412, 414, 438, 441, 459, 463, 485, 496, 519-20, 526, 537-8, 554, 585, 587-8, 702, 709-10, 717, 726-7, 733, 771, 779, 781, 816, 819, 823, 834, 846-7, 856-8, 862-3, 881, 891, 930, 943-4, 951, 955, 957, 965-7, 989-90, 992, 1002, 1032, 1034, 1037, 1059, 1063, 1072, 1083, 1085, 1100-2, 1104-5, 1112-4, 1120, 1134-6.

1055. **Van Leer, Ella Wall,** comp. Van Leer genealogy; compilation of genealogical and historical information on the Van Leer (von Lohr) families. *Gainesville, Fla., 1937.*

75 ff. 28 cm. Photocopied from typewritten copy; original at the Chester County Historical Society. Pages 51-52 not consecutive. [10c/109]

1056. **Venditio facta [in] Nomine Ducalis Camerae,** dominus Petro Martini et Francisco, filliis . . . domini Martini Zanardi de Placentia (sales document concerning property [vineyards?, etc.] "in loco Altanelli"; notarized by Joannis Antonius de Taegio). *Milan?, 13 January, 1497.*

Vellum document, measuring ca. 92 × 34 cm., 2 sheets sewn together. Decorated initial I on upper left, intricate composite letter S, L?, M?, V in upper center; notarial signet. Few holes. In gilt, decorated red leather folder with the arms of Pope Pius IX. Mention of Prince Ludovicus Maria Sfortia (Sforza), on lines 4-5, identifies the camera ducalis (Milan). − Letter of transmittal from S (or T) Kirby to a Mrs. Reynolds, Rome, 1879 laid in.   *[n.c.]*

1057. **Venice. Magistrato di Sanità.** Documents relating to remedies (secreti) produced and distributed by Giuseppe Maria Felice Scutellio and his successors, under the authority of the Magistrato and the Collegio dei Medici Fisici. *Venice, 1703-69.*

1 v. ([12] ff.). 38.5 cm. Manuscript on vellum, illuminated. Contents: Lettera . . . all' ill.^mo et ecc.^mo sig.^r podestà, e capitanio in Treviso (concerning "dodeci vasi . . . di balsamo . . . del Cauag.^r Scutellio), 1706 (2 ff.). − Approval and renewal of the 1703 permission granted by the Collegio dei Medici "nelli figlii dell' auttore [Scutellio]" and their associate Antonio Cimolin, 1720 (2 ff.). − Renewal granted to Cimolin, 1769 (2 ff., 2nd blank). − Patent for 4 "balsami", 3 "polveri", "vino medicato" and an "empiastro" by the Magistrato di Sanità, 1703 (6 ff.). − Gift of E.B. Hodge, Jr.   *[Z 10/43]*

1058. **[Volkmann, Richard von, 1830-1889].** Twenty-eight letters to, and one letter by, R. von Volkmann. *V.p., 1867-89.*

1 envelope. 37.5 cm. The collection is accompanied by the following items (typewritten, both originals and carbons): F.T. Callomon's Statement on the collection (2 × 4 ff.); English translations of letters (2 × 34 ff.); Commentary (2 × 12 ff.) − Most letters were published in *Janus*, v. 43, 45 (1939, 1941); Dr. Callomon lists the 10 letters not included in Janus. Alphabetical list of correspondents attached. The letter by Volkmann deals with cancer and is draft of a letter to H.T. Butlin.   *[n.c.]*

1059. **Wadsworth, William Scott,** 1868-1955, comp. Scrapbooks. *Philadelphia, 1898?-1948?*

24 v.; illus. (incl. portraits). 25.5-35.5 cm. Vols. 1-13, 17-18, 23, portraits, illustrations, and other printed materials. − Vols. 14-16, 19-22 deal with Alpha Mu Pi Omega Fraternity, Univ. of Penna. chapter; Medical Jurisprudence Society of Philadelphia; Aesculapian Club of Philadelphia; Medical Club of Philadelphia; Univ. of Penna. Department of Medicine, Historical Club. − Gift of the compiler.   *[Z 10/223]*

1060. **Wagner, Frederick Balthas,** b. 1916. The founding fathers and centennial history of the Philadelphia Academy of Surgery. *Philadelphia, 1979.*

21 ff.   28 cm.   At head of title: Annual oration for 1979.   Mimeographed in few copies with signed author's note "this manuscript is unfinished" (p. 21).   *[n.c.]*

1061.   **Waldschmidt, Johann Jakob,** 1644-1689.   Institutiones medicinae ad mentem recentiorum et imprimis Joh. Jacob Waldschmit[!] . . . accomodatae (223 pp.). — *With* Albinus, Bernard. Collegium theoretico-practico medicum, sive Explicatio morborum ac eorum causarum, quibus adjecta est earum cura juxta mentem . . . Doctoris Bernhardi Albini . . . 1688, ex Ethmullero expromptum fuit thema, *inc.:* Praxis secundum Ethmullerum, est vel volgaris ordinaria, vel extraordinaria (155, 252 pp.). — Chirurgia medica, *inc.:* Chirurgia duplex est . . . (two parts: Chirurgia medica, 38 pp.; Chirurgiae manuales operationes, 54 pp.). — [Loosely inserted:] Vehr, Irenaeus.   Excerpta ex publicis lectionibus D. Doct. Vehr . . . De simptomatibus parturientium et puerpuerarum, *inc.:* Ubi foetus nosdum . . . (4 ff., last blank).   *Germany, end of 17th cent.*

1 v. (contemp. pagination, with errors).   20 cm.   Ad Waldschmidt: Compiler unnamed.   Divided into 4 parts, the first without heading; 2.   Pars pathologica; 3.   Pars semiotica; 4.   Hygieina.   Incl. references to chemists (e.g. Boyle), philosophers (Descartes) as well as to many medical authorities (from Galen to Ettmüller).   Addenda on pp. 219-20, Observatio facta Bredae . . . 1691 (pp. 221-24). — Pencilled on the title of Albinus, the Collegium Francof. ad Viadr (Frankfurt a.d. Oder) where Albinus taught.   Separate indexes for each part (pp. 153 and 249-52). — Two indexes for the Chirurgia (pp. 37-8 and 53-4); Annotata in paracentesin (1 f.) inserted between pp. 26-7.   Some corrections throughout.   Few inserts. — "Presented by Sam.[l] Betton M.D. to Joseph Hartshorne" on 2nd prel. f.   Gift of Edward Hartshorne.   *[10a/114]*

1062.   **Wallace, Ellerslie,** 1819-1885.   Women and children from Wallace.   *Philadelphia, 1876-77.*

Title page, 60 pp., [2 blank] ff.   27 cm.   Lectures on obstetrics at Jefferson Medical College; scribe not identified. — Presented by Charles Rosenberg.
                                                                                    [10a/491]

1063.   **Walsh, Joseph Patrick,** 1870-1946.   Papers, incl. correspondence, reports, memorabilia, printed items, photographs, etc.*V.p., 1895-1940.*

16 v., 2 boxes; illus.   31 cm.   Contents: v. 1.   White Haven Sanatorium, 1905-11, incl. minutes, reports, financial statements. — v. 2.   Phipps Institute, 1905-10, incl. bills, reports, financial statements. — v. 3.   National Association for the Study and Prevention of Tuberculosis, 1904-12, incl. minutes and nominations. — v. 4.   Fifth to Ninth International Conferences on Tuberculosis, 1906-10, and International Congress on Hygiene and Demography, 1912; largely printed items and photographs. — v. 5.   International Congress on Tuberculosis, Washington, D.C., 1908; largely minutes and correspondence of

the Committee on Arrangements. — v.6. Laënec Society, 1926–40, incl. membership lists, meeting of TB specialists, lecture notes, etc. — v. 7-9. Material relating to Dr. Walsh as captain, U.S. Medical Corps, 1918-19, enlistment, activity of General Hospital no. 17, Markleton, Pa., statistics, etc. — v. 10-11. Trips to Europe and the Near East, 1896-1924, incl. various reports on areas visited, photographs, bills, etc. — v. 12. 40th reunion of the medical class, Univ. of Penna., '95. — v. 13. Largely personalia, incl. bibliography, also biographical accounts of various personalities, among them Sister Mary Borromeo of St. Agnes Hospital of Philadelphia, Drs. Henry M. Fisher, S. Weir Mitchell, and Lawrence F. Flick. — V. 14-16 and Boxes 1-2. Photographs, photostats, illustrations, slides, and papers on Galen.   [Z 10/185]

————. See also nos. 324-5, 451, 519.

1064.   **Walton, Juliet Coates.** Book of notions. *Philadelphia, 1848-66.*

64 ff. 20 cm. Miscellany of recipes, remedies, household hints, prayers, etc. With clippings and some inserts.   [n.c.]

1065.   **Wang, Ch'i,** fl. ca. 1760, ed. [Ta Sheng Pien]. The Tat Shang Pin, or midwifery made easy, a translation ... by John G. Kerr ... *Canton, China, 187—?*

[2], 44 ff. 21 cm. "For the Am. Journal of Med. Sci." at head of title. Published in the *Annals of Gynaecology and Paediatry*, v. 7: 326-33 (1893/94). John G. Kerr (M.D. Jefferson 1847), medical missionary in China from 1854 until his death, translated many medical works into Chinese, opened one of the first insane asylums, etc. The Ta Sheng Pien was translated into English a number of times, under a variety of titles (Ta Sheng P'ien and Ta Sheng Pieng, etc.), among these in the *Dublin Journal of Medical Science*, v. 20: 332-69 (1842) and in *Annals of Medical History*, v. 5: 95-9 (1923). — Entry and title courtesy of G.C.C. Chang (East Asia Coll., Univ. of Penna.).   [10a/509]

1066.   ———— ————, transcribed by Robert P. Harris ... *Philadelphia, 1881.*

111 pp.; illus. 12.5 cm. Copied for the Samuel Lewis Library. The medical ideas of the Chinese (pp. 108-11) and Chinese ideal anatomy by R.P. Harris added at end of volume.   [(L)C3]

1067.   **Warthin, Aldred Scott,** 1866-1931. On the occurrence of numerous large giant cells in the tonsils and pharyngeal mucosa in prodromal stage of measles. *Ann Arbor, 1931.*

[13 (and 1 half)] ff. 28 cm. Report of 4 cases, published in *Arch. Path.*, v. 11: 864-74 (1931). — Letter of transmittal, C.V. Weller to E.B. Krumbhaar, enclosed.   [n.c.]

1068.   **Watson, Douglas Chalmers,** 1870-1946. The importance of diet; an experimental study from a new standpoint, by "the Gleam." An unpublished essay submitted in competition for the Alvarenga Prize, College of Physicians. *Philadelphia, 1905.*

50 ff.; plates. 27.5 cm. Typewritten; captions for plates handwritten. — Pasted on flyleaf letter (1905, Nov. 23) to C.P. Fisher, from T.R. Neilson, secretary, depositing this manuscript which won the Alvarenga Prize.

[10a/53]

1069.   **Waugh, William Francis,** 1849-1918. Practice of medicine; notes on lectures delivered at the Medico-Chirurgical College ... *Philadelphia, 1888-89.*

128 pp. 25.5 cm. Incomplete; p. 128 ends in midsentence. Note-taker unidentified.   *[10a/240]*

— — — — —. See also nos. 649, 651.

1070.   **Webb, Reynold,** 1791-1856. Day book, commenced August 24, 1829. *Madison, Conn., 1829-35.*

1 v. ([3], 178, [2] ff.). 31 cm. Name on flyleaf. Webb's personal expenses, 1830-35, at end. — Gift of Charles E. Rosenberg.   *[Z 10a/15]*

1071.   **Weick, John Michael,** 1803-1880. Papers. *V.p., 1823-79.*

1 v. (loose-leaf). 35.5 cm. Manuscript with typewritten translations, commentaries, etc. Includes photograph of Weick family genealogy, baptismal certificate (Rhodt, Bavaria), letters from teachers certifying attendance of various courses; diploma (M.D.) Heidelberg, 1823; semester-certificates of professors and diploma from Royal Surgical School at Bamberg, 1825-28; Vereins-Diploma, Hydropathischer Gesundheits-Verein, 1835(?); certificate of competence in hydropathy from Prof. Dr. Oertel of Ansbach, June 27, 1836; citizenship paper, Philadelphia, 1855; will, November 20, 1879, Philadelphia; transcript of biographical notice in Cleave, 1873, and photocopy of obituary from *Hahnemannian Monthly,* Apr. 1880. Weick came to Philadelphia ca. 1846 to study homeopathy, settling in Clinton County, Iowa, and returning to Philadelphia where he practiced most of his remaining life. — Gift of Clara Ethel Potts.   *[Z 10/238]*

1072.   **Weidman (Wiedenman), Frederick De Forest,** 1881-1956. Notes on physiological chemistry and materia medica (v. 1) and diseases (v. 2); lectures at the University of Pennsylvania. *Philadelphia, 1905-06.*

2 v. 26 cm. Printed sheets on urine tests, tipped in at end of v. 1.   *[10a/467]*

1073.   — — — — —. Student notebooks. *Philadelphia, ca. 1900-08.*

5 v.; illus. 20-23 cm. Contents: v. 1. American history, 1760-ca. 1865. — v. 2. Physics. — v. 3. Bacteriology. — v. 4. Zoology no. 2 — Botany (with label F.D. Wiedenman on cover). — v. 5. Histology. — Family photograph laid in v. 1.   *[10a/488]*

1074.   **Wenrich, David Henry,** 1885-1968, comp. Leidy material deposited at the College of Physicians of Philadelphia. List of letters and other documents relating to ... Joseph Leidy (1133 items). — Correspondence and notes of Dr. Joseph Leidy II concerning biographical material (deposited *ibid.*; 53 items). — Miscellaneous biographical items (38). *Philadelphia, n.d.*

[5, incl. 1 blank], 42, [7, incl. 1 blank] ff.   30.5 cm.   *[Z 10/207]*

1075. **West Philadelphia Medical Society.** Constitution, by-laws, and members' signatures to June 7, 1888. *Philadelphia, 1881-88.*

[17] pp.   21.5 cm.   Contains amendments, with references to corresponding entries in the society's Minute-book. — In the handwriting of the society's secretaries, James Hendrie Lloyd and Guy Hinsdale.   *[10a/140]*

1076. —————. Minutes, April 1, 1881 to June 10, 1890. *Philadelphia, 1881-90.*

101 pp.   27 cm.   In the handwriting of the Society's secretaries.   Deposited by Guy Hinsdale.   *[10a/141]*

1077. **Westcott, Thompson Seiser,** 1862-1933. Abstract of a memoir of Louis Starr, . . . read before the College of Physicians. *Philadelphia, 1926.*

7 ff.   33 cm (in envelope).   Typewritten (carbon copy) with manuscript corrections.   More complete memoir appeared in *Trans. & Stud.*, ser. 3, v. 48: lxxi-lxxvi (1926). — Gift of Mrs. Westcott.   *[10d/35]*

1078. —————. A case of acetanilid poisoning in an infant. *Philadelphia, 1897.*

5 ff.   19 cm.   Fragile.   Presented by the author.   *[10a/244]*

1079. —————. Clinic notes from the University of Pennsylvania, the Almshouse, and the Children's Hospitals. *Philadelphia, 1885-86.*

146 pp.   21 cm.   Professors and instructors include William Osler, William F. Norris, William Goodell, H.W. Stelwagon, H.C. Wood, John Ashhurst, William Pepper, William L. Taylor, B.A. Randall, J. William White. — Gift of Mrs. Westcott.   *[10a/220]*

1080. —————. Notebooks of lectures, clinical cases and laboratory work. *Philadelphia, 1883-86.*

15 v. in 2 boxes; illus.   22 cm (boxed).   Notes entered beginning at end as well as in front of volumes.   Lectures by D.H. Agnew (vols. 3, 5, 14), Harrison Allen (1-2, 4-7, 9-10), John Ashhurst (10), H.F. Formad (3-4, 13-15), William Goodell (7, 9-12), Joseph Leidy (1), John Marshall (3-4), A.W. Miller (1), W.F. Norris (11), William Osler (11, 13, 15), A.F. Penrose (4, 7), William Pepper (3-10, 14-15), N.A. Randolph (1), Louis Starr (15), George Strawbridge (11), James Tyson (1, 3, 14-15), J.W. White (3), De Forrest Willard (11, 15), H.C. Wood (3, 6, 10, 13) and T.G. Wormley (3-9).   Lectures from the Department of Medicine

and Hospital of the University of Pennsylvania, the Almshouse and perhaps other Philadelphia hospitals. — Gift of Mrs. T.S. Westcott. *[10a/245]*

1081. — — — — —. A simple method of calculating the proportions of cream and whole milk required to make any percentage formula for home modification. *Philadelphia, 1897.*

[39] ff. 24 cm. Draft of paper read before Philadelphia Pediatric Society, October 12, 1897, and published in *Arch. Pediatrics*, v. 15: 21-28 (1898). Paper fragile. — Presented by the author. *[10a/295]*

1082. — — — — —. Volume containing notes from the lectures of James Tyson and Henry F. Formad, commencing with Oct. 2nd, 1885. *Philadelphia, 1885-86?*

1 v. 23 cm. Inscribed on page 1 T.S. Westcott, Medical Department, Univ. of Penna. *[10a/445]*

— — — — —. See also no. 1035.

1083. **[Whistler, William MacNeill,** 1836-1900]. Documents relating to W.M. Whistler. *V.p., 1867-94.*

1 envelope. 67 × 38 cm. Three diplomas: Royal College of Surgeons of England, 1871, Royal College of Surgeons, London, 1876, Société française d'otologie, de laryngologie et de rhinologie, 1893; one certificate from the Medical Dept. of the Univ. of Penna., 1869, and 3 printed biographical items (2 in photostat). *[Z 10c/39]*

1084. **White, Angela.** An index of obituaries published in the *Medical Register* of New York, New Jersey and Connecticut, 1862-95. *N.p., 1943.*

32 ff. 22 cm (oblong). Typewritten and photocopy. *[10d/85]*

1085. **White, James William,** 1850-1916. Notes on surgical lectures, incl. observation of cases, recorded by E.B. Krumbhaar. *Philadelphia, 1907-08.*

1 v. 24 × 13 cm. Includes brief notes on lectures by Maurice Ostheimer, and Barton C. Hirst. Ward schedule and class roster tipped in. *[10b/52]*

— — — — —. See also nos. 623, 1079-80.

1086. **Whitmer, Benjamin F.,** 1838-1914. Register and book of prescriptions. *Goshen, Ind., 1867-92.*

[5 prel.], 186 pp. (p. 103 repeated). 19 cm. Laid or pasted in stationery, professional cards of Whitmer, clippings of recipes and pharmaceutical order blank. Index, primarily of ailments, on prel. pages. Cover-title: Register and prescription book. *[10a/476]*

087. **Wills Eye Hospital,** Philadelphia. General rules and regulations for the management and supervision of the Wills Hospital for the indigent lame and blind. By-laws of the Board of Managers. Election of managers by the Philadelphia Common Council. *Philadelphia, 1833.*

6 ff. 32 cm.   [n.c.]

————. See also no. 730.

088. **Wilson, Frank Norman,** 1890-1952. Lectures on electrocardiography. *Ann Arbor?, 194—.*

7, 241 ff.; illus. 29 cm. Typescript. "Outline . . . written from notes taken during the course given by Dr. Frank N. Wilson . . . at the Univ. of Michigan . . ." (cf. Preface).   [10a/477]

089. **Wilson, James Cornelius,** 1847-1934. Revisions of the text of the fifth edition of N.P. Potter's and Wilson's *Internal Medicine* (Philadelphia, etc., 1919), in preparation of the sixth edition (*ibid.*, 1923). *Philadelphia, 1922?*

Several hundred ff., handwritten and carbon copies. Various sizes (ca. 17-28 cm, boxed). The revisions are mainly to volumes II-III, all by J.C. Wilson who was responsible for the 6th edition.   [n.c.]

————. See also no. *185.13.*

090. **Wistar, Caspar,** 1761-1818. Lecture notes. *Edinburgh, 1784-85.*

3 v. 24 cm. With additions and corrections; in a different hand? Contents: V. 1. Midwifery (lecture of William Lowder?). — v. 2. Chemistry, lectures of Joseph Black, 1784 (incl. primitive drawings). — v. 3. "Extracts from [James or John] Rae's lectures on the teeth," followed by "Anatomical observations by Dr. Monro, Nov. 10th, 1785," (195 pp., with additions on preceding pp. A-K[-L]; 1 p. "Anatomical observation by Mr. Cline" interspersed. V. 2-3 with index. "From Dr. Caspar Wistar's medical library, presented to the College of Physicians in the name of Dr. Mifflin Wistar."   [10a/115]

091. **[————].** Collection of Wistar related letters and documents, presented to the College of Physicians in 1897 by Wistar's daughter-in-law, Mrs. Mifflin Wistar. *V.p., 1786-1802[-1897].*

11 ff. Various sizes, in leather container, 41 cm. Contents: Letter from William Cullen on animal and vital functions, opium and blistering, with a postscript on Benjamin Franklin, dated Jan. 6, 1786. — Brief letter of transmittal, by Cullen, July 27, 1786. — Charles Stuart on Cullen's death, dated Jan. 27, 1790. — Document informing Wistar of his election to the Société de Medicine of Bordeaux, 30 fructidor, an 9 (1802), signed by the president (F.A. de Grassi and the secretary Capelle). — Diploma of membership, 25 fructidor,

an 9, signed by de Grassi and others. — Letter by de Grassi, incl. suggestion to acknowledge the receipt of the diploma, July 24, 1802. — Letter from H.M. Fisher to George C. Harlan, transmitting Mrs. Wistar's gift, May 14, 1897.

[Z 10/28]

— — — —. See also nos. 73, 114, 269, 445, 448, 693, 1026, 1127.

1092.   **Wistar, Caspar,** 1801-1867. Letters to Isaac Jones Wistar. *Philadelphia, 27 June 1837-20 Sept. 1846.*

32 letters. 25 cm. Letters from the father, and some from his mother, to their son at boarding school and with relatives (cf. I.J. Wistar's Autobiography, pp. 24-6; photocopy enclosed). — Presented by Mrs. Robert F. Norris.   *[10c/124]*

— — — —. See also no. 1112.

1093.   **Wolf, Joseph A.** Lecture admission cards, Pennsylvania College, Medical Department. *Philadelphia, 1844-45, 1847-48.*

16 cards in box, 14 × 10 cm. According to Abrahams, *Extinct Medical Schools...,* p. 106, Wolf graduated in 1848, after writing a thesis on typhus fever.   *[n.c.]*

1094.   **Wolff, Kaspar Friedrich,** 1733-1794. Discursus ... von Erzeugung der Menschen und Thiere. *Berlin?, ca. 1760.*

180 ff. (ff. 177-180 blank). 20 cm. Text in German and Latin. Contains references to a large number of authors, among them R. de Graaf (ff. 5v, 6r, 25r-v, 44r, 68r, 72v, 73r, 74r, 84r), Descartes (11r, 124r), Harvey (2r, 36v, 37v, 67r-v, 68r-v, 70r, 74r, 75r, 77v, 81v, 90v, 92r, 98v), Leeuwenhock (32r, 34r, 36v, 37r, 38r, 74r, 106r, 107v), Leibniz (125v), Littré (79v, 81r, 83r), Malebranche (116v, 117v, 118r, 119r, 120v, 123r, 124v, 127v), Malpighi (90r, 92r-v, 94v, 95r, 101v, 105r, 106r), Swammerdam (101v) and Verheyen (7r, 9v, 10r, 12r, 13v, 36v, 38r-v, 39v, 52v, 62v, 63v, 68r, 73r, 119v, 143r). Name Samuel Gottlieb Scholtz in contemporary hand on prel. blank f. — From the J. Stockton Hough Collection.   *[10a/163]*

1095.   **Woman's Medical College** of Pennsylvania. Department of Preventive Medicine. Annual reports. *Philadelphia, 1954-60.*

5 folders. 29 cm. Carbon copies (annual reports), mimeographed (appendices), few typewritten special reports. The appendices represent the largest part of the folders, and contain reports on lectures, meetings, conferences, etc.   *[n.c.]*

— — — —. See also nos. 829, 869-74, 885.

1096.   **Wood, Alfred Conrad,** 1863-1959. Notes on anesthesia. *Philadelphia, 1890-1910.*

1 envelope. 30 cm. Miscellaneous notes on odd sheets of paper, including a 4-page typewritten essay, evidently intended for delivery at a commemoration of the 50th anniversary of Wells' use of nitrous oxide (1844).   *[10b/45]*

1097.   – – – – –. On the prevention of cancer. *Philadelphia, n.d.*

14, 20 ff. 21.5, 28 cm. Typescripts. 2 copies of the same paper, one heavily corrected by the author, the other a clean copy with few annotations.   *[n.c.]*

1098.   **Wood, George Bacon,** 1797-1879. Address delivered before the Athenian Institute [Atheneum of Philadelphia], Jan. 23, 1839. *Philadelphia, 1839.*

[47] ff. 25 cm. "The subject of the lecture . . . is British India," p. [1].
[Z 10/153]

1099.   – – – – –. Case book. *Philadelphia, 1818-28[-34].*

217 (vero 218) pp., followed by numerous blank and 2 text leaves. 21 cm. Among the cases is a lengthy report on yellow fever (pp. 36-72) and another on erysipelas (pp. 99-113, 138-42). Beginning on p. 143 cases are summarized in "Account of my practice," 1826-28. In the back 3 pp. listing of pupils in the course on materia medica in the College of Pharmacy, 1833-34. Notes from Dr. Irvine's Treatise (on the yellow fever), written in Charleston in 1820, laid in (4 ff.).   *[10a/23]*

1100.   – – – – –. Catalogue of pupils attending the lectures on materia medica and pharmacy in the University of Pennsylvania in the winter of 1840-41 [-1848-9]. *Philadelphia, 1840-49.*

122 ff. (f. 10 removed, ff. 37, 58 and 121-22 blank). 19 cm. Contains, beginning in the back (f. 120), expenditures and income, 1840-49 (ends f. 90v), entering under the former salaries and wages, cost of printing syllabi and tickets, paintings and specimens, funeral expense, etc., and under the latter tuition payments.   *[10a/200]*

1101.   – – – – – – – – –, in the session of 1855-6 [and 1859-60]. *Philadelphia, 1855-60.*

92 pp., [24] ff. (ff. 1-8 blank). 20 cm. Contains, beginning in the back (f. 24), expenditures and income, 1855-60 (ends f. 9), entering under the former wax models from Guys Hospital, London ($509.53; $501.76 and $500.05), besides salaries and wages, printing, student and commencement parties, and cleaning.   *[10a/201]*

1102.   – – – – –. Comparative state of the class each year, commencing one week before introductions, 1835-1858. *Philadelphia, ca. 1858.*

[2] ff. 32 cm.   *[n.c.]*

1103.   – – – – –. Correspondence; largely letters to G.B. Wood, but also including several by him. *V.p., 1813-75.*

26 envelopes in 2 boxes. 30 cm. Contents: Box 1, envelopes 1-8: Letters dealing with medical and pharmaceutical topics, and the Dept. of Medicine of the Univ. of Penna., Wood's own publications, the American Philosophical

Society, slave trade, the Civil War, etc. Among the many correspondents are D.H. Agnew, P.P. Broca, Charles Brown-Séquard, Joseph Carson, Robert Christison, Edward Hartshorne, Isaac Hays, Thomas Hodgkin, W.E. Horner, T.S. Kirkbride, Joseph Leidy, C.D. Meigs, S.W. Mitchell, T.D. Mütter, J.H. Packard, Isaac and Joseph Parrish, William Pepper, R.E. Rogers, F.G. Smith, Alfred Stillé, W.H. Van Buren and Caspar Wistar. — Env. 9-10: Correspondence with Franklin Bache. — Env. 11-12: Draft of letter from the American Medical Assoc. to the Senate and House on Copyright Law. — Box 2, envelopes 1-14: Family correspondence.   *[ZZ 10a/20, boxes 1-2]*

1104.   —————. Documents and papers, I. *Philadelphia, 1835-1873?*

9 envelopes. 30-38 cm. Contents: Documents relating to the University of Pennsylvania, Board of Trustees, 1836-1873? (env. 1); relating to the University of Pennsylvania Hospital, 1837-1846 (env. 2); relating to the University of Pennsylvania Medical School, 1835-1852 (env. 3); history of materia medica, 1855 (env. 4); docs. relating to the College of Physicians, 1836-1856 (env. 5); relating to the Pharmacopoeia, from the first revision of 1831 to 1850 (env. 6-9). Summary description without analysis of individual items.
                    [ZZ 10a/20, box 3]

1105.   ———— —————, II. *Philadelphia?, ca. 1825-1860.*

7 envelopes. 27-38 cm. Contents: Envelope 1. Deeds, etc., and letters (by G.B. Wood, G.M. Wharton, S.W. Mitchell, Thomas Mütter, J.M. Da Costa) relating to the Mütter Museum, 1856-58. — 2. Four notebooks listing students enrolled at the Dept. of Medicine, Univ. of Pennsylvania, 1837-43, and list of students and physicians invited. — 3. Bills delivered, 1849-60. — 4. Girard College papers, n.d. — 5. Two valedictory lectures, n.d. — 6. Three lectures on natural history, specifically botany, n.d., and Notebook, 1841-42. — 7. Lectures on miscellaneous pharmacological topics.   *[ZZ 10a/20, box 4]*

1106.   —————. First and last, a poem intended to illustrate the ways of God to man. *Philadelphia, 185—?*

57 pp. 24 cm (boxed). Except for minor corrections, the text duplicates about one-third of the printed version, issued anonymously (London, Longman, Green, Longman, and Roberts, 1860; Philadelphia, J.B. Lippincott & Co., 1864). The circumstances of publication are explained in a typewritten note, signed by H.C. Wood, pasted in the front of the College of Physicians' copy of the London edition and in the note by Wm. Osler on the title-page.   *[10c/34]*

1107.   —————. Journals. *V.p., 1817-29, 1836-49.*

v. 1 and 3. 20 cm. Topics incl. Wood's practice, his teaching career, his association with Dr. Joseph Parrish, work on the *U.S. Pharmacopoeia*, trips to New York and New England, Girard College, Philadelphia Dispensary, and controversy with Dr. Rush. Vol. 3 with partial table of contents. — Bequest of G.B. Wood to Richard Wood, presented by Mrs. G.B. Wood and Harold B. Wood.   *[10c/63]*

1108.   ———— —————, July 20, 1837-45, 1848, 1851-55, 1860-62. *V.p., 1837-62.*

5 folders (1837-38; 26 cm); 13 bound vols. (travels in Europe, Great Britain, etc.; 17-23 cm); 14 note books (1860-61; 21-26 cm); 1 folder (cover only; 1844).   *[10c/108]*

09.   — — — — —. Lectures on materia medica and pharmacy . . ., summer of 1827; notes taken by William W. Gerhard. *Philadelphia, 1827.*

[1], 63 ff. 20 cm. Lectures dated April 29-July 9, 1827.   *[10a/116]*

10.   — — — — —   — — — — — and autopsy and Memorial address on James Blythe Rogers. Valedictory address at the University of Pennsylvania (1860), etc. *Philadelphia, 1845-65?*

2 boxes. 31.5 cm. Partly interleaved with pages of printed versions.
                                                                              [10a/437]

11.   — — — — —. Ledger. *Philadelphia, 1831-52.*

304 pp. 33.5 cm. Contains index, by patients' names.   *[Z 10/102]*

12.   — — — — —. List of medical students at the University of Pennsylvania [1822], 1830-1854[-1857] (pp. 2-11, 76-81). — List of Wood's students registered in various courses or attached to hospitals, 1837-1855 (pp. 13-74). *Philadelphia, 1830-56.*

101 pp. (pp. 82-101 blank), 1 f., 56 pp. 19 cm. Contains, beginning in the back (56 pp.), expenditures and incomes in connection with medical instruction or internships, 1830-56. Courses entered include those of Drs. W.W. Gerhard, J.K. Mitchell, F. Bache, W.E. Horner, W. Pepper, H.H. Smith, E. Parrish, J. Leidy, C. Wistar, H. Hartshorne and many others, and assignments to the Pennsylvania Hospital and the Philadelphia General Hospital.
                                                                              [10a/205]

13.   — — — — —. Lists of physicians in the United States, by counties, as known to his students at the University of Pennsylvania Medical School. *Philadelphia, 1836.*

1 box. 37.5 cm. Consists of 1, a paper-covered, thumb-indexed notebook with names listed by the students; 2, the students' lists, on single sheets of varying size, some signed by the student compilers; entries mainly from Eastern states. See also Wm. Gibson's similar, more complete, compilation of the same year.   *[Z 10a/9]*

14.   — — — — —. Lists of students received, University of Pennsylvania. *Philadelphia, 1837-45.*

2 v. 19 cm. With lists of medical students and physicians invited to commer   ment parties, 1837-41. Includes names from the classes of 1838 through   45. — Presented by George B. and Horatio C. Wood.   *[10a/274]*

1115.   —————. Miscellany I. *V.p., 1815-1866.*

7 envelopes. 30-38 cm. Contents: Envelope 1. Engraved portraits of J.D. Godman, John Grigg and G.B. Wood; estate of David C. Wood (2 ff. ms., n.d., post 1848); 18 photographs, mostly by Disdéri, Paris, collected in 1862. — 2. Memoir of Dr. Parrish, presented to the College of Physicians, 4 May 1841 (16 ff.); account of the case of the late Dr. Joseph Parrish (8 ff., 1840?); statement concerning the sanity of John Zimmerman, made at the College of Physicians, 7 Dec. 1824 (1 f.); professional and social aspects in the life of Dr. Parrish, notes for Dr. Wood by unnamed person (6 ff.). — 3. Poem for Dr. Wood by B.H. Coates (2 ff., 1847), and another by C.H. Wood (2 ff., 1847); remembrance of Thomas Hodgkin (6 ff., 1866). — 4. Address to stockholders of the Schuylkill Navigation Company (23, vero 24 ff., n.d.). — 5. Printed and ms. material, 3 on railroads, 1847-48; receipts; printed invitation; Dr. Wood's report for the Committee on copyright of the AMA, 1849; indenture, 1815; printed circular of the Building Committee of the College of Physicians, and another of the Citizens Volunteer Hospital Assoc. — 6. Letters introducing Dr. Wood (C.D. Meigs, J.H. Griscom, S.G. Morton). — 7. Memoirs of Franklin Bache for the College of Physicians (63 ff., 1865) and the American Philosophical Society (26 ff., 1865?).   *[ZZ 10a/20, box 5]*

1116.   ———— ————— II. *V.p., ca. 1830-ca. 1865.*

8 folders. 27-31 cm. Contents: Envelope 1. Lecture on metals (zinc, cobalt, arsenic, etc.), no. 46 (n.d., [1], 23 ff.). — 2. Lecture on antimony, no. 47 (n.d., 24 ff.). — Diuretics (n.d., 46 ff., ff. 34-46 blank). — 4. Introduction to pharmacology (n.d., [1], 59 ff.) and preface to second edition (1833, 2 ff., 2nd blank). — 5. Newspaper clippings on various subjects, not chronologically arranged (pasted in booklet, 1850-61). — 6. Map of Italy (mounted, in slip case; 1861). — 7. Account book of payments, largely for work on and inside various properties (1860-62, 6 ff. incl. blank f.). — 8. Notes towards a biography of Franklin Bache in 2 booklets (both ca. 1864; 3 pp., ff. 4-20 [1 f. removed following p. 2]; 16 ff., ff. 15-16 blank); genealogical table and 2 letters of genealogical interest from T. Hewson Bache (1864).   *[ZZ 10a/20, box 6]*

1117.   —————. Notebook containing "engagements" (i.e. cost of journal subscriptions), contributions, debts, sums to be collected, memoranda (generally of a financial nature), etc. *Philadelphia, 1849-55.*

80 ff. (ff. 12, 22, 63-66 and 77 blank; 1 f. each removed between ff. 6-7, and 16-17). 21 cm. Contains, beginning at the back (f. 80), addresses, list of dinners (1843-52), evening parties (1848-55), gentlemen to be invited, invitations to club, Wistar Party (1850-55), and delivery of the Centenary Hospital Address (1852).   *[10a/317]*

1118.   —————. Notes on clinical cases, under the direction of Drs. Wood, Norris, etc. *Philadelphia, 1857-59.*

1 v. (unpaged, few ff. removed). 15 cm. Autograph of student, Robert Blake Cruice (M.D. — 1859, Univ. of Penna.), on flyleaf. Cases treated primarily by

G.B. Wood, George W. Norris, Edward Peace, William Pepper, and James Jones Levick. — Inscription of presentation to Blencome Eardley Fryer on flyleaf.   *[10a/427]*

9.   — — — — —. Notes on materia medica and pharmacy delivered by Dr. G.B. Wood in the University of Pennsylvania. *Philadelphia, 1837.*

5 v. 19-19.5 cm. Notes by Joseph Carson. Contents: V. 1. Six short lectures and notes on astringents. — V. 2. Tonics, bitters, aromatics. — V. 3. Mineral tonics, stimulants, narcotics. — V. 4. Narcotics, sedatives, mercury. — V. 5. "Medicine which acts upon the functions."   *[10a/117]*

0.   — — — — —. Notes on the lectures of George B. Wood, special physics and the practice of medicine. *Philadelphia, 1859-60.*

2 v. ([2] ff., 145, 170 pp.; pp. 427-558); illus. 25-32 cm. Notes taken by Jacob da Silva Solis-Cohen (M.D., Univ. of Penna., 1860). According to a pencilled note on the first prel. f., in the hand of Dr. Solis-Cohen, there should be another volume, measuring 25 cm.; it would have covered pp. 171-426, now missing. — Presented by Myer Solis-Cohen.   *[Z 10/95]*

1.   — — — — —. Notes on the subject of Christianity in India. *Philadelphia, n.d.*

v. 1. 20 cm. Apparently intended to be longer, but never completed (see *Trans. & Stud.*, ser. 3, v. 5: xliv-xlv [1881]). Engraved frontispiece carrying legend paraphrasing Ps. 136:4. — Gift of Horatio C. Wood.   *[10d/151]*

2.   — — — — —. Thirty-three autograph letters to his wife Caroline, largely from *Philadelphia*, but also from *Detroit* (May 4-8, *1856*, meeting of the American Medical Association), *Greenwich, N.J.* (April 5, *1857*; April 11, *1858*) and *Washington, D.C.* (May 3-7, *1858*).

142 pp. 18-25 cm. Beyond personal and family matters these letters contain references to a large number of physicians and other information of medical interest, e.g. meeting of the American Medical Assoc., 1856. Contents: 1856, May 4-Nov. 6; 17 letters. — 1857, April 5-Oct. 24; 9 letters. — 1858, April 11-Oct. 7; 7 letters.   *[10d/151]*

— — — — —. See also nos. 114, 148, 164, 171, *185.13*, 257, 382, 587, 589, 623, 765, 787-8, 790, 1032.

3. **Wood, George Bacon,** 1871-1954. The Horatio C. Wood clan and some of their antics [by] George Bacon Wood and Helen Foss Wood. *Philadelphia, 1950.*

1 v. (loose-leaf); illus. 25.5 cm. "In honor of Horatio C. and Eliza Huldah Longacre Wood. . . ," p. [iii].   *[10d/145]*

1124.   **Wood, Horatio C.,** 1841-1920.   Notes on the lectures on therapeutics (and nervous diseases) delivered to the medical class of the University of Pennsylvania.   *Philadelphia, 1891-93.*

> 2 v., 1 envelope. 21 cm. Notes taken by John M. Swan. Vol. 1, dated 6 Oct. 1892-18 Feb. 1893. On last sheet, a humorous poem in pencil, dedicated to "Pop" Wormley (Theodore G. Wormley, Prof. of chemistry and toxicology), signed J.F. Hamilton (a classmate of Swan's). Added 32 ff. of notes on therapeutics headed "Wood", dated 15 Oct. 1891-14 Jan. 1892. — V. 2: "Notes on the clinics on nervous diseases . . . by Horatio C Wood 1892-1893" (sixteen cases), and continuation of notes in v. 1, dated 4 Mar.-1 Apr. 1893. V. 2 mostly blank.   *[10a/333]*

————. See also nos. 137, *185.13,* 623, 675, 834, 1079-80, 1106, 1123.

1125.   **Woodhouse, James,** 1770-1809.   Notes from lectures on chemistry delivered in the University of Pennsylvania.   *Philadelphia, ca. 1807.*

> 2 v. ([6], 236, [5]; [2], 256, [7] ff.). 21 cm. Notes probably by Samuel Benezet (cf. v. 2, f. 19v; M.D. — Univ. of Penna., 1808). Lectures 2-59; lecture 1 (on the utility of chemistry to other fields) consists of a one-paragraph summary on f. 1, followed by lecture on the origin and progress of chemistry (ff. 1-8). Table of contents on preliminary ff. of v. 1. Each volume has alphabetical topical index. References to earlier and contemporary scientists throughout, incl. Robert Boyle, Joseph Priestley and Antoine Laurent Lavoisier. Faint pencilled name Geo. Hamilton on flyleaves of both volumes. — Bookplate of Dr. Samuel Washington Woodhouse, Jr. in both volumes. Gift of Mrs. S.W. Woodhouse.   *[10c/53]*

1126.   **Woodruff, Charles Edward.**   Letters to Colonel John Page Nicholson on Japanese death rates (with mention of extraneous matters) during the Russo-Japanese War (Aug. 15, 1911) and fatalities (Dec. 24, 1911), and on the health of French (vs. German) soldiers (March 4, 1914).   *N.p., ca. 1915.*

> 1 envelope. 37.5 cm. Printed items and clippings included, e.g. Woodruff's "Death rates in the Japanese War," *Medical Record,* April 8, 1911.   *[n.c.]*

1127.   **[Yellow Fever I].**   Letters, documents and some printed items, primarily on yellow fever.   *Philadelphia, etc., 1787-1820.*

> 1 v. 46 cm. 56 items, mounted in scrapbook, on the origin, history, diagnosis and progress of yellow fever (incl. few references to tetanus and typhus) in Philadelphia (1747, 1793-98, 1820), Virginia (1741), New Jersey (1793-99), New York (1793-1803, 1805), New Haven (1796, 1803), the West Indies, and on board the ships *Arethusa, Deborah, Hind* and *Iris.* Involves a large number of medical and lay persons, including several letters by, or pertaining to, William Currie, Samuel Powell Griffitts, David Hosack and Caspar Wistar. Two items concern the Academy of Medicine of Philadelphia (pp. 85-6; 1798, 1800) and

the last item (p. 165; 1820) is a communication from the Select and Common Council on the Means of Preventing Malignant Fever, addressed to Thomas Parke, president of the College of Physicians of Philadelphia, signed by the chairman John R. Coates. Among clippings and other printed items is a broadside of the Society for Bettering the Condition of the Poor, London, entitled *Heads of the Plan for the Extermination of Infectious Fever*, dated 7th May, 1802 and inscribed to the College of Physicians of Philadelphia, with manuscript corrections. Compiler or early owner not identified. — Analytical contents with alphabetical index filed with the volume. *[Z 10/15]*

28. **[Yellow Fever II].** Reports, letters and dissertations on yellow fever, etc., collected by John Kearsley Mitchell. *V.p., 1822-56.*

1 v. 27 cm. Contents: Memoranda and extracts of reports on the yellow fever on board the frigate *Macedonia*, 1822, involving the Bureau of Medicine and Surgery, the Board of Commissioners of the U.S. Navy Department, and the surgeons B. Washington and C.B. Hamilton (10 ff.). — Yellow fever at Bristol, Pa., G. Emerson's letter to J.K. Mitchell, 1825 (8 ff.). — Yellow fever on board the *Hornet* (1821 or 1822), 2 letters from J. Shubrick and 2 from Thomas Harris to Mitchell (1 enclosing copy of letter from Waters Smith to T. Harris), 1845-46 (10 ff.). — Sickness (not yellow fever) on board the *Caledonia*, etc., letter from E.M. Donaldson to Mitchell, 1846 (2 ff.). — Yellow fever on the steamer *Alleghany*, Robert Woodworth to Mitchell [Jefferson Medical College], 1847 (1 f.). — Copy of letter from fleet surgeon B.F. Bache to T. Harris on cases of yellow fever, 1850 (3 ff.). — Dissertations: A.N. Bell, Yellow fever, 1849 (66 ff.); W.J. Deupree, Congestive fever, Jefferson Medical College, 1848 (24 ff.); J.M. Lazzell, Typhoid fever, *ibid.*, for J.K. Mitchell, ca. 1850 (1, 17 ff.); John Newcomer, Typhoid fever, *ibid.*, 1852 (20 ff.). — Charles Peirce's weather reports (with a few references to yellow fever), 1780-1844 (16 ff.). *[10a/302]*

29. **[Yellow Fever III].** Treatment of yellow fever; unsigned (incomplete) letter to H.U. Onderdonk in New York. *Philadelphia?, ca. 1810.*

4 pp. 25 cm (envelope, 31 cm). *[n.c.]*

30. **Young, Thomas,** d. 1783. Lectures on midwifery . . . notes taken by John McMorran. *Edinburgh, 1782-83.*

2 v. in 1 ([8], 206 pp.). 18 cm. Bookplate of H. Lenox Hodge. *[10a/119]*

31. —————. Notes on lectures on midwifery. *Edinburgh, 1777?*

[2], 314 pp. 23 cm. Pages 46-50, 76-91, 160-81, 226-48, 263-71, 307-13 torn out. *[10a/120]*

—————. See also no. 111.

32. **Young, William.** Medical and household recipes, incl. paint, cosmetics, alcoholic drinks, horse medicines, etc. *Philadelphia, ca. 1837.*

[1] f., 107 pp., [30] ff. 16 cm. Owned by "William Young M.D. Philadelphia Sept. 11ᵗʰ/37." Pasted inside front cover 2 newspaper clippings and inside back cover printed "Dr. William Stoy's cure for the bite of a mad dog," blank spaces filled in by hand. Alphabetical index at end of volume. — Gift of William Pepper.   *[10a/349]*

1133. **Zentmayer, William,** 1864-1958. Memoir of Dr. Posey. *Philadelphia, 1934.*

8 ff. 28 cm. Typescript, signed. Printed in *Trans. & Stud.*, ser. 4, v. 2: xxiii-xxviii (1934).   *[n.c.]*

1134. —————. The theory and practice of ophthalmoscopy; notes of the lecture course . . . Dept. of Ophthalmology . . ., University of Pennsylvania. *Philadelphia, 1934.*

[2], 99, [1], 12 ff. (f. 13 lacking). Spring binder, 29.5 cm. Mimeographed. Title of final leaves: Medical ophthalmology. Based on J. Bjerrum's Introduction to the use of the ophthalmoscope. — Bookplate of F.H. Adler on prel. leaf.   *[ZZ 10d/16a]*

1135. ———— —————. *Philadelphia, 1934.*

[2], 99, [1], 13 ff. 28.5 cm. Typewritten (carbon), with many handwritten and some typed additions. Title of final 13 leaves: Medical ophthalmology.
                                                                          [ZZ 10d/16]

1136. ———— —————. *Philadelphia, 1938.*

[2], 94 ff. 38 cm. Mimeographed, with corrections, and handwritten and typed additions. "Presented to the author by the group in ophthalmology, Graduate School of Medicine, University of Pennsylvania, 1938-39" (front cover), with letter from K.L. Roper pasted inside and signatures of members of the group on fly-leaf. Zentmayer's review in *Am. Jour. of Med. Sc.*, v. 210: 262 (1945) inserted before f. 59.   *[ZZ 10d/16b]*

1137. **Ziegler, Samuel Lewis,** 1861-1926. Papers. *V.p., 1906-1926.*

5 boxes. 32 cm. Contents: Box 1. Translations of text of a. Félix Terrien, *Chirurgie de l'oeil* (Paris, 1902) and chapts. 1-5, 2d ed. (Paris, 1921); b. *Encyclopédie française d'ophthalmologie* by Lagrange & Valude, v. 9 (Paris, 1910). — Box 2. Materials for his unpublished work, *The Surgery of the Eye.* — Box 3. Typescripts, drafts, etc. of papers (as far as available in reprints, marked MS on list filed at beginning of box). Beyond these it contains: Extract of an immature cataract; Tubercular cyclitis; Fox's capsular advancement; Practical problems in the surgery of trachoma; Daviel's original memoir on cataract extraction; Mikulicz's disease (abstract); V-shaped iridotomy . . .; Dr. Ziegler's surgical photophore; Technic of bilateral sclero-choriotomy; Inquiry into the functions of maxillary antrum; Ocular signs . . . associated with intranasal lesions; Technique of refraction; Hay fever; Discussion on accessory sinus disease; Discussion of trachoma; Partial and complete tenotomy for the relief of heterophoria; Medical philanthropy; Successful removal of a piece of steel . . .; Total blindness from . . . wood alcohol with recovery . . . under electricity;

Excision of lacrimal sac; Hemophilic extrarasation. . .; Discussion of Dr.
Schwenk's paper (on keratoconus); Of Dr. Thorington's case of chronic simple
glaucoma; On electro-therapeutics; Electrolysis-cataphoresis; Electric modali-
ties . . . — Boxes 4-5. Translations, transcriptions, etc. of articles and chapters
by a variety of specialists, among them J.B.M.E. Aubaret, C.J. Carron du
Villards, G.A. Critchett, Wilhelm Czermak, A.P. Demours, L.A. Desmarres,
Henri Dor, Camille Fromaget, Xaver Galezowski, P.F. Lagrange, Edmund
Landolt, Ernest Motais, G. Pellier de Quengsy, Charles Saint-Yves, Victor
Stoeber, Albert Terson; also case histories, correspondence and miscellany.
Descriptive items on contents of boxes 4-5 filed at end of box 5.   *[Z 10/161]*

—————. See also no. 245.

38.   **Ziem, Constantin Heinrich,** 1850-1917. Plague and nose.
Danzig, 1911?

4 ff. 28.5 cm. Typewritten; fragile. With typewritten signed letter (in
German) to [J. da S.] Solis-Cohen requesting him to present it to the American
Laryngological Association, and to seek publication in an American journal
(apparently unpublished). Translation of "La peste et le nez," *Rev. hebdomad.
de laryngologie,* v. 1: 705-12 (1911).   *[10d/82]*

39.   **Zimmerman, Mason Woodward,** 1861-1956. Children's Aid
Society's ophthalmologic cases. *Philadelphia, 1891-1909, 1911-
19.*

Pp. 11-200. 27 cm. Pp. 119-99 by Dr. B. Chance. Pp. 1-10 missing. Name
index on pp. 198-200.   *[ZZ 10a/6]*

Index I

List of persons, institutions and organizations, and of selected titles appearing in the descriptions of the catalogue. This list excludes the entries found in the alphabetically arranged main section.

Abbe, Robert Waldo (1851-1928), 185.*632*, 678

Abbott Laboratories, 244

Academie des Sciences, Paris, 698

Academy of Medicine of Philaelphia, 1127

Academy of Natural Sciences, Philadelphia, 42, 589

Adler, Lewis Harry (1864-1934), 77

Aesculapian Club of Philadelphia, 1059

African Church, Philadelphia, 919

Agassiz, Alexander Emanuel (135-1910), 589

Agassiz, Louis Jean Rodolphe (1807-1873), 113

Agnew, Cornelius Rea (1830-1888), 1024

Aiken, Robert (1734-1802), 931

Albertson, Henry Walter (1875-1955), 701

Alden, C.U., 251

Alexander, Ashton (1772-1855), 200

Alibert, Jean Louis Marc (1766-1837), 507

Alison, Francis (1751-1813), 891

Alison, Pulteney, 111

Alison, Robert (d. 1854), 51, 204, 925

Allen, Joshua Gibbons (1832-1903), 226

Allen, William (1810-1900), 36

Allerman, Julia, 371

Allibone, Samuel Austin (1816-189), 270

Allis, Oscar Huntington (1836-1921), 837

Allison, John, 243

Alpha Mu Pi Omega, 1059

Ambrose, Anthony, 238

Ambulance Hospital, Paris, 943

American Academy of Political and Social Science, 185*2226*

American Association for the Advancement of Science, 529

American Board of Pathology, 520

American Climatological Association, 982

American College of Physicians, 529, 934

American College of Surgeons, 253

American Congress of Internal Medicine, 934

American Dermatological Association, 58

American Heart Association, 523

American Laryngological Association, 981, 1138

American Medical Society, Philadelphia, 789, 805d, 938-39

American Neurological Association, 676

American Philosophical Society, 185.*62*, 271, 361, 487, 671, 1103, 1115

American Society for Experimental Pathology, 520

Anaxagoras (d. 428 B.C.), 35

Anderson, Hyrum Andrew (1868-1952), 85

Andrews, Thomas Hollingsworth (1843-1918), 588

Apostolis, Giovanni (17th cent.), 183

Archer, Benjamin (fl. 1804-36?), 908

Archer, John (1741-1810), 29

Archer, John (1777-1830), 904

Ariosto, Francesco (d. 1492?), 632

Armstrong, Charles (1886-1967), 246

Armstrong, John (1709-1779), 111

Arnemann, Justus (1763-1806), 629

Aronson, Joseph David (1887-1958), 534

Artzneybüchlein, 40

Aschoff, Karl Albert Ludwig (1866-1942), 545

Ash, Rachel (1893-1977), 769

Ashmead, William (1801-1888), 223, 443, 762

Ashton, Thomas George (1867-1933), 228

Association of Military Surgeons, 227, 780

Atkins, Dudley (1798-1845), 795

Atlee, Walter Franklin (1828-1910), 213

Aubaret, Jean Baptiste Marie Edmond (b. 1874), 1137

Audubon, John James Laforest (1785-1851), 113

Austin, James Harold (1883-1952), 185.*14, 34*

Avicenna (980-1037), 647, 877

Avila, Juan Antonio de, 666

Babinski, Joseph François Félix (1857-1932), 669

Bache, Thomas Hewson (1826-1912), 185.*63,* 1116

Backus, William, 884

Baillie, Mattias (1761-1823), 183

Baird, Spencer Fullerton (1823-1887), 589, 591-92

Bamberger, Ira Leon, 244

Banester (or Banister), John (1533-1610), 719

Banks, Joseph(1743-1820), 307

Banting, Frederick Grant (1891-1941), 507

Bard, Samuel (1742-1821), 705, 931

Barker, Benjamin F. (1819-1891), 679

Barker, J.J., 821

Barnes, Robert (1817-1907), 739

Bartholin, Caspar (1585-1629), 9

Bartholin, Thomas (1616-1680), 645

Bartlett, Elisha (1804-1855), 112

Barton, Edward, 145

Barton, William (fl. 1775-1815), 45

Bartram, John (1699-1777), 329

Bauhin, Caspar (1560-1624), 9

Baum, Charles (1855-1938), 779

Baumann, Gustave A., 425

Bayer Co., New York, 886

Bayle, Gaspard Laurent (1774-1816), 605

Beaumont, William (1785-1853), 42

Beck, D.R., 806

Bedner, William, 94

Beebe, Silas Palmer (b. 1876), 883

Beecher, Abraham C.W. (1845-1893), 495

Bell, Agrippa Nelson (1820-1911), 1128

Bell, Charles (1774-1842), 111

Bell, John (1796-1872), 112, 806

Bell, Whitfield Jenks (b. 1914), 16, 705

Bellows, Horace Martin (1839?-1912), 1041

Bensel, Carl, 40

Berger, David Hendricks (1860-1937), 623

Berks County Medical Society, 1036

Bernard, Claude (1813-1878), 507

Besnier,Ernest Henri (1831-1909), 841

Betton, John Price, 818, 914

Betton, Samuel (1786-1850), 2, 55, 1061

Beyers, James (1733-1817), 703

Bheden, M.S., 341

Biddle, John Barclay, 875

Billings, John Shaw (1838-1913), 36, 454, 679, 685, 1050

Billroth, Christian Albert Theodore (1829-1894), 317

Binaschi (or Binachi), Ambrosio, 647

Bird, Robert Montgomery (1806-1854), 112

Birkhaug, Konrad Elias (b. 1892), 1051

Bjerrum, Jannik (1851-1920), 1134-36

Blackwell, Elizabeth (1821-1910), 801

Blake, John Ballard (b. 1922), 16

Blane, Gilbert (1749-1834), 494

Blayney, Richard Stone, 76

Blume, Carl Albert (1860-1938), 633

Blumstein, George Issac (b. 1904), 185.*13*

Boardman, Andrew, 42

Boceffey, L.D.A., 580

Boerhaave, Hermann (1668-1738), 182, 697

Bonaparte, Charles Lucien Jules Laurent (1803-1857), 113

Bond, Phineas (1717-1773), 84

Borelli, Giovanni Alfonso (1608-1679), 697

Borrows, Dr., 82

Bos (or Bosch), Cornelius (1506?-1556?), 941

Boston, Leonard Napoleon (1871-1931), 652

Boston City Hospital, 581

Bouret, Auguste, 1020

Bowditch, Henry Ingersoll (1808-1892), 450

Boyd, George Melick (1861-1939), 940

Boyer, Alexis (1757-1833), 269

Boyle, Robert (1627-1691), 9, 645, 1125

Bradner, Albert H., 90

Bridges, Robert (1806-1882), 42

Brinton, Daniel Garrison (1837-1899), 37

Brinton, Ward (1874-1935), 185.*63*

Broca, André (1863-1925), 92

Brockenbrough, Austin, Jr., 805a

Brodie, Benjamin Collins (1783-1862), 183

Brooks, John Wallis (b. 1762), 177

Broom, Jacob, 924

Brown, John (1735-1788), 640

Brown, William (1692-1774), 931

Browne, Harriet H., 737

Browne, Thomas (1605-1682), 687

Brownley, Joseph, 805b

Bryan, James (1810-1881), 650

Bryant, Joseph Decatur (1845-1914), 491

Burke, Bernard, 219

Burney, Leroy Edgar (b. 1906), 351

Burns, Michael Anthony (1855-1938), 212

Burr, Aaron (1756-1836), 339, 706

Burwell, Charles Sidney (1893-1967), 529

Bush, Jacob, 806

Bush Hill Hospital, Philadelphia, 573

Butler, James R., 821

Butlin, Henry Trentham (1845-1912), 1058

Butterfield, Lyman Henry (b. 1909), 559

Butterworth, Thomas (b. 1904), 942

Byron, George Gordon Noël (1788-1824), 395

Cabot, Richard Clarke (1868-1939), 188

Cahoon, Dr., of Chambersburg (Pa.), 181

Caldwell, S., 721

Callomon, Fritz Thomas (1876-1964), 1058

Calmette, Léon Charles Albert (1863-1933), 487

Cannon, Walter Bradford (1871-1943), 486, 507

Capello, Arcadio, 685

Carasquilla, Juan de Díos (1833-1908), 37

Cardano, Girolamo (1501-1576), 645

Carnegie, Andrew (1835-1919), 679

Carpenter, Howard Childs (1878-1955), 356

Carrel, Alexis (1873-1944), 486-87, 507

Carron du Villards, Charles Joseph (1800-1860), 1137

Carson, John (1752-1794), 9

Carson, Joseph (1808-1876), 875

Castiglioni, Arturo (1874-1953), 541

Cattell, Henry Ware (1867-1936), 1013

Cayol, Jean Bruno (1787-1856), 172, 605

Cenas, A.W., 330

Chain, Ernst Boris (1906-1979), 801

Chambers, Rhuhammah, 181

Chancellor, William (fl. 1761-1763), 111

Chapman, Nathaniel (1780-1853), 631

Chaptal, Jean Antoine Claude (1756-1832), 805g

Chase, Heber, 804, 806

Chaveas, William Francis (b. 1922), 185.*18*

Chervin, Nicholas (1783-1843), 42

Cheselden, William (1688-1752), 117

Cheston, C. Morris (d. 1898), 965

Cheston, Daniel Murray (1843-1919), 781, 965

Cheston, James, 965

Chew, Benjamin (1722-1810), 339

Cheyne, George (1671-1743), 111

Chicago Medical Society, 253
Children's Aid Society of Pennsylvania, 1139
Children's Hospital, Philadelphia, 34
Chirurgia medica, 1061
Chisholm, Colin (1755-1825), 573
Chittenden, Russell Henry (1856-1943), 678, 970-71
Chovet, Abraham (1704-1790), 749
Christophorus B. (scribe, 15th cent.), 618
Churchill, John, 42
Cimolin, Antonio (18th cent.), 1057
Citizens Volunteer Hospital Association, Philadelphia, 1115
Clark, Alonzo (1807-1887), 390
Clark, John Goodrich (1867-1927), 496
Clark, John Yardley, 261
Clark, Leonardo Street (1847-1932), 431
Clark, Micajah (1788-1849), 921
Clarke, John (1761-1815), 751
Cleveland, Grover (1837-1908), 253, 491
Cleveland Dermatological Society, 180
Clifton, Ann Maria, 920
Clio Medica, 517
Coates, Benjamin Hornor (1797-1881), 4, 481, 805j, 1115
Coates, John Reynell (1777-1842), 1127
Coates, Lawrance, 4
Cohen, Herman Bernard (b. 1891), 802
Coke, Samuel, 805c
Cokes (Kokkes?), Dr. (16th cent.), 66
Colden, Cadwalader (1688-1776), 114, 671
College of Physicians and Surgeons, New York, 390-92. See also Lectures and Lecture notes, New York
Coller, Frederick Amasa (1887-1964), 562
Columbia University, 390, 479, 744
Compendium medicinae, 40
Comroe, Julius Hiram (b. 1911), 879
Conant, James Bryant (1893-1978), 514
Conklin, Edwin Grant (1863-1952), 486

Conover, Sophia Stevens, 185.*2110*, 678
Constable, Cuthbert (d.1746), 170
Cook, Alexander Bennett, 77
Cooke, James 150
Coolidge, Calvin (1872-1933), 238, 501
Cope, Porter F., 208, 776
Cornell University, 949
Corner, George Washington (1889-1981), 514, 519
Corti, Alfonso Giacomo Gaspar (1882-1876), 185.57
Coues, Elliott (1842-1899), 589
Councill, Malcolm S. (1868-1930),356
Cowell, Benjamin (d. 1771), 177
Coxe, William Griscom, 859
Craft, John Peter, 931
Crawford, John Barclay (1845-1925), 304
Critchett, George Anderson (1845-1925), 1137
Crocker, Henry Radcliffe (1845-1909), 841
Croll, Oswald (1580-1609), 9, 134
Croxton, Arthur, 306
Cruice, Ellen J., 218
Cruice, James P., 219
Cruice, Robert Blake (1838-1899), 932
Cruice, Sarah, 219
Cuming, William (1714-1788), 111
Cumming, John, 805d
Cummings, William (fl. 1815-1820), 106
Curie, Marie Sklodowska (1867-1934), 185.*51*, 487
Curie, Pierre (1859-1906), 185.*51*
Currie, James (1756-1805), 183
Currie, William (1754-1828), 573, 1127
Cushing, Harvey Williams (1869-1939), 253, 507, 593, 687
Custer, Richard Philip (b. 1903), 562
Cutbush, Edward (1772-1843), 806
Cutler, Elliott Carr (1888-1947), 529
Cuvier, Frederick Georges (1773-1838), 113
Czermak, Wilhelm (1856-1906), 1137

Da Costa, Charles Frederic, 229
Da Costa, John Chalmers (1863-1933), 253

Dalton, John Call (1825-1889), 679
Dana, Edwin Salisbury, 593
Dana, James Dwight (1813-1895),
    113, 592
Darlington, William (1782-1863), 113,
    815, 907
Darrach, James (1828-1923), 298, 311,
    691
Darrach, William (1796-1865), 298,
    646, 822
Dartmouth College, 196
Darwin, Ersmus (1731-1802), 805a
Daviel, Jacques (1693-1762), 1137
Davis, Edward Parker (1856-1937),
    1014
Davis, Eugene, 486
Davis, F.A., publisher, 934
Davis, Gwilym George (1857-1918),
    32, 499, 972
Day, Henry (1814-1881), 679
De Benneville, George (1759?-1850),
    242
De Berdt, Dennys, 931
Deckard, Park Austin (b. 1881), 341
De cura sterilitatis, 28
Deems, Frank M., 395
De infirmitatibus occulorum, 28
Del Gaizo, Modestino (1854-1921),
    685
De Markley, A., 861
Demours, Antoine Pierre (1762-1836),
    1137
Denman, Thomas (1733-1815), 751
Dercum, Francis Xavier (1856-1931),
    669
De regimine et principum, 5
Desault, Piere Joseph (1744-1795),
    269
Descartes, René. (1596-1650), 1094
Desmarres, Louis Auguste (1810-1882),
    1137
Deupree, William J., 1128
Deutsches Lyceum, Pottsville (Pa.),
    90
Devon and Exeter Hospital, 931
Devèze, Jean (1753-1829), 573
De Voto, Bernard Augustine (1897-
    1955), 89
Dewees, William Potts (1768-1841),
    459, 471, 750
Diepgen, Paul (1878-1966), 515
Dietarius optimus, 643

Dix, Dorothea Lynde (1802-1887),
    368
Dixon, Samuel Gibson (1851-1918),
    680, 772
Donaldson, E.M., 1128
Dor, Henri (1835-1912), 1137
Dorsey, (d. 1833?, estate), 255
Dorsey, Robert Ralston, (d. 1869), 461
Dorsten, Theodore (d. 1552), 393
Douglas, Patrick, 805e
Douglas Hospital, Washington (D.C.),
    729
Drabkin, David Lion (1899-1980), 879
Drake, David (1785-1852), 112
Drake, Emma Frances (Angell) (b. 1849),
    986
Drysdale, Thomas (1770-1798), 200
Du Bois, Eugene Floyd (1882-1959),
    519
Dubois, Paul (1795-1871), 758
Duckworth, Dyce (1840-1928), 679
Duffield, Benjamin (1753-1799), 689
Duke University, 679
Duncan, Garfield George (b. 1901),
    533
Duncan, James Matthews (1826-1890),
    739
Dunglison, Richard James (1834-1901),
    275
Dunlap, J.B., 861
Durand, Elias (1794-1873), 113
Durant, Thomas Morton (1905-1977),
    185.*13*, 351
Dyer, William Wallace (1906-1970),
    185.*18*

Earle, Edward, stationer, 892
East Tennesee Medical Association,
    637
Easton, James, 442
Eaton, Amos (1776-1842), 113
Eaton, Darwin G., 391
Eberle, John (1787-1838), 384, 843
Echaverría, Juan de, 665
Echeverría, Manuel Gonzales, 679
Ecker, Enrique Eduardo, 1051
Edinburgh. Royal Infirmary, 427
Edinburgh Univeristy, 275, 689-90,
    709, 931, 1130-31
Egbert, Seneca (1863-1939), 652
Ehrenfried, Albert (1880-1951), 593

Ehrich, William Ernst (1900-1967),
	879
Ehrlich, Paul (1854-1915), 840, 1013
Eisenhart, Luther Pfahler (1876-1965),
	553
Eisenhower, Dwight David (1890-
	1969), 455
Ellicott, Valcoulon Le Moyne (b. 1893),
	597
Ellis, Henry Havelock (1859-1939),
	346
Ellis, R.G., 330
Elmer, William (1788-1836), 47, 819
Elzevier, printer-publishers, 550
Emergency Medical Service, Pennsyl-
	vania Zone 3, 423
English, Peter, 324
Enos, DeWitt C. (d. 1867), 391
Episcopal Hospital, Philadelphia, 34,
	963
Erdmann, John Frederick (1864-1954),
	491
Erlangen University, 275
Este, Ercole I (1431-1505), 632
Ettmüller, Michael (1644-1683), 1061
Eustice, William (1753-1825), 706
Eve, Paul Fitzsimmons (1806-1877),
	521
Ewing, James (1866-1943), 521
Ewing, James Hunter (1798-1827),
	481
Eyre, Manuel, 924
Ezickson, William Julius (b. 1892),
	296

Fabbri, Giovanni Battista (1806-1874),
	739
Faber, Erwin Frank (1866-1939), 254
Fahnestock, George, 294
Far Eastern Association of Tropical
	Medicine, 411
Faraday, Michael (1791-1867), 271
Farbwerke-Hoechst Co., 244
Farmer, Benjamin, 494
Federation of American Societies of
	Experimental Pathology, 520
Federation of American Societies for
	Experimental Biology, 523
Felton, Lloyd Derr, 1051
Ferriar, John (1761-1815), 82, 928
Ferrier, Paul, 805a

Field, Charles J., 23
Finlay, James, 706
Fishbein, Morris (1889-1976), 520
Fisher, Charles Perry (1857-1940),
	185.*611*, 641, 675, 1068
Fisher, Mary (d. 1787), 931
Fitzpatrick, Philip, 932
Flexner, Simon (1863-1946), 486-87
Flint, Austin (1812-1886), 390-91
Fludd, Robert (1574-1637), 877
Forbes, William Smith, (1831-1905),
	87
Fordyce, John Addison, (1858-1925),
	58
Fordyce, William (1724-1792), 111
Formad, Henry F. (1847-1892), 936,
	1013, 1035, 1037, 1080, 1082
Forsey, F.E., 592
Fothergill, John (1749-1800?), 706
Foulke, Thomas S., 589
Fouquier, Pierre Éloi (1776-1850),
	172
Fownes, George (1815-1849), 42
Fox, George (1806-1882), 721, 795
Frampton, Algernon (1766-1842), 743
Franklin, Benjamin (1706-1790), 84,
	114, 615, 625
Franklin and Marshall College, 394
Franklin Medical College, Philadelphia,
	67
Fraser, G.B., 185.*632*
Frederick Douglas Memorial Hospital,
	Philadelphia, 1034
Freeman, James Phillips (d. 1819), 54
Freeman, Strickland, 638
Freudenberger, Katrina (1860-1922),
	873
Frick, Charles (1823-1860), 112
Frické, Albert (1815-1898), 589
Friedenwald, Harry (1864-1950), 138
Friedrich I, king of Prussia (1701-
	1713), 9
Friedrich, Martin, 776
Fromaget, Victor Camille (1869-1928),
	1137
Fryer, Blencome Eardley, 1118
Fryer, Grace, 521
Fuchs, Alfred (1870-1927), 547
Fuchs, Ernst (1851-1930), 247, 313
Fulton, John Farquhar (1899-1960),
	514-15, 519-20, 541, 564

Gale, Thomas (1507-1587), 325

Galezowski, Xavier (1832-1907), 245, 1137

Galilei, Galileo (1564-1642), 877

Gallinger, Jacob Henry (1837-1918), 486-87

Galton, Francis (1822-1911), 395

Gardiner, John G., 640

Garrett, Philip C., 595

Garrison, Fielding Hudson (1870-1935), 138, 450, 507, 515, 519, 593

Gates, Frederick L., 515

Gay-Lussac, Joseph Louis (1778-1850), 42

Geikie, Archibald (1835-1924), 593

Gerardus of Cremona (1114-1187), 323

Gerhard, Benjamin (1812-1864), 42

Gershon-Cohen, Jacob (1899-1971), 953

Ghon, Anton (1886-1936), 547

Gibbon, John Heysham (1871-1956), 185.*13*

Gibbon, John Heysham (1903-1973), 185.*13, 511*

Gibbons, Henry (1840-1911), 729

Gibson, James Edgar (1875-1953), 889

Gilbert, Newell Clark (1880-1953), 552

Gilbridge, John J., 652

Gilfillan, William, 391

Girard College, Philadelphia, 1105, 1109

Girardi, Mario, 685

Glover, Thomas Joseph (b. 1887), 521

Goetze, Johann Cristoph (1688-1733), 31

Goldschmidt, Jules (b. 1843), 37

Gomoiu, Victor (1882-1960), 520

Gooch, John, 494

Good, William Harmar (b. 1909), 726

Goodman, Henry Ernest (1836-1896), 67

Gorgas, William Crawford (1854-1920), 486, 1025

Gould, Augustus Addison (1805-1863), 592

Gould, Sylvester Emanuel (b. 1900), 539

Graaf, Regnerus de (1641-1673), 1094

Grant, William Robertson (1811-1852), 773

Grassi, Candide Fréderic Antoine de (1753-1815), 1091

Gratz, Simon (1838-1925), 444

Gravesande, Willem Jacob Storm van s' (1688-1742), 653

Gravisi, Girolamo, 685

Gray, Asa (1810-1888), 113

Gray, William, 919

Gray and Bowen, publishers (London), 271

Great Britain. Army, 178, 183

Green, Ashbel (1762-1848), 855

Green, Jacob (1790-1841), 384, 388

Green, Louis David (1883-1937), 352

Green, Mary, 842

Green, Traill (1813-1897), 589

Gregg, Amos, 805h

Grier, Richard (d. 1808), 816

Griffin, Corbin (d. 1813), 931

Griffith, Robert Eglesfield (1798-1850), 155, 171?, 775

Griffiths, Elijah (d. 1847), 905

Grove, Robert (1634-1696), 687

Guy's Hospital, London, 484, 1101

Gye, William Ewart, 515

Gynecean Hospital, Philadelphia, 742

Haen, Antonius de (1704-1776), 269

Hahnemann, Samuel Christian Friedrich (1755-1843), 367, 615

Hahnemann Medical College, Philadelphia, 699

Halberstadt, George Howell (1855-1921), 726

Hall, Asaph (1829-1907), 877

Hall, Douglas, 747

Hall, Elisha (1754-1814), 918

Hall, William (fl. 1706), 114

Halsey, R., 515

Halsted, William Stewart (1852-1922), 346

Hamey, Baldwin (1568-1640), 687

Hamilton, George, 1125

Hamilton, James (1749-1835), 427, 1048

Hamilton, James Francis (d. 1902), 1124

Hamilton Hahn, Eugen (1839-1900), 317

Hammond, Frank Clinch, (1875-1941), 934

Hammond, William Alexander (1828-1900), 464, 679

Hancock, Richard, 924

Handy, Harry Tucker (b. 1874), 85

Hare, Francis Washington Everard (1851-1932), 346

Hare, Hobart Amory (1862-1931), 356

Hare, Robert (1781-1858), 42, 114, 169, 459

Harlan, George Cuvier (1835-1909), 1091

Harris, H.W., 806

Harris, Robert Patterson (1822-1899), 1066

Harris, Thomas (1784-1861), 721, 806, 1128

Harrison, John, 805i

Harrison, John Pollard (1796-1849), 825

Hartford (naval vessel), 194

Hartshorne, Edward (1818-1885), 439, 765

Harvard University, 42, 85, 196, 513, 542, 655

Harvey, William (1578-1657), 185.55, 300, 564, 645, 678, 687, 899, 1094

Hasbrouck, Ferdinand, 491

Hasson, Henri Marie (1772-1853), 805t

Hastings, Charles (1794-1866), 183

Hausheer, W.C., 962

Hayden, Ferdinand Vandeveer (1829-1887), 589, 592

Hays, Issac (1796-1879), 257, 470, 750, 775

Hays, Randall Burrows (1878-1938), 943

Headington, Richard Clement, 743

Heaviside, John (1748-1828), 440

Heberden, William (1710-1801), 183

Heidelberg University, 1071

Helmont, Jean Baptiste van (1577-1644), 645, 958

Hemmeter, John (1863-1931), 593

Hemphill, Joseph, 89

Henry, Frederick Porteous (1844-1919), 592

Henry, Joseph (1799-1878), 113

Henry Phipps Institute, Philadelphia, 206, 522

Heraty, E.J., 932

Herter, Christian Archibald (1865-1910), 669

Hewish, Edgar M., 853

Hickling, Daniel Percy (b. 1863), 670

Higgins, Charles Michael (b. 1854), 776

Hillary, William, 573

Hine, Elmore Charles (d. 1895), 431

Hinrichs, J.N., 424

Hirschler, Rose (1876-1940), 874

History of Science Society, 185.62

Hitzig, Eduard (1838-1904), 669

Hobart, Robert E. (fl. 1868), 173

Hodge, John (graduated 1769), 702

Hodgen, John Thompson (1826-1882), 711

Hodgkin, Thomas (1798-1866), 1115

Hoeber, Paul B. (publisher), 517

Hoffman, Clarence, 185.63

Holland, Henry (1788-1873), 271

Hollingwirth, William V., 304

Hollopeter, W.C., 652

Holloway, Lisabeth Marie Feind, 185.62

Holloway, Thomas Beaver (1872-1936), 519

Holmes, Oliver Wendell (1809-1894), 112

Holyoke, E.A., 446

Home for Friendless Children, Reading (Pa.), 429

Hope, John (1725-1786), 931

Hope, Thomas Charles, 111

Hôpital de Charité, Paris, 758

Hôpital des Enfants Malades, Paris, 331

Hôpital St. Louis, Paris, 758, 841

Hopkins, John, 219

Horner, William Edmonds (1793-1853), 250, 264, 588, 765, 791, 795, 806, 916, 1052, 1112

Horsley, Victor (1857-1916), 669

Hôtel Dieu de Paris, 758

Howard, Benjamin (1841-1901), 282

Howell, Abraham (d. ca. 1834), 243

Hubbard, John Perry (b. 1903), 185.13

Hubbard, LeRoy Watkins (1857-1938), 949

Hughes, Samuel (b. 1732), 691

Hughes, Samuel, Jr., 691

Hull, Cordell (1871-1955), 507

Hunt, William (1825-1896), 588

Huston, Robert M. (1794-1864), 388
Hutchinson, James (1752-1793), 573
Hutchinson, James Howell (1834-1889), 36, 765
Hutchison, Joseph Chrisman (1827-187), 390-91
Huxley, Thomas Henry (1825-1895), 183.*591*
Hyrtl, Joseph (1811-1894), 185.*632*

Ibn al-Jazzar (d. 1009), 190
Ingersoll, Charles E. (1920-1982), 185.*18*
Institute for the Control of Syphilis, Philadelphia, 420
International Congress of Dermatology, 1907, 58
International Congress of Otolaryngology, 1957, 22
International Congress on the History of Medicine, 1935, 529
————, 1959, 544
International Congress on Hygiene and Demography, 1912, 1063
International Leprosy Conference, 1897, 37
International Physiological Congress, 13th, 518
International Society of Surgeons, 32
Irvine, Matthew (ca. 1755-1827), 1099
Irwin, William F., 821
Ives, Eli (1779-1861), 596
Ives, Sarah Edith (1873-1957), 871
Ivy, Andrew Conway (b. 1893), 473

Jackson, Edward, 943
Jackson, George Thomas (1852-1916), 58
Jackson, James (1777-1867), 330
Jackson, John Hughlings (1834-1911), 669, 679
Jackson, Robert, 573
James, Isabella, 173
James, Robert Ruston (1881-1959), 138
Jameson, Robert, 11
Jameson, Thomas, 805l
Janssen van Ceulen, Cornelius (1593-1664?), 687
Jarcho, Saul Wallenstein (b. 1906), 16
Jefferson, Thomas (1743-1826), 275, 844
John XXI, pope (1226-1277), 643

Johnson, Robert (d. 1793), 851
Johnson, Samuel (1787-1872), 791
Johnstone, John (1607-1675), 111
Jones, Absalom, 919
Jones, J. Levering (b. 1851), 678
Jordan, Henry Dowling (1874-1959), 784
Jordanus de Turre (fl. 1335), 28
Jouenne, François, 1020

Kalodner, J.E., 341
Kaposi, Moritz (1837-1902), 313
Kaufman, Harry M., 511
Kearsley, John (1684-1772), 200
Keating, John, 821
Keating, John Marie (1852-1893), 834, 994
Keeting, William H., 775
Keitel, A., 629
Kelly, Aloysius Oliver Joseph (1870-1911), 885
Kelly, Howard Atwood (1858-1943), 404
Kennedy, John Pendleton (1795-1870), 270
Kepler, Johannes (1571-1630), 877
Kern, Richard Arminius (1891-1982), 185.*13*
Kerr, John Graham (1824-1901), 1065-6
Ketch, Samuel (1855?-1899), 865
Kety, Seymour Solomon (b. 1915), 879
King, W.S., 932
Kircher, Athanasius (1602-1680), 958
Kirkpatrick, Thomas Percy Claude (1869-1954), 346
Kneass, Samuel Stryker (1864-1928), 312
Kokkes, Dr. (16th cent.), 66
Kuhl, Marcus Hillegas (fl. 1786-1792), 570

Lacaze, Louis (fl. 1831), 172
Laënnec Society, 1063
Lagrange, Pierre Felix (1857-1928), 1137
Lake, M.J. (Mrs.), 737
Lamarck, Jean Baptiste Antoine de Monet (1744-1829), *591*
Lambert, Aylmer Bourke (1761-1842), 113

Lambert, Samuel Waldron (1859-1942), 486

Landis, Henry Robert Murray (1872-1937), 299

Landolt, Edmund (1846-1926), 245, 1137

Lansing, Dorothy I., 1029

Laplace, Ernest (1861-1924), 784

Larice, Albina, 521

Laub, C.H., 845

Lavater, Johann Caspar (1741-1801), 183

Lavoisier, Antoine Laurent (1743-1794), 386, 1125

Lawrance, Benjamin Hornor, 4

Lawrance, Jason Valentine, 4

Lazzell, James McLane (b. 1824), 1128

Lea, Issac (1792-1886), 89

Lea and Febiger, publishers, 516

Leake, Chauncey Depew (b. 1896), 514

Lee, Arthur, 931

Lee, Benjamin (1833-1913), 776

Lee, Roger Irving (1881-1965), 514

Leeds, Gideon (?), 814

Leeuwenhoek, Antony van (1632-1723), 697, 1094

Le Fanu, William Richard (b. 1904), 138

Lehman, George F. (fl. 1810-1859?), 915

Leib, Michael (1761-1822), 114

Leibniz, Gottfried Wilhelm (1646-1716), 1094

Le Moyne, Francis Julius (1798-1879), 167, 597, 823

Lettsom, John Coakley (1744-1815), 111, 494

Levan, George Kistler (b. 1877), 341

Levengood, Howard Wilson (b. 1882), 341

Levering, John, 762

Levick, James Jones (1824-1893), 213, 439, 1118

Levis, Richard J. (1827-1890), 248

Lewis, Francis Park (1855-1940), 943

Lewis, Margaret Adeline (Reed) (b. 1881), 534

Lewis, Samuel (1813-1890), 44, 61, 111, 185.*13, 34, 613*, 446, 582, 604, 679, 1066

Lewis, Warren Harmon (1870-1964), 520, 534

Library Company, Philadelphia, 889, 896

Lind, James (1716-1791), 573, 900

Lippincott, Henry C., 776

Lipscomb, William (1754-1842), 640

Littré, Maximilien Paul Émile (1801-1881), 1094

Lizars, Alexander Jardine, 111

Lloyd. assistant surgeon (1865-1866), 1042

Lloyd, James Hendrie (1853-1932), 1075-76

Lobstein, Johann Friedrich Daniel (1777-1840), 804

Locatelli, Giacomo, 1027

Lodi, Pierre, pseud., see Viaud, Julien

Lodewick, Christopher, see Ludwick, Christopher

Long, Esmond Ray (1890-1979), 515

Long, John Wesley (1859-1927), 1008

Long Island College Hospital, Brooklyn, 390-91

Longaker, Daniel Carel (1858-1949), 940

Longcope, Warfield Theobald (1877-1953), 507, 514-15, 519-20, 529

Loomis, Joseph Griswold (1811-1853), 699

Lorimer, John (b. 1722), 111

Loutfian, John Ludwig (1875-1939), 341

Lovell, Joseph (1788-1836), 42

Lowenburg, Harry (1878-1943), 652, 769

Loyola University, Chicago, 253

Lucas, Prosper (1815-1885), 395

Ludwick, Christopher, 896

Ludwig, Christian Friedrich (1751-1823), 367

Lyon, Bethuel Boyd Vincent (1880-1953), 79

Macalister, Alexander (1862-1938), 940

McCall, Edwin LeRoy, 805n

MacCallum, William George (1874-1944), 507

McClellan, George W. (1796-1847), 251, 384

McClellan, John (1762-1846), 695

McClenahan, William Urie (b. 1899), 767

MacCormac, William (1836-1901), 36

McCoy, George Walter (b. 1876), 244

McCrae, Thomas (1870-1935), 753

McDowell, Augustus William (d. 1878), 1042

McGill University, 1, 752

McHenry, James, 268

McIntyre, Donald (fl. 1767-1769), 111

Mackenzie, Morell (1837-1892), 317

McKenzie, Robert Tait (1867-1938), 185.*632*, 507

McMorran, John, 1130

Macrae, James W.F., 825

Macreight, Daniel C., 112

McWilliam, William, 955, 1049

Magendie, François (1783-1855), 4

Magill, Edward Hicks (1825-1907), 589

Mallory Institute of Phatology, 581

Malpighi, Marcello (1629-1694), 697, 1094

Marburg, Otto (1878-1948), 547

Marcellini, Joannes Petrus A., 648

Marcotte, Oscar, 776

Margarita, queen of Spain, 643

Maris, Richard (1808-1891), 461

Markoe, Thomas Masters (1819-1901), 390

Marshall, John (1855-1925), 540, 630, 1080

Martin, Edward (1859-1938), 265, 799

Martin, John S., 805m

Martin, Samuel, 931

Martinet, Louis (1795-1875), 242

Martini, Petrus and Franciscus (fl. 1497), 1056

Masini, Giulio, 633

Massey, Anne, 634

Mattioli (Matthiolus). Petro Andrea (1500-1577), 393

Mauthner, Ludwig (1840-1894), 313

Mayo, Charles Horace (1865-1939), 253

Mayo, William James (1861-1939), 487

Mayo Clinic, Rochester, 32

Mays, Ralph Whiteman (1907-1976), 167

Mead, Kate Hurd, 185.*239*

Mead, Richard (1673-1754), 177, 269

Mease, James (1771-1846), 479

Medical Club of Philadelphia, 1059

Medical Documentation Service, Philadelphia, 185.*611*

Medical Examiner, 330

Medical Institute of Philadelphia, 141

Medical Jurisprudence Society of Philadelphia, 1059

Medical News, 875

Medical Register of New York, New Jersey and Connecticut, 1084

Medical Society, Edinburgh, 931

Medical Society of Ohio, 69

Medical Society of the State of Pennsylvania, 523, 1039

Meek, Fielding Bradford (1817-1876), 592

Meigs, Arthur Vincent (1850-1912), 185.*13*

Meigs, Charles Delucena (1792-1869), 112, 289, 765, 795

Meigs, Joe Vincent (1892-1963), 514

Meigs, John Forsyth (1818-1882), 625, 765

Meltzer, Samuel James (1851-1920), 486

Mencken, Henry Louis (1880-1956), 89

Mercurialis, Hieronymus (1530-1606), 959

Merrill, Ayres Phillips (1793-1873), 579

Merritt, Anna Lea (1844-1930), 588

Mesue Damascenus, Johannes (ca. 777-857), 647

Mettler, Lee Harrison, 651

Metz, Herman A. (1867-1934), 244

Mewhinney, James C. (1859-1933), 1037

Meyer, Adolf (1866-1950), 670

Meyer, Willy (1858-1932), 235

Michael, F. Robert, 185.*18*

Mid-Eastern Regional Medical Library Service, 185.*611*

Mifflin, C., 806

Mifflin family, 84

Military Order of the Loyal Legion of the United States, 217

Mill, Henry, 481

Miller, Edward (1760-1812), 112

Miller, Thomas Grier (1886-1981), 185.*13*, 455, 863
Mills, Harry Brooker (1869-1947), 652
Minot, George Richards (1885-1950), 514-15, 520
Minot, Henry J. (b. 1887), 748
Minsky, Henry J. (b. 1895), 247
Miskjian, Hagore G. (b. 1887), 748
Mitchell, Albert Graeme (1889-1941), 356
Mitchell, John S., 45
Mitchell, Mary Cadwalader (d. 1914), 185.*2110*
Mitchell, Samuel Latham (1764-1831), 114
Mitchell, Thomas James, 675
Mohican (naval vessel), 195
Mombreloz, de (Reverend), 189
Montaña, Aloysius, 695
Montgomery, James, 894
Mooney, Herbert C., 346
Moore, John, 932
Moore, John Percy, 590
Morand, Sauveur François (1697-1773), 698
Moreau, Jacques Louis (1771-1826), 805t
Morehouse, George Read (1829-1905), 684
Morozzo, count, 39
Morris, J. Cheston (1831-1923), 965
Morris, Henry, 185.*63*
Morris, John (1759-1793), 575
Morris, Malcolm Alexander (1849-1924), 841
Morris, Robert (1823-1913), 185.*63*
Morrison, Albert C., 177
Morse, Elliott How (b. 1916), 185.*611*
Morse, Samuel Finley Breese (1791-1872), 113
Morton, Thomas George (1835-1903), 397
Morton, William James (1845?-1920), 346
Morton, William Thomas Green (1819-1868), 91
Moseley, Benjamin (1742-1819), 573
Moseley, William, 825
Mosher, Thomas Bird (1852-1923), 346
Motais, Ernest (1845-1913), 1137
Mott, Valentine (1785-1865), 112

Mount Sinai Hospital, New York, 466
Moyer, Elizabeth, 185.*63*
Mudd, Emily Hartshorne (b. 1898), 856
Mudd, Harvey Gilmer (1857-1933), 711
Mudd, Henry Hodgen (1844-1899), 711
Muhlenberg, Henry A. (1753-1815), 113
Mulgrave, John, see Sheffield, John, Duke of Buckingham
Muller, George Paul (1877-1947), 185.*13*
Mundall, John H., 850
Murphy, John Benjamin (1857-1916), 238
Murray, Charles, 477
Musschenbroek, Petrus van (1692-1761), 653
Myers, Leonard S., 242

Nancrède, Charles Beylard Guerard de (1847-1921), 36
Nariskin, lady, 1005
National Library of Medicine, 780
Neff, Joseph Seal (1854-1930), 354
Neidhard, Charles (1809-1895), 699
Neill, John (1819-1880), 161, 185.*218*
Neilson, Thomas Rundle (1857-1939), 185.*13*, 1068
Nelli, Giovanni Battista Clemente (1725-1793), 877
New York City. Board of Health, 795
New York Medical Society, 934
New York Surgical Society, 796
New York World's Fair, 528
Newbold, Mary Scott, 185.*236*
Newcomer, John, 1128
Newton, Issac (1642-1726), 625, 653
Nicholson, John (d. 1800?), 919
Niemeyer, Felix von (1821-1871), 1034
Nightingale, Florence (1820-1910), 113
Nobl, Gabriel, 58
Norris, Charles Camblos (1877-1961), 726
Norris, Henry (1875-1941), 726
Norris, Issac (1834-1918), 84
North, Edward Washington (1778-1843), 805o

North American Medical and Surgical Journal, 481
Norwalk General Hospital, 706
Nott, Josiah Clark (1804-1873), 589
Nuttall, Thomas (1786-1859), 113

Oeconomiae historicus, 40
Oertel, Dr. (Ansbach, Germany), 1071
Oliver, Charles Augustus (1854-1911), 728, 1024
Ontyd, Coenraad Gerard (1776-1844), 494
Ord, George (1781-1866), 185.*613*
O'Reilly, Robert Maitland (1845-1912), 491, 679
Ostheimer, Maurice (1873-1954), 1085
Otis, George Alexander (1830-1881), 36

Packard, Francis Randolf (1970-1950), 138, 185.*13*, 253, 519, 626, 671, 726, 780
Packard, Frederick Adolph (1862-1902), 700
Packard, John Hooker (1832-1907), 589, 765, 1034
Paget, James (1814-1899), 679
Pallis, Bertha, 647
Pan American Congress, 1892, 867
Pancoast, Henry Khunrath (1875-1939), 356
Pancoast, Joseph (1805-1882), 112, 185.*216*, 271, 397, 439
Pancoast, William Henry (1835-1897), 12, 701
Pannel, John, 624
Paracelsus, Theophrastus (1493-1541), 9, 958
Paré, Ambroise (1510?-1590), 333
Paris, Collège de France, 577
Paris, John Ayrton (1785-1856), 183
Parke, William Ernest (1862-1944), 940
Parker, Frederic (b. 1890), 581
Parker, John, 805p
Parker, Willard (1800-1884), 390
Parkman, George (1790-1849), 242
Parrish, Edward (1822-1872), 1112
Parrish, Issac (1811-1852), 185.*218*, 464, 765
Paschall, Joseph, 179
Pasteur, Louis (1822-1895), 864

Pasteur Institutes, 487
Patten, W. (fl. 1555), 66
Patterson, Robert (1743-1824), 45
Patterson, Robert Maskell (1787-1854), 112
Pattison, Granville Sharp (1792-1851), 271, 388
Paul, Joseph W. (d. 1842), 760
Pavia, Nosomio, 1027
Pearce, Richard Mills (1874-1930), 930
Pearson, Abiel (1756-1827), 446
Peers (Petrus?) of Salerno, 643
Pellier de Quengry, Guillaume (1750-1835), 1137
Pemberton, Israel (1715-1779), 339
Pemberton, Ralph (1877-1949), 185.*238*
Pemberton Family, 84
Pendergrass, Eugene Percival (1895-1980), 529
Penington, E., 446
Pennsylvania. General Assembly, 42
Pennsylvania. National Guard, 515
Pennsylvania State Quarantine Board, 185.*16*
Penrose, Charles Bingham (1862-1925), 742
Penrose family, 84
Pepper, William (1874-1947), 356, 519, 780
Percival, Thomas (1740-1804), 150
Pereira, Jonathan (1804-1853), 112
Perrot, Émile, 582
Peterson, Frederick (1859-1938), 670
Petrus de Barulo, 643
Petrus de Salernia, 643
Petrus de Trano, 632
Petrus Hispanus, 643
Pew, Joseph N., Jr., 185.*2116*
Pfahler, George Edward (1874-1957), 701
Philadelphia. Board of Education, 420
Philadelphia. Board of Guardians of the Poor, 38
Philadelphia. Board of Health, 243, 287
Philadelphia Almshouse, 72
Philadelphia College of Medicine, 71, 168, 349, 583, 786, 950, 984
Philadelphia College of Pharmacy and Science, 118-19, 1099
Philadelphia Dental College, 701

Philadelphia Dispensary, 1107
Philadelphia Heart Association, 523
Philadelphia Insane Asylum, 594-95
Philadelphia Journal of the Medical and Physical Sciences, 17
Philadelphia Lying-in Charity Hospital, 226
Philadelphia Marriage Council, 856
Philadelphia Medical College, 42, 185.*215*
Philadelphia Nurses Home, 226
Philadelphia Obstetrical Society, 185.*2210*, 492
Philadelphia Polyclinic, 1025
Philadelphia Psychiatric Society, 368
[Philadelphia] Select and Common Council on. . .Preventing Malignant Fever, 1127
Philip IV, king of France (1285-1314), 5
Phillips, Thomas, MS. 9402, 442
Phrenological Society of Calcutta, 764
Phrenological Society of Philadelphia, 764
Physiological Review, 518
Pick, Walther (1874-1932), 547
Pierce, Louise, 520
Pillmore, George Utley (1892-1961), 421
Pinel, Philippe (1745-1826), 605
Pinel, Pierre Louis, 1020
Pitcairn, John, 37
Plinius Secundus, Caius (23-79), 958
Polakowsky, H., 37
Pomeroy, Eduard P., 812
Porrée, Victor, 1020
Posey, William Campbell (1866-1934), 886, 1129
Pott, Percival (1713-1788), 269, 479
Potter, Nathaniel Bowditch (1869-1919), 1089
Potts, Jonathan (1745-1781), 173
Powel, Mary Edith, 593
Power, D'Arcy (1855-1941), 138, 507, 679, 687, 1015
Preston, Francis F. Cleveland, 491
Preston, Jonas (1764-1836), 838
Pridgeon, Lily G.H. (b. 1872), 872
Priestly, Joseph (1733-1804), 39, 114, 183, 1125
Princeton University, 389, 894
Pringle, John (1707-1782), 892, 899

Pringle, John James (1855-1922), 841
Priscianus, Theodorus (4th cent.), 618
Proctor, William (1817-1874), 790

Radcliffe College, Cambridge (Ma.), 856
Ramón y Cajal, Santiago (1852-1934), 669
Ramsay, Henry A., 875
Randall, Alexander, 185.*632*
Randolph, Jacob (1796-1848), 721
Randolph, John Field (d. 1880), 213
Randolph, Nathaniel Archer (1858-1888), 1080
Randolph Macon Medical College, Prince Edward (Va.), 657-58
Ravdin, Isidore Schwaner (1894-1972), 514
Raymundus de Moleriis (fl. 1335), 28
Read, John (fl. 1758), 10
Red Cross, U.S., 488
Reed, Walter (1851-1902), 679, 801
Regeneration de l'homme, 30
Regimen sanitatis, 27, 643
Research Institute of Cutaneous Medicine, Philadelphia, 244
Revere, John (1787-1847), 388
Rhees, Benjamin Rush (1798-1831), 384
Rhett, Henry J., 837
Rhoads, Jonathan Evans (b. 1907), 185.*13*
Rhoads family, 84
Ribot, Théodule Armand (1839-1916), 395
Richardson, Maurice Howe (1851-1912), 238
Richardson, Robert Pryor, 262
Richardson, William, 471
Riehl, Gustav (1855-1943), 58
Riesman, David (1867-1940), 253, 356, 507, 519
Ritchie, Thomas Hendry (1801-1836), 766
Rivers, William Cabell (1793-1868), 270
Rivinus, Edward Florens (1801-1873), 112
Robert, A. Sidney, 865
Roberts, Norman (b. 1876), 346
Roberts, Sidney, 949

Robertson, Robert (1742-1829), 573

Robinson, George Canby (1878-1960), 507, 515

Rockefeller Institute (University), New York, 652

Rodenheiser, Edwin William (b. 1890), 423

Rodman, William Louis (1853-1916), 623, 652, 784

Rogers, Frank Bradway (b. 1914), 16

Rogers, James Blythe (1802-1852), 1110

Rogers, Robert Empie (1813-1884), 589, 1032

Rogers, Will (1879-1935), 1025

Roosevelt, Franklin Delano (1882-1945), 507

Roosevelt, Theodore (1858-1919), 253

Rosemond, George Parrott (b. 1910), 185.*13*

Rosenberger, Emil, 776

Rossander, Carl Jacob (1828-1901), 282

Rous, Francis Peyton (1879-1970), 507

Rowley, William (1742-1806), 1027

Royal College of Physicians, London, 275

Royal College of Surgeons, 1015, 1083

Rudolf II, emperor (1576-1612), 80

Rufz de Lavison, Étienne (b. 1806), 330

Rush Hospital for Consumption. . ., Philadelphia, 1036

Russell, Alexander (1715?-1768), 111

Russell, Frederick Fuller (1870-1960), 558

Russell, Patrick (1727-1804), 111

Ruston, Thomas (Mrs.) (d. 1797), 931

Rutherford, Daniel (1749-1819), 427

Rutledge, Edward (1712-1780?), 706

Ryff, Walter Hermann (16th cent.), 941

Sänger, Max (1853-1903), 739

Sailer, Joseph, 715

St. Agnes Hospital, Philadelphia, 742, 1063

St. George's Hospital, London, 426

St. Louis Dermatological Society, 370

St. Martin, Alexis (1794-1880), 42

St. Thomas Hospital, London, 177

Saint Yves, Charles de (1667-1736), 1137

Sajous, Louis Theo de Médicis, 934

Saliceto Placentinus, Guliemus de (1210-1280), 423

Sanctorius Sanctorius (1561-1636), 685, 877

Saranac Lake Medical Society, Osler Club, 991

Sargent, Fitzwilliam (1820-1889), 463

Sargent, Winthrop (1753-1820), 446

Sarton, George Alfred Léon (1884-1956), 507

Saunders, W.B. Co., publishers, 356

Sayre, Lewis Albert (1820-1900), 36

Schaeffer, Jacob Parsons (1878-1970), 185.*13*

Schamberg, Jay Frank (1870-1934), 244, 776

Scheie Eye Institute, Philadelphia, 396

Schenck, Harry P. (1894-1978), 185.*63*, *631*

Schireson, Henry Junius, 602

Schively, Mary Alice, 869

Schlumberger, Hans Georg (b. 1913), 608

Schmidt, Henry D. (1823-1888), 589

Schofield, Frederick Sewall (1895-1963), 770

Scholtz, Samuel Gottleib, 1094

Schoonover, Ezekiel, 243

Schrick, Michael (d. 1472), 31

Schulz, Theodor, 113

Schwarz, Frigyes, 292

Schwenk, Peter Nathaniel Klinger (1854-1934), 1137

Science de la conaissance des maladies, 189

Scientific Chemical Company, New York, 244

Scripps, Robert Paine (1895-1938), 89

Scutellio, Antonio (18th cent.), 1057

Segal, Meyer (b. 1890), 341

Selden, Henry (1818?-1855), 462

Semon, Felix (1849-1921), 981

Sewall, Thomas (1787-1845), 42

Seybert, Adam (1773-1825), 607

Shallcross, Morris Cadwalader (1846-1898), 129

Sharswood, George (1810-1883), 406

Shattuck, George Cheyne (1813-1893), 251

Sheffield, John, duke of Buckingham (1648-1721), 165
Sherrington, Charles Scott (1857-1952), 669
Shippen, Joseph (1732-1810), 1048
Shippen, Joseph Galloway (d. 1857), 909
Shivers, Thomas, Jr., 260
Shoemaker, John Veitch (1852-1910), 784
Short Character of Charles ye Second, 165
Shryock, Richard Harrison (1893-1972), 371
Sigerist, Henry Ernest (1891-1957), 529
Sigma Xi, 518
Siler, Joseph Franklin (b. 1875), 558
Silliman, Benjamin (1779-1864), 42, 114
Silva, Donato, 618
Sims, Francis (1823-1880), 699
Singer, Charles Joseph (1876-1960), 507, 563
Sinkler, Wharton (1845-1910), 185.34, 737
Slaughter, W.B., 213
Smibert, Williams, 706, 931
Smith, Edgar Fahs (1856-1928), 590
Smith, Ellsworth Fayssoux (1825-1896), 711
Smith, Ellsworth Stricker (1864-1940), 711
Smith, G. Robert, 330
Smith, John Mark (1812-1871), 141
Smith, Maria Wilkins, 860
Smith, Theobald, 515
Smith, William (1727-1803), 706
Smith, William Bowers (b. 1893), 558
Société des Medicine de Bordeaux, 1091
Société française d'Otologie, de Laryngologie et de Rhinologie, 1083
Société Médicale d'Observation, Paris, 330
Society for Bettering the Condition of the Poor, London, 1127
Society for the Improvement of Medical Knowledge, London, 931
Society for the Protection of Scientific Research, 523
Society of Apothecaries, London, 271

Solis-Cohen, Solomon (1857-1948), 346
Somervail, Alexander (1758-1833), 112
Sommer, John (fl. 1810), 911
Southern Dispensary for the Medical Relief of the Poor, 42
Sower, Chistopher, Jr. (1721-1784), 619
Spare, Aristoph, 784
Spalding, Lyman (1775-1821), 450
Spector, Benjamin (1893-1976), 560
Spencer, Herbert (1820-1903), 395
Spitzka, Edward Anthony (1876-1922), 593
Springs, Andrew Wilton (1869-1944), 801
Spurzheim, Johann Christoph (1776-1832), 183
Stahl, Georg Ernst (1660-1734), 697
Stanley, Edward (1791-1862), 112
Starr, Louis (1849-1925), 765, 1077, 1080
State of His Late Majesty's Body [Charles II], 165
Stefanie Children's Hospital, Budapest, 81
Stejskal, Karl ritter von (b. 1872), 547
Stelwagen, Henry Weightman (1853-1919), 1079
Stephenson, Sydney (1862-1923), 346
Stevens, Alexander Hodgdon (1789-1869), 795
Stewardson, Thomas (1807-1878), 330
Stewart, Samuel?, 805s
Sieglitz, Julius Oscar (1867-1937), 244
Stillé Society Library, 26
Stockton, Elias Boudinot (d. 1818), 928
Stoeber, Victor (1803-1871), 1137
Stout, Samuel Hollingsworth (1822-1903), 413
Stoy, Henry William (1726-1801), 1132
Strawbridge, George (1844-1914), 1080
Strotz, Charles Martin, 341
Stroud, William Daniel (1891-1959), 538
Stuart, Charles, 1091
Stuart, David, 223
Stuart, Edwin S., 185.2216
Suesserott, Jacob Louis (1829-1886), 371

Swaim, William, 804, 806

Swammerdam, Jan (1637-1680), 697, 1094

Sweet, Joshua Edwin (1876-1957), 556

Sydenham, Thomas (1624-1689), 9, 899

Ta Sheng Pien, 1065-66

Taft, William Howard (1857-1930), 507

Tanner, Benjamin Tucker (1835-1923), 701

Taylor, Alfred Bower (1824-1898), 129

Taylor, Samuel, bookbinder, 84

Taylor, William, 271

Taylor, William Long (1853-1931), 779, 1079

Temkin, Owsei (b. 1902),559-60

Temple University. School of Medicine, 41, 244, 503-3, 934

Terson, Albert (1867-1935), 1137

Thayer, Stephen Henry (1839-1919), 346

Thayer, William Sidney (1864-1932), 687

Thomas, Arthur H. Company, Philadelphia, 509

Thompson, Samuel, 450

Toles (Towles?), John (?), 805t

Trenton Community Chest, 288

Trinder, William Martin, 494

Tri-County Medical Society (Pa.), 849

Tri-State Medical Association, 26, 236

Trumbull, Jonathan (1740-1809), 706

Trumbull, Jonathan (1844-1919), 346

Tryon, George Washington (1838-1888), 588

Tucker, Aaron B. (d. 1839), 820

Tuke, Daniel Hack (1827-1895), 669

Tully, William (1785-1859), 596

Tunstall, C., see Constable, Cuthbert

Turner, Edward (1798-1837), 42

Turner's Lane Hospital, Philadelphia, 684

Tyson, Ralph Maguire, 769

Underwood, Edgar Ashworth (b. 1899), 563

Union Benevolent, Philadelphia, 276

United States Army. Base Hospital, Le Tréport, 530, 756

————. Base Hospital, Nantes, 32

————. Bureau of Medicine and Surgery, 1128

————. Camp Upton, 483

————. General Hospital, Chester (Pa.), 35

————. Headquarter's Hospital Center, Kerhouan, 1008

————. Medical Corps, 956

————. Medical Library, see National Library of Medicine

————. Officers Reserve Corps, 528

————. Veterans Volunteers, 1042

United States Navy, 251

————. Marine Hospital Service, 327

United State Board of Medical Examiners, 867

United States Pension Examining Surgeons, Annual Meeting, 1910, 230

United States Radium Corporation, 521

United States Senate, 244

University of Edinburgh, 13, 73-75, 111

————. See also Lectures and Lecture notes, Edinburgh

University of Ghana, 185.*16*

University of Illinois, 473

University of Maryland, 275

University of Michigan, 32, 1088

University of Pennsylvania, 432, 1110

————. Medical Department, Medical School, and Subdivisions are combined as *see also* references following no. 1054, except

————. Graduate School of Medicine, 420, 526, 879-80

————. Hospital, 526, 730, 1010, 1014

————. Library, 50

————. School of Dentistry, 522, 623

University of Virginia, 275

Upton, George, 1042

Ushakoff, Vasily Gavrilovich (b. 1865), 487

Valeri, Gaetano (1818-1882), 112
Vander Veer, Henry (1792-1874), 49, 151
Van Dyke, Henry (1852-1933), 346
Van Dyke, Rush (1813-1882), 464
Vaughen, Victor Clarence (1851-1929), 776
Vehr, Irenaeus (d. 1710), 1061
Veitch, Mary (fl. 1758), 10
Venice. Collegio dei Medici Fisici, 1057
Venn, John (1834-1923), 687
Viaticum, 190
Viaud, Julien (1850-1923), 346
Vieussens, Raymond (1641-1715), 697
Villa, Jacquin, 695
Vinci, Leonardo da (1452-1519), 452
Vir Publishing Company, 986
Virchow, Rudolf Ludwig Karl (1821-1902), 37, 317
Viviani, Vincenzio (1622-1703), 877
Vogt, Adolf, 776
Von Mikulicz-Radecki, Johannes (1850-1905), 1137

Wade, Ella Nora (b.1892),185.*631*
Wagoner, George W. (1896-1957), 526, 529
Waldenburg, Louis (1837-1881), 286
Waldeyer, Heinrich Wilhelm Gottfried (1836-1921), 317
Walker, Arthur Meeker (1896-1955), 546
Wallace, James Westwood Mason (d. 1833), 825
Wallace, William S. (fl. 1821-1824), 202
Ward, H.K., 1051
Ward, Townsend (1817-1885), 446
Warner, Andrew F. (d. 1825), 969
Warren, John Collins (1778-1856), 42
Warren, John Collins (1842-1927), 36
Warren, Joseph Weatherhead (1849-1916), 623
Warren, Stafford Leak (b. 1896), 235
Warrington, Joseph (1805-1888), 804
Washington, Bailey (1787-1854), 1128
Washington, George (1732-1799), 954
Washington, Margaretta, 730
Washington, Mary, 918

Washington Medical College, Baltimore, 656, 659
Waterhouse, Benjamin (1754-1846), 443
Waters, W.N.B., 251
Watts, John (1785-1831), 15
Watts, Robert (1812-1867), 390
Webster, John White (1793-1850), 42
Wecker, Hans Jacob (1524-1586), 393
Weiss, Charles, 1051
Welch, William Henry (1850-1934), 346-47, 486, 507, 848, 1025
Welch, Henry Miller (1827-1921), 776
Weller, Carl Vernon (b. 1887), 1067
Wells, Horace (1815-1848), 1096
Wenzel, Mary, (d. 1936), 870
WFIL, radio station, 801
Wharton, Henry Redwood (1853-1925), 837
Wharton, Thomas (1735-1778), 84
Whilldin, John Galloway (1797-1824), 481
Whisten, William (1667-1752), 653
White, A.M., 721
White, Andrew Dickson (1832-1918), 346
White, James Clarke (1833-1916), 36, 58
White, James William (1850-1916), 837
White, William Hale (1857-1949), 484
White Haven Sanatorium, 207, 1063
Whitehouse, Henry Howard (b. 1864), 970-71
Whitmore, Eugene Randolph (b. 1874), 558
Wien (Vienna) University, 547
Wikoff, George H., 41
Wilhelmi, K., 716
Willard, De Forrest (1846-1910), 1080
Williamson, Walter (1811-1870), 699
Wills, William Le Moyne (1853-1933), 823
Willson, Robert Newton (1873-1916), 776
Wilson, Julius Lane (b. 1897), 726
Wilson, Samuel (1803-1832), 481
Winchilsea, earl of Finch, 687
Wintrobe, Maxwell Myer (b. 1901), 534

Wistar, Caspar (1761-1818), 84
Wistar, Issac Jones (1827-1905), 588, 1092
Wistar, Richard (1727-1781), 84
Wistar Institute, Philadelphia, 421
Witman, Henry, 631
Wolff, Ludwig (b. 1860), 282
Wolman, Irving Jacob (b. 1905), 769
Wood, C.H., 1115
Wood, Caroline (Mrs. George Bacon W.) (1805-1865), 1122
Wood, Casey Albert (1856-1942), 138
Wood, David C., 1115
Wood, Eliza Huldah Longacre (1837-1912), 1123
Wood, Emlen (b. 1889), 858
Wood, Francis Carter (1869-1951), 185.*13*, 521
Wood, Helen Foss (b. 1872), 1123
Wood, Horatio Charles (1874-1958), 652
Wood, Leonard (1860-1927), 680
Wood, Robert Crooke (1800-1869), 98
Woods, Edward A., 776
Woodson, Robert Scott (b. 1865), 680
Wormley, Theodore George (1826-1897), 623, 936, 1080, 1124
Worthington, Wilmer (1804-1873), 149

Wright, Edith Armstrong (b. 1906), 665
Wright, William, 446
Würdemann, Henry Vanderbilt (1865-1938), 346
Wyman, Jeffries (1814-1874), 592, 679
Wynn, L.G., 806

Yale University, 275, 596, 679, 969-71
Yeates, Jasper (1745-1817), 45
Yellowly, John (1774-1842), 444
Young, Arthur (1741-1820), 394
Young, John Richardson (1782-1804), 623

Zanardi, Martinus (fl. 1497), 1056
Zanetti, Joannes Hieronymus (18th cent.), 685
Ziegler, Ernst (1849-1905), 864
Ziegler, Jacob Lindemuth (1822-1906), 237
Zinsser, Hans (1878-1940), 515
Zoelle, P.A., 341
Zulatti, Angelo (18th cent.), 1027
Zulick, Howell Shoener, 652
Zumbusch, Leo ritter von (1874-1920), 547

Index II

Topical index of subjects

Abnormalities. See Anomalies
Acetanilide, 1078
Adenocarcinoma, 981
Air, 39
Alchemy, 513, 630
Alcohol, effects of, 78
Allergies, 755
Amblyopia, 946
Amputation, 177
Anatomy
   Early, to 1800, 133, 268, 283, 295,
   399-400, 447-49, 689-90, 692-94,
   955
   Post-1800, 185.229, 231, 340, 363,
   365, 391, 425, 440, 471, 475, 484,
   489, 540, 577, 588, 743, 784-85,
   812, 825, 827, 941, 970, 1052
Anemia, 316, 581, 960
Anesthesia, 42, 91, 1009, 1096
Aneurysm, 94, 709
Ankle, 93
Anomalies, anatomical, 70, 110, 279,
   293, 309, 319, 403, 441, 506, 623,
   717, 847, 967
Anoxia, 376
Anthrax, 864
Antimony, 1116
Aphasia, 186-87, 1036
Aphorisms, medical, 172, 406
Apoplexy. See Cerebral hemorrhage
Apothecaries, France, 7
Appendicitis, 239
Appetite, 473
Arsenic, 834, 1020, 1116
Arsphenamine, 244
Arteries, 447, 846
Arthropyosis, 938
Astrology, 948
Atomic theory, 42
Autopsies,165, 331, 358, 508, 526,
   536, 754, 1020, 1040

Bactericides, 174
Bacteriology, 503, 864, 1013, 1051,
   1073
Bees, 999
Beriberi, 65
Bibliography, medical, 977. Biblio-
   graphies of individual authors are
   listed under their names
Bile, 129
Biography, 211, 270, 1084
Bilious remitting fever. See Malaria
Biochemistry, 540, 616
Biology, 340, 589-92. See also Botany,
   Zoology, etc.
Birth control, 61
Bladder, 744
Blind, 271
Blood, 278, 291, 376, 392, 438, 447,
   587, 864, 979
Blood circulation, 4, 697, 878
Blood cells, veterinary, 535
Blood diseases, 528, 993
Blood vessels, 225, 295. See also Arte-
   ries; Cardiovascular system; Veins
Bloodletting, 185.214
Body fluids, 133
Bohemia, 80
Bone marrow, 561
Bone growth, 12, 234, 373, 421
Book club, medical, 804
Botany, 113, 377, 618-19, 1073, 1105
Breast, cancer, 372, 918
Brunonian system, 42, 922

Cancer, 543, 944, 952, 1058. See also
   specific organs.
————. Case histories, 327, 605
————. Etiology, 235, 281, 418
————. Research, 521
————. Prevention, 1097
————. Treatment, 109

Cardiovascular diseases, 1, 171, 230, 299, 539a-b, 881, 935, 994
Cardiovascular system, 4, 994
Case records, 276, 287, 290, 327, 416, 427, 437, 439, 480, 482, 536, 639, 651, 700, 721-22, 757-58, 768, 774, 794, 798, 830, 936, 1009-10, 1023, 1027, 1041, 1118
Catheters, 251
Cats, fear of, 678
Cerebral hemorrhage, 31, 140, 291, 638, 899
Certificates, 111
Cervix uteri, cancer, 832
Charities, medical, 38, 330, 932
Chemistry, 42, 73-75, 169, 185.*14*, 193, 283, 380, 386, 391-92, 467, 513, 628, 639, 702, 704, 825, 891, 936, 971, 979-80, 1072. See also Biochemistry
Childbirth. See Obstetrics; Labor
Cholera, 42, 71, 171, 185.*214*, .*2211*, .*2214*, 330, 390, 416, 465, 646, 791, 795, 805n, s
Chorea, 993
Chyle, 660
Circumcision, 44
Climate, medical aspects, 307, 893, 900, 982
Clubfoot, 865
Conception. See Pregnancy
Colic, 105
Confidence, professional, 185.*2218*
Convulsions, 213
Copaiba, 123
Copyright, 892, 1115
Corporal punishment, 251
Correspondence, 58, 104, 112-14, 130, 138, 181, 205, 271, 303, 332, 339, 346-47, 356, 361, 416, 423, 429, 450, 466, 481, 485, 494, 514-19, 532, 546, 580, 589, 592-93, 614, 623, 669, 678-80, 705-6, 732, 864, 867, 895, 930, 934, 986, 1005, 1016, 1091-92, 1103, 1105, 1122
Crises, 323, 645
Crural arch, 604
Cysts, 609
Cytology, 548

Deafness, 22
Death certificates, 1007

Dentistry, 447, 644
Dermatology, 58, 180, 265, 310, 370, 1054
Diabetes, 171, 1036
Dictionaries, medical and scientific, 134, 653 (Latin)
Diet, 418, 615, 632, 647, 1068. See also Nutrition
Digestion, 615
Digitalis, 805a
Diphtheria, 951
Directories, 336, 407, 813, 1113
Diseases, contagious, 185.*2221*, .*2223*, 291, 805d. See also specific diseases
Diseases, parasitic, 385, 387. See also specific diseases
Diuretics, 1116
Dogs, experiments on, 374
Dreams, 89
Drugs, 7, 127
Drunkenness, 78
Dry gripes, 105
Dupuytren's contracture, 490
Duodenum, 953
Dyes, 174
Dyspepsia, 171
Dystocia, 408. See also obstetrics

Echinochrome, 615
Echinococcus, 387
Eclampsia, puerperal, 126
Education, medical, 20, 185.*224*, .*64*, 273, 694, 706, 773, 843-44, 889, 930, 992, 1034, 1112. See also individual medical schools
Electricity, 471, 864, 897
Electrocardiography, 55, 792, 1088
Electro-therapy, 25
Embryology, 313, 363, 537, 828
Emetics, 118
Emphysema, 42
Endocarditis, 178
Endocrine glands, 89, 933
Environment, 42
Epidemics, 86, 142, 185.*2212*, 360, 701, 864. See also specific diseases, e.g. Cholera, etc.
Epilepsy, 31, 464
Epiphysis, 234
Eriometer, 548
Erysipelas, 35, 1099
Erythromelalgia, 753

Esophagus, 978
Etherization, 1009
Ethics, medical, 185.*2218*, 416, 998
Evolution, 252
Explosives, 96
Eye, 59, 247, 848, 864
Eye, diseases, 28, 191, 241, 247, 313-14, 338, 352, 468, 479, 500, 730, 733, 943, 1015, 1023, 1025, 1137, 1139. See also Ophthalmology

Fees, medical, 76, 84, 91, 106, 185.*223*, 215-16, 218, 255-56, 258, 378, 624, 842, 861, 884, 920, 937, 1006, 1070, 1111
Fermentation, 771, 805g
Fever, 579, 707, 761, 926, 959
Fibrin, 438
Fingers, 993
First aid, 335
Fistula lachrymalis, 177
Fluorine and fluorine compounds, 615
Food, inspection, 304
Food poisoning, 755
Forceps, 742
Forensic medicine, 274, 1059
Forensic psychiatry, 613, 670, 1019
Formularies
    Early to 1800, 31, 40, 84, 96, 183, 294, 300, 308, 444, 597, 638-39, 648, 763, 833, 850-51, 884, 924, 947, 1027
    Post-1800, 82, 90, 96-99, 112, 135, 137, 183, 218, 276, 294, 305, 342, 371, 382-83, 416, 464, 597, 612, 631, 638-40, 647, 672, 708, 850-53, 884, 886, 924, 957, 1064, 1086, 1132
Fractures, 32, 234, 266, 582, 718
Fruit, 632

Gall bladder, 1034
Galvanism, 62
Gastric juice, 42
Gastrointestinal diseases, 108, 142, 236, 715, 761, 978
Gastrointestinal system, 953
Gentian violet, 174
Geriatrics, 185.*611*
Glaucoma, 64
Goiter, 89, 615-16

Gonococcus, 770
Gout, 291, 640
Gynecological diseases, 25, 226, 242, 343, 409, 417, 496, 778, 794, 959, 1014, 1027
Gynecology, 183, 185.*46*, 343, 409, 586, 644, 829. See also Labor; Obstetrics; Stillbirth; Uterus

Halometer, 548
Head injuries, 647
Health insurance, 14, 62, 600
Health services, 288
Heart, 805q
Heart, diseases. See Cardiovascular diseases
Heat, 386
Herbs, 619
Heredity, 395
Hepatitis, 171, 291
Hernia, 177, 805j, 993
Histology, 357, 511, 537, 828, 970, 1053, 1073
History, medical, 81, 116, 120, 180, 185.*2230*, .*47*, .*62*, 211, 237, 315, 326, 334, 370, 396, 505, 508, 519, 542, 563, 585, 591, 619, 690, 720, 839, 886, 1039
Hodgkin's disease, 335
Hookworm disease, 26
Homeopathy, 849, 1071
Hormones, 328
Horses, diseases, 242
Hospital administration, 197, 932
Hospital surveys, 288
Hospitals, 332, 431, 734, 775, 791, 809, 831, 837-38, 932, 1087
Humerus, 12
Hydrogen, 42, 150
Hydropathy, 1071
Hydrophobia. See Rabies
Hygiene, personal, 27, 133, 185.*2228*, 864, 888
Hymen, 277
Hyperthyroidism, 483, 616

Immortality, 683
Impotence, 928
Infant mortality, 95
Inflammations, 35, 204, 269
Influenza, 86, 349, 701
Injections, 483, 644

Inoculation, 233, 488, 640, 805k
Iris, surgery, 245
Insanity, 595, 670, 674, 926, 1019. See also Psychiatry
Instruments and apparatus, 286, 320, 461, 499, 548, 555, 586, 742, 877, 1134-36
Internships and residences, 185.2229
Intestines, 362-63
Iodine, 616

Jaundice, 31, 389, 581
Johnstown disaster (1889), 185.2213
Joint diseases, 938

Kidneys, 545, 608

Labor, 126, 408
Laryngitis, 335, 950
Laryngology, 185.42, 452, 802, 1083
Larynx, cancer, 981
Lead poisoning, 105
Lectures and lecture notes, 413, 635-66, 749-50
    Ann Arbor, 1088
    Baltimore, 79
    Cambridge (Ma.), 85, 196
    Dartmouth (N.H.), 196
    Edinburgh, 13, 73-75, 222-24, 268, 353-54, 427, 689, 691-94, 1130-31
    Hanover, (Ger.), 424
    Heidelberg, 716
    Holland, 1018
    Leipzig, 367
    Leyden, 9
    London, 2, 177, 192, 220-21, 232, 295, 400, 426, 443, 445-49, 479, 484, 607, 743, 751
    Mexico, 695
    New Haven, 969-70
    New York, 390-91, 430, 479, 1021
    Paris, 21, 577, 605, 758, 826
    Pavia?, 959
    Philadelphia, 41, 45-48, 50-55, 67, 72, 83, 101, 117-19, 121, 124-25, 127-28, 141, 143, 145-62, 171, 193, 201-4, 212, 226, 228, 257, 260-62, 272-73, 291, 329, 337-38, 365, 388, 412, 414, 425, 439, 459, 461-63, 467, 470-71, 476, 485, 502, 540, 566-67, 568-76, 588, 649, 652, 668, 673, 702, 704, 707, 714, 733, 759-

61, 777-79, 781-84, 815-24, 828-29, 857-88, 864, 879-80, 891, 901-17, 921, 925, 930, 936, 955, 961, 963-66, 979-80, 989-90, 993-94, 1013-14, 1032, 1035, 1037-38, 1062, 1069, 1072-73, 1079, 1082, 1085, 1105, 1109-10, 1116, 1119-20, 1124, 1134-36
    Vienna, 313, 748, 1001
Legislation, medical, 351, 1025
Leprosy, 37
Libraries, medical, 35, 185.213,.2227, .61-.614, 384, 416, 432-34, 478, 641, 728, 740, 793, 800, 807
Licensing, physicians', 243, 665-66, 866
Ligaments, 604
Lithotomy, 177, 654, 661
Liver, 923
Longevity, 307, 442, 458
Lung diseases, 390, 595
Lungs, 982
Lymph glands, 363
Lymphatic system, 399

Macula lutea, 59
Magnetism, 150
Malaria, 68, 241, 291, 579, 627, 805e, i, s
Malnutrition, 984
Manuals, nursing, 215
Materia medica
    Early to 1800, 9, 13, 134, 150, 232, 242, 283-84, 298, 393, 568-70, 712, 948, 1049
    Post-1800, 45-48, 55, 72, 121, 124-25, 127-28, 145, 151-52, 154, 198-99, 201, 203, 214, 257, 260-63, 329, 367, 461, 476, 587, 596, 629, 635-36, 668, 816, 825, 1072, 1105, 1109, 1119. See also Formularies
Maxillofacial development, 254
Measles, 204, 1067
Medical schools. See individual institutions
Medicine, clinical and practical
    14th to 17th cent., 66, 1061
    18th cent., 10, 170, 222-24, 283, 285, 291, 354, 567, 571-72, 759, 811, 899, 901-6, 925, 938, 1027, 1049
    19th cent., 49, 51, 54, 83, 104, 141, 143, 146, 148-50, 153, 155-62, 171, 194, 215, 228, 260, 272-73, 329,

331, 353-55, 379, 390-91, 427, 430, 437, 439, 459, 462-63, 482, 577, 605-66, 631, 673, 695, 760-61, 781-83, 825-26, 890, 899, 907-17, 921, 928, 964-65, 969, 980, 1014, 1032, 1037, 1069, 1079-80, 1082, 1099, 1101, 1110, 1118, 1120, 1124
20th cent., 185.*145*, 215, 389-91, 455, 622, 652, 715, 880, 936, 989, 1089
Medicine, history. See History
Medicine, industrial, 185.*48*
Medicine, military. See Miliatry medicine
Medicine, naval. See Naval medicine
Medicine, preventive, 185.*2114*, *.48*, 612, 1095
Medicine, tropical, 411
Medicine andphilosophy, 366, 472
Medicine, proprietary, 1057
Memoranda book, medical, 34
Meningitis, 246
Mental health, 185.*64*
Metals, 63, 1116
Microbiology, 616
Microscopy, 79, 302, 358, 970-71
Midwifery, 192, 470-71, 607, 825, 1065-66, 1130-31. See also Obstetrics
Military medicine, 32, 91, 120, 173, 175, 183, 213, 217, 227, 253, 456, 488,
530, 546, 601, 614, 680, 684, 686, 725, 729, 732, 756-57, 772, 845, 956, 988, 1008, 1042-46, 1063, 1126. See also U.S. Civil War; War of 1812; War of Independence; World War I and II
Milk, 1081
Mind and body, 167
Muscular diseases, 490
Museums, medical, 185.*218*, 518
Music, 578
Mustard gas, 536
Myasthenia gravis, 541
Myelitis, 144
Myocardial infarct, 881

Nail diseases, 805p
Narcotics, 131. See also Opium
Natural history, 50, 731, 1094

Naval medicine, 194-95, 251, 741, 882, 1047, 1128
Neoarsphenamine, 244
Nervous system, 424, 669, 675, 684, 1000
Nervous system diseases, 328, 614, 898, 993-94, 1124
Neuralgia, 163, 348, 470, 864
Neurology, 669, 676, 808, 985
Neuroma, 944
Neurosurgery, 315, 974, 985
Neurotic disorders, 614, 677, 595, 898
Nosology, 42, 283, 430, 1004
Nurses' training, 35, 185.*2112*, 214, 369, 408, 1034
Nutrition, 697

Obituaries, 112
Obstetrics, 28, 31, 43, 69, 226, 333, 343, 401, 408, 413-15, 470-71, 586, 607, 645, 716, 739-40, 750-51, 758, 777, 784, 830, 875, 940, 961, 979, 1021, 1049, 1061-62. See also Forceps; Gynecology; Labor Pregnancy
Ointments, 928
Ophthalmology, 138-39, 185.*41*, 209, 214, 313-14, 345-46, 396, 414, 697, 746-47, 775, 943, 946, 1024, 1087, 1134-37. See also individual characteristics
Opium, 798, 1091
Orthopedics, 499, 809, 949
Osteology, 295
Osteonecrosis, 12
Osteopathy, 797
Otolaryngologic diseases, 282, 341, 475, 975-76, 981, 983
Otolaryngology, 185.*42*
Otology, 452, 775, 1083
Ovaries, 493, 609
Oxide, nitrous, 1096

Pain, 709
Palate, 254
Pancreas, 107
Paracentesis, 177, 399
Paralysis, 595, 978
Paranoia, 942
Paraplegia, 993
Parasitology, 503

Parathyroid glands, 132. See also Thyroid gland
Paronychia, 805p
Patent medicines, 804
Pathology, 21, 41, 43, 154, 185.*218*, 212, 283, 365, 374, 440, 485, 518, 520,
539, 539a-b, 563, 622, 697, 710, 758, 765, 885-86, 914, 936, 962, 996, 1001, 1013, 1018, 1035, 1037-38, 1053, 1072. See also Neuropathology
Pathology, cardiovascular, 94, 709
Pediatrics, 19, 43, 81, 172, 242, 331, 334, 596, 712, 769, 778, 849, 860, 959,
1014
Pelvis, 608
Personality, 102
Phallicism, 495
Pharmacology, 40, 119, 121, 182, 185.*14*, 203, 300, 351, 476, 636, 647, 1100, 1105, 1109-10, 1119. See also Drugs, Formularies, Materia medica
Pharmacopoeias, U.S., 42, 185.*211*, .*611*, 787-90, 1104, 1107
Phlegmasia alba dolens, 69
Phrenology, 758, 764
Physicians, Black, 1034
Physicians, Jewish, 713
Physics, 42, 150, 471, 625, 1049, 1073
Physiognomy, 102, 146
Physiology, 11, 85, 133, 147-48, 154, 269, 283, 363, 402, 425, 443, 467, 484, 518, 554, 567, 615, 691, 697, 749, 758, 805n, 810, 857-58, 917, 921, 933, 936, 953, 963, 965-66, 971, 1049, 1120
Physiology, animal, 971
Pigmenation, 1001
Pituitary gland, 556
Plague, 31, 29, 625, 839, 1138
Platinum, 42
Pneumatometry, 286
Pneumonia, 605, 759
Podophyllum (May apple), 805h
Poisons and poisoning, 338, 682, 755, 835, 1020, 1078
Pollution, 185.*2228*
Polygraph, 555
Portraits, 111-12, 183
Potassium iodite, 993

Pregnancy, 213, 292, 316, 611, 618, 963, 987, 1003. See also Obstetrics; Labor
Prescriptions. See Formularies
Prizes, Alvarenga Prize (College of Physicians), 78, 107-8, 132, 174, 185.*232*, 186, 210, 233, 241, 254, 278, 328, 363, 373, 385, 387, 405, 457, 493, 497, 621, 627, 767, 770, 848, 946, 953, 1068; William Osler Medal (A.A.H.M.), 29
Prostatectomy, 1017
Psychiatry, 101, 196, 291, 368, 595, 613, 670, 798, 809, 897-98, 926. See also Insanity
Psychology, 512, 758, 917, 1916
Public health, 42, 185.*2114*, .*2212*, .*2217*, .*48*, 502, 528, 930, 986, 1012. See also Hygiene; Sanitation
Publishing, medical, 185.*217* 396. See also names of publishing firms
Pulse, 133, 242, 877
Purgation and puratives, 118, 805h

Quackery, 804, 806, 866

Rabies, 114, 150, 267, 1132
Radiology. See X-ray
Radium poisoning, 521
Raynaud's disease, 753
Recipies. See Formularies
Rectum, 431
Religion in India, 1121
Reproduction in animals and plants, 731, 1094
Respiration, 269, 805r
————. Artificial, 282
Respiratory diseases, 152, 269, 282, 286, 414
Retina, 296
Rheumatic fever, 767
Rhinology, 452, 802, 1083
Rickets, 638
Russo-Japanese War (1911), 1126

Salvarsan, 244
Sanitation, 185.*2215*. See also Hygiene
Scarlatina, 185.*214*, 583
Schistosomiasis, 385
Science (General), 879
Sclerosis, 230
Scrofula, 655, 842

Selenium, 169
Septicemia, 178
Skull, 266, 718
Sleep, 89
Small pox, 42, 185.227, 291, 680, 724,
    776, 805k, 940, 1022
Small pox, vaccination, 23-24
Snake bite, 805l
Societies, nurses', 737-38
Societies, medical, 15-16, 18-19, 38,
    326, 407, 410, 428-29, 475, 481,
    862. see also names of specific
    societies
Sphincters, 108
Spinal cord, 144
Spiritualism, 30
Spleen, 511, 551, 562
Splenomegaly, 581
Staining, 840
Statistics, obstetrical, 875
Statistics, vital, 435, 584
Sterility, female, 28
Stillbirth, 31
Stethoscope, 461
Stomach, 264
Stroke, 31
Superstition in medicine, 546
Surgery
    Early, to 18th cent., 177, 220-21, 259,
        295, 400, 445, 479, 692-93, 810,
        1061
    19th cent., 2, 6, 35-36, 43, 52, 67,
        185.216, .43, .44, .511, 192, 248,
        250, 259, 329, 337-38, 361-62, 379,
        397, 412, 426, 587, 602, 647, 656,
        659, 664, 711, 714, 721-23, 743,
        762, 768, 784, 794, 796, 815-26,
        837, 869-74, 949, 968, 980, 1037,
        1058
    20th cent., 32-33, 35-36, 210, 240,
        711, 784, 1085
Symmetry and assymetry, 313
Syphilis, 419-20, 422, 502, 504, 595,
    776, 840
Syringomyelis, 405

Testicles, 357
Tetanus, 144, 623, 776, 1127
Tetanus, antitoxin, 185.2224
Theraputics, 31, 115, 117, 185.14, 338,
    358, 391, 630, 639, 784, 849, 914,
    995, 1124

Thermometers, 877
Thorax, 271, 399
Throat, 317, 975-76
Thrombophlebitis, 69
Thyroid gland, 132, 883. See also Hyper-
    thyroidism; Parathyroid glands
Tissue, culture, 565
Tobacco, use of, 185.221, 805c
Tokology. See Obstetrics
Tonics, mineral, 329
Tonsils, 1067
Trachea, 282
Tracheotomy, 976
Travels, medical and scientific, 32,
    289, 364, 707, 888, 936, 1063, 1108
Trephening (Incas), 231
Treponemiases, 420
Tuberculosis, 303, 331, 497-98, 605,
    610, 786, 983, 993, 1031, 1063
Tumors, 417, 608, 621, 623, 805o, 944
Twins, Siamese, 557
Typhoid, 233, 488, 558, 605
Typhus, 291, 663, 928, 1033, 1093,
    1127-28
Tyrotoxicosis, 616

Ulcers, 236, 243
Ultrasonics, 22
United States. Bicentennial, 185.59,
    .510
————. Civil War, 91, 175, 217,
    304, 684, 686, 729, 732, 845, 988,
    1042, 1045, 1103
————. Spanish-American War
    (1898), 680
————. War of Independence
    (1775-1783), 120, 129, 173, 601,
    615, 706
Ureter, 608
Urethra, 662
Uric acid, 1034
Urology, 133, 189, 242, 265, 645, 661,
    805o. See also Catheters; Genito-
    urinary organs
Uterus, 446, 611, 832, 1017

Vaccination, 23-24, 42, 185.227, 208,
    339, 477, 599, 776, 805t
Vagina, wounds and injuries, 77
Varicose veins, 398
Varioloid, 724
Veins, 4

Venereal diseases, 31, 419-20, 422, 424, 445,836, 1033
Viscera, 922
Viscus, 374
Vitamins, 373
Vivisection, 185.*14*, 486-88, 603

Water, 939
William Osler medal, 29
Women in medicine, 940
World War I, 32, 178, 253, 456, 475, 483, 488, 509, 530, 536, 614, 725, 756-57, 772, 835, 1008, 1063

World War II, 423, 475, 1043-44

X-ray, 93, 457, 528, 556

Yellow fever, 42, 104, 168, 179, 185.*12*, 200, 291, 297, 301, 330, 339, 359, 494, 573, 579, 623, 634, 671, 688, 839, 854-55, 899, 923, 1025, 1099, 1127-29

Zoology, 50, 340, 377, 1073